The No-Diet Weight Loss Solution!

EAT
THIS
NOT
THAT!®

NEW! EXCLUSIVE EDITION

BY DAVID ZINCZENKO
WITH MATT GOULDING

GALVANIZED

No book can replace the diagnostic expertise
and medical advice of a trusted physician.
Please be certain to consult with your doctor before
making any decisions that affect your health,
particularly if you suffer from any medical condition or
have any symptom that may require treatment.

Published in the United States by
Galvanized Books,
a division of Galvanized Brands, LLC, New York

Galvanized Books is a trademark of Galvanized Brands, LLC

ISBN 978-0696-30218-3

Printed in the United States of America on acid-free paper

246897531

Book design by George Karabotsos with Laura White

GALVANIZED

Dedication

To the 8 million men and women who have made *Eat This, Not That!*
a publishing phenomenon and who have spread the word to friends
and relatives about the importance of knowing what's really in our food.
Because of your passionate efforts, food manufacturers and restaurant
chains are waking up to the fact that more and more of us demand
good, solid information about our food, and healthy choices that will let
us drop pounds and stay lean for life.

And to the men and women working in America's fields, farms,
and supermarkets, waiting tables, and toiling in kitchens everywhere:
It is because of your hard work that Americans have so many options.
This book is designed to help us choose the best of what you've created.

—Dave and Matt

Acknowledgments

This book is the product of thousands of meals, hundreds of conversations with nutritionists and industry experts, months of intensive research, and the collective smarts, dedication and raw talent of dozens of individuals. Our undying thanks to those who have helped to make this book a possibility:

The team at Galvanized, an extraordinary collection of men and women who have come together to create a business, establish an empire, and change the way a media company thinks. Your hard work and dedication is an inspiration to all our partners.

Sara Vigneri, Heather Hurlock, James Carlson, Ashley Ross, Amelia Harnish, Tara Long, Jeff Harris, Dan Engongoro, and many others who contributed directly to the success of this project.

Steve Lacy and the team at Meredith; David Pecker and the crew at American Media; Dave Freygang and the squad at Bonnier Corp., and the other media executives who have seen the potential of *Eat This, Not That!* and gotten behind the movement in a huge way.

The folks at Penguin Random House, in particular Gina Centrello, Libby McGuire, Bill Takes, Marnie Cochran, Jennie Tung, Richard Callison and Nina Shield, for their ongoing support of our book efforts.

Barbara Fedida, Robin Roberts, George Stephanopoulos, Lara Spencer, Jen Ashton and the team at Good Morning America for their love of a good food swap.

Jennifer Rudolph Walsh, Jon Rosen, Andy McNicol, and the brilliant minds at WME.

Dan Abrams, Christine Cole, Floyd Cardoz, and the team at White Street— thanks for keeping us lean!

Larry Shire, Eric Sacks, and Jonathan Erlich for their invaluable counsel.

Mehmet Oz, Travis Stork, Strauss Zelnick, Steve Gilbert, Joe Armstrong, Amy Rhodes, Malcolm Netburn, David Carey, and the many friends and colleagues who continue to inspire us with their wisdom and insight.

And to the best families two men could be blessed with.

—Dave and Matt

Contents

INTRODUCTION **Welcome to the Future!** page 1
PLUS 8 new superfoods you should eat every day, and the *Eat This, Not That!* Hall of Fame

CHAPTER 1 **Food Right Now** page 36
The best and worst developments across the food industry landscape.
PLUS The *Eat This, Not That!* Awards and the worst new foods

CHAPTER 2 **The Truth About Your Food** page 50
20 top nutrition myths—busted!
PLUS Secrets the diet industry doesn't want you to know, and the 20 worst foods in America

CHAPTER 3 **The All-New Menu Decoder** page 94
From the local frozen yogurt shop to those juice bars popping up all over, learn how to make smart choices no matter what trendy cuisine you're enjoying.

CHAPTER 4 **At Your Favorite Restaurants** page 112
The newest picks and pans from the most popular fast-food and sit-down chains

CHAPTER 5 **At the Supermarket** page 230
Learn to stock your pantry, fridge and freezer with world's best packaged foods

CHAPTER 6 **Little Kids Versus Big Food** page 296
Our kids are under attack from a food industry intent on making them fat. Here's how to stand up to the bullies!

CHAPTER 7 **Cook This, Not That!** page 312
Delicious breakfast, lunch and dinner recipes that could strip more than a pound a week off your frame

Index page 334

Introduction

WELCOME TO THE FUTURE.

If a coterie of science fiction writers got into a room 40 years ago and imagined what our current decade would look like, what would they have thought up?

Flying cars? We're not there yet. Teleportation? Still waiting. Cure for the common cold? They're working on it. Food appearing out of nowhere at the touch of a button?

Ahh. Bingo. The time it takes to go from "I'd like a hamburger" to "That was a delicious hamburger" has shrunk exponentially from the time of our great-grandparents, who had to tramp through snow to the butcher shop, lug home a pound of chuck, grind it, and fry it up themselves. Even our own parents, back in the dark ages of the last millennium, had to rummage around for a menu, make a phone call (from their house!), and then wait 40 minutes for dinner to show up. Today, you can accidentally butt dial a burger from your GrubHub app. Problem solved!

But one person's paradise is another's purgatory, and all the super-convenient food delivery apps and restaurant reservation sites and proliferating juice and smoothie bars—where food is reduced to the most quickly consumed form possible—have only served to speed the race of calories into our bodies. I envy Great-Grandma and the muscles she built grinding that chuck steak and chopping those vegetables. Today, we just drink our lunch—and then go to the gym to work up some calorie burn because life is so damn convenient.

Consider this: When I wrote the *Eat This Not That! Restaurant Survival Guide*, in 2010, I reported on how Americans were getting 33 percent of their calories from outside the home—up from less than 20 percent in the 1980s. And it's not just because we're spending more time in restaurants.

The Great Recession changed the way we eat. When everyone was too worried about the future to book that trip to the Bahamas, we instead looked to little indulgences to feed our passions. And one of the places we indulged ourselves was food. Look at how our food is behaving differently:

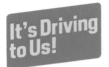

The food truck industry has grown by 12 percent each year since 2009—again, perhaps in part as a response to the recession. Eating indulgent food, eating more local, and eating on the go—especially when lunch hours are squeezed and bosses are angsty—are three trends that coalesce around the idling food truck. In 2014, America's 3,900 food trucks took in $804M in revenue, but some analysts see this as a $2.7B industry within the decade.

Numbers Munching

867 people just like you responded to the most recent *Eat This, Not That!* poll and shared what was going on in their heads—and in their bellies. The surprising facts? Almost half of us are on a diet, yet more than half of us have no idea how many calories were in our last meal....

Does it count as "food shopping" if you go to a supermarket and buy a takeout dinner there, instead of at a takeout joint? More and more, supermarkets aren't selling us fixin's, they're selling us food that's already been fixed. Every year, Americans swing by the grocery store and pick up 450 million rotisserie chickens; in 2012 alone, Costco sold 68 million of them.

That's a trend that's only going to grow. According to one survey, 78 percent of millenials brought home prepared foods from the supermarket in the last month. Only 57 percent of seniors did the same. As our cooking skills erode, so too does our ability to control exactly what it is we're eating.

It's Coming at Us Through Our Phones!

Sixty-nine percent of Americans have used a mobile device to order delivery food. The growth of GrubHub and other delivery apps

Foods prepared by restaurants, caterers, and other sources now account for 43% of our calories, up from 33% just five years ago. On any given day, a third of Americans have eaten at a restaurant. In the 1980s, only 20% of our calories came from outside the home.

When was the last time you ate a meal at a restaurant?

Last 24 hours **33%**
Last week **46%**
Last month **14%**
More than a month ago.. **7%**

Do you know how many calories were in your meal there?

Yes **28%**
No **71%**

Are you concerned with counting calories?

Yes **73%**
No **26%**

Are you currently on a diet?

Yes **46%**
No **53%**

has made ordering takeout so simple that there's no reason to go through the hassle and inconvenience of trekking to the grocery store and buying food—even if someone's already cooked it for you.

And Then Going Back out Through Our Phones!

Sharing and collecting images of our meals has become a national pastime—one in four Americans say they photograph their meals. In a one-month survey of social media users in 2014, 29 million Americans posted a photo of their meal at a restaurant. Pinterest reports that food-related content is its top category, with 57 percent of users posting food shots. One food industry report showed that over a two-week period, Instagram users posted 48,000 photos from just 30 of the nation's top restaurants. And once our friends start sharing their awesome restaurant meals, it makes us wonder why we should bother slaving over a hot stove.

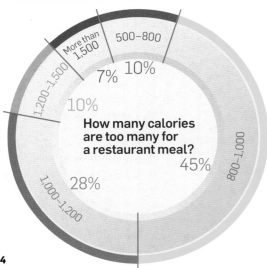

How many calories are too many for a restaurant meal?

More than 1,500 — 7%
500–800 — 10%
1,200–1,500 — 10%
800–1,000 — 45%
1,000–1,200 — 28%

In a recent study in the *Journal of the American Medical Association*, researchers looked at the nutrition facts of a typical breakfast, lunch, and dinner from 19 chain restaurants. Their findings were pretty stunning. While only 45 percent of respondents in our poll say they're okay with a restaurant meal that tops 1,000 to 1,200 calories, the average restaurant meal (and remember, this includes breakfasts!) contains:

1,128 CALORIES	2,269 mg SODIUM	58 g FAT
or about 56 percent of a person's daily calorie intake	or 95 percent of a person's daily intake	or 89 percent of a person's daily intake

It's Showing Us to Our Tables Faster

Gone are the days when you had to call five different restaurants to find an open reservation, and then slip the maître d' 20 bucks to get a decent table. Today, one in five restaurant reservations are made online, up from just 12 percent a few years ago. Fifteen million people use OpenTable.com every month. By taking the stress, guesswork, and fear of rejection out of dining out, sites like OpenTable are also removing one more reason to stay at home and cook.

OMG It's Naked

One of the reasons customers see supermarket-prepared foods as healthier is that they don't meet our preconceived notion of "prepared" foods. If it's not in a plastic bag or cardboard box, we see it as more natural. And that's sparked a new trend in food packaging: When LaraBar switched to a clear wrapper in early 2014, customers told

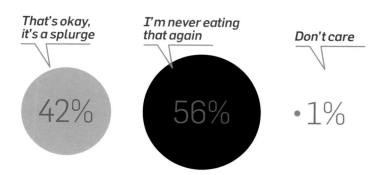

You've just learned that your favorite restaurant meal contains more calories than you should eat in an entire day. Your reaction is:

That's okay, it's a splurge — 42%

I'm never eating that again — 56%

Don't care — 1%

A 2013 survey of foods at popular restaurants found dishes at Perkins, On the Border, Cheesecake Factory, Friendly's, Applebee's, Bertucci's and Uno Pizzeria & Grill that exceeded 1,800 calories per serving—the total number of calories an adult woman should eat in an entire day.

surveyors the bars felt less artificial and seemed fresher. Nothing had changed on the company's notoriously sparse ingredient list. Yet, their bars were perceived as more wholesome. Even packaged goods now look more like food delivery!

So how dramatically have food delivery apps and reservation services and the growth of food trucks and prepared foods changed our lives? In less than five years, the percentage of our calories that come from food outside the home has risen to 43 percent—the highest since the USDA began tracking such statistics. To put that in perspective, the average man now eats about 2,700 calories a day—500 more than he should. And 1,161 of those calories come from restaurants, mini marts, and prepared foods. (The average woman eats 799 calories a day from foods prepared outside the home.)

In a 2014 study in the journal *Public Health Nutrition*, people were asked

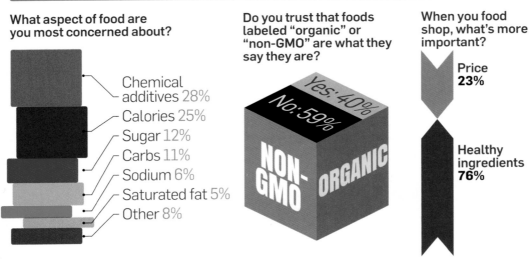

What aspect of food are you most concerned about?

Chemical additives 28%
Calories 25%
Sugar 12%
Carbs 11%
Sodium 6%
Saturated fat 5%
Other 8%

Do you trust that foods labeled "organic" or "non-GMO" are what they say they are?

Yes: 40%
No: 59%
NON-GMO
ORGANIC

When you food shop, what's more important?

Price
23%

Healthy ingredients
76%

to report their food intake over the course of 48 hours. Those who ate at a restaurant during that time took in an average of 200 calories per day more than those who prepared all of their own meals. (Those who ate in sit-down restaurants actually consumed slightly more calories than those who ordered from fast food joints.) It takes 3,500 calories to create a pound of body weight; so according to that study, our eat-in, take-out, anywhere-but-my-own-kitchen culture is adding just under 21 pounds of extra fat to our bodies every year. Is it any wonder shows like *MasterChef* are so popular? They're like cooking porn for the culinarily repressed.

It all adds up to one essential truth: Understanding what's in our food is harder than ever. Getting accurate nutritional information is harder than ever. And *Eat This, Not That!* is going to be working harder than ever to keep you informed about the clientele in the most exclusive joint in the whole world—your belly.

What promises on food packaging are most likely to get you to pick up a product?

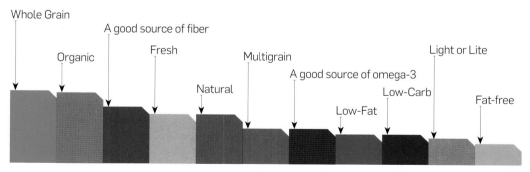

Look for "100% whole grain" on the label; even a "healthy" bread like Pepperidge Farm Light Style Soft Wheat is made with a mix of whole wheat and white flour. Same holds true at restaurants: Panera's Whole Grain Loaf and Whole Grain Baguette are primarily enriched white flour.

8 SUPERFOODS YOU SHOULD EAT EVERY DAY

We all want to eat a "balanced" diet. But what does that mean in an era of 1,759-calorie burgers? (Your Pretzel Burger is not a good buy, Ruby Tuesday!) Or soups with three days' worth of sodium? (P.F. Chang's Hot & Sour—yep, we're pretty hot and sour!) Or coffee drinks with the equivalent of 42 sugar packets? (That's not cool, Dunkin' Donuts Vanilla Bean Coolatta!)

Eating a balanced diet in today's food landscape means that when you're surrounded by bad, you've got to maximize the good. We've chosen eight of the best foods to build your pantry around—a belly-filling, metabolism-revving, nutrient-maximizing mix of classic health-food favorites and 21st century superfoods.

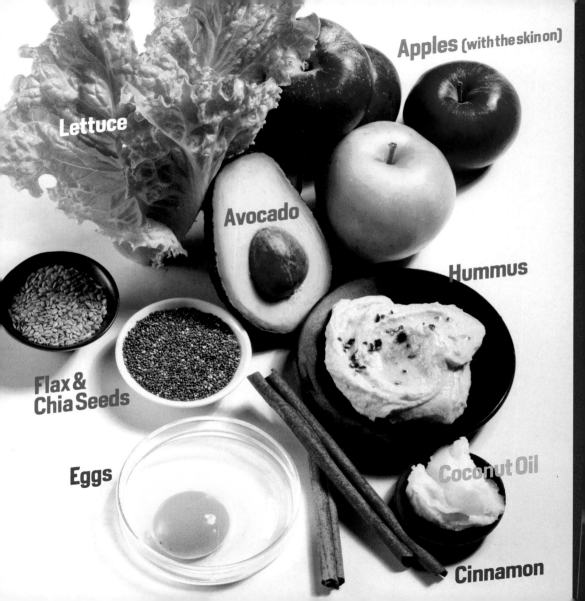

1 Coconut Oil

One study from the *American Journal of Clinical Nutrition* found that subjects who ate coconut oil lost overall weight and belly fat faster than a group consuming the same amount of olive oil. The secret is in coconut's medium-chain triglycerides. Unlike the long-chain fatty acids in most oils, coconut oil is broken down immediately for use rather than stored, and has been found to speed up the metabolism. That's right—your body has trouble storing the calories in coconut oil, and revs up its metabolism to burn them instead. Coconut oil's high smoke point makes it great for just about every dish from eggs to stir-fries, and a delicious substitute for butter when baking.

2 Flax and Chia Seeds

One of the hallmarks of a balanced diet is to have a good ratio of omega-6 fatty acids to omega-3s. A 4:1 ratio would be ideal, but the modern American diet is more like 20:1. That leads to inflammation, which can trigger weight gain. But while eating a serving of salmon every day isn't exactly convenient, sprinkling these two seeds—among the most highly concentrated sources of omega-3s in the food world—into smoothies, salads, cereals, pancakes, or even desserts is as easy a diet upgrade as you can get. Animal studies suggest a chia-rich diet can lower harmful LDL cholesterol and protect the heart, and a recent study in the journal *Hypertension* found that daily consumption of flaxseed-fortified bakery products reduced blood pressure in patients with peripheral artery disease. Best absorbed when ground, flax adds delicious nuttiness to oats, cereal, smoothies, and baked goods.

Eggs

Eggs are the single best dietary source of the B vitamin choline, an essential nutrient used in the construction of all the body's cell membranes. Two eggs will give you half your day's worth; only beef liver has more. (And believe us, starting your day with a slab of beef liver does not make for a great morning.) Choline deficiency is linked directly to the genes that cause the accumulation of belly fat. Eggs can solve the problem: Research has shown dieters who eat eggs for breakfast instead of high-carb bagels have an easier time losing weight due to eggs' satiety value. At about 70 calories, a hard-boiled egg also makes an easy afternoon snack ... just don't tell your coworkers; according to a personality analysis by the British Egg Industry Council, boiled-egg consumers tend to be disorganized! (Other findings: fried egg fans have a high sex drive and omelet eaters are self-disciplined.)

Apples (with the Skin On)

A medium-sized apple, at about 100 calories and 4.5 grams of fiber per fruit, is one of the best snack options for anyone looking to slim down—but especially apple-shaped folks. A recent study at Wake Forest Baptist Medical Center found that for every 10-gram increase in soluble fiber eaten per day, visceral fat (that's dangerous belly fat) was reduced by 3.7 percent over five years. Participants who paired their apple-a-day habit with 30 minutes of exercise two to four times per week saw a 7.4 percent decrease in the rate of visceral fat accumulation over the same time period. But don't peel your apple if you want to peel off the pounds: A study conducted at the University of Western Australia found that the blushing varieties (such as Pink Ladies) had the highest level of antioxidant phenols, most of which are found in the skin. Apple sauce isn't a worthy substitute.

Cinnamon

It may be the easiest nutrition upgrade of all: Put cinnamon on your toast. According to researchers, cinnamon contains powerful antioxidants called polyphenols proven to improve insulin sensitivity and, in turn, our body's ability to store fat and manage hunger cues. A series of studies printed in the *American Journal of Clinical Nutrition* found that adding a heaping teaspoon of cinnamon to a starchy meal may help stabilize blood sugar and ward off insulin spikes.

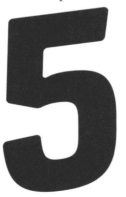

Avocado

A scoop of guacamole is one of the most effective hunger-squashers known to man. In a study published in *Nutrition Journal*, participants who ate half a fresh avocado with lunch reported a 40% decreased desire to eat for hours afterward. At only 60 calories, a 2-tablespoon serving of guacamole (on top of eggs, salads, grilled meats, etc.) can provide the same satiety benefit with even more of a flavor punch. Just be sure when buying store-bought guac that avocados actually made it into the box (many are made without the real fruit)! We love Wholly Guacamole as a store brand.

Lettuce.
Yep, Lettuce

Move over, King Kale. In a new William Paterson University study that compared the 47 top superfoods by nutrient volume, the trendy green came in a respectable—but unremarkable—15th on the list. Ranking higher: watercress, spinach, leafy green lettuce and endive. Make yourself a bowl of simple leafy greens and splash on some olive oil. According to a Purdue University study, as little as 3 grams of monounsaturated fat can help the body absorb vegetables' carotenoids (those magic molecules that protect you from chronic diseases like cancer and heart disease). Pairing your lettuce with a scant tablespoon of olive oil–based vinaigrette is your best bet.

Hummus

A recent study published in the journal *Obesity* found people who ate a single serving a day of garbanzo beans or chickpeas (which form the basis of hummus) reported feeling 31 percent fuller than their beanless counterparts. Packed with fiber and protein, garbanzo beans have a low glycemic index, meaning that they break down slowly and keep you feeling full. The secret is to avoid hummus varieties made with tahini; sourced from sesame seeds, tahini has a high omega-6-to-omega-3 fatty acid ratio. Look for hummus that's olive-oil based.

HOW
EAT THIS, NOT THAT!
CHANGED THE WORLD!

Here's how hard it is to change American culture:

In 2007, the year the first *Eat This, Not That!* was released, the top 20 most popular movies of the year included *Transformers*, *Hot Fuzz*, and *Teenage Mutant Ninja Turtles*. In 2014, the top 20 most popular movies included *Transformers: Age of Extinction*, *Let's Be Cops*, and yes, *Teenage Mutant Ninja Turtles*.

But while some things stay the same, one thing is very, very different: We all have a better idea of what we are eating.

When the first *Eat This, Not That!* was released, there was no way to know how many calories were sandwiched into your Subway sandwich, how much fat and salt a Denny's Grand Slam slams you with, or how much totally unnatural sugar, hydrogenated oil, and preservatives were in Wendy's "Natural-Cut" Fries. The ingredients—even the number of calories—in the foods Americans ate every day remained one of the great mysteries of modern society, right up there with Google's algorithm and Justin Beiber's ongoing celebrity.

But in those ensuing seven years, everything about the way we eat has changed.

Today, thanks to the outcry unleashed by *Eat This, Not That!*, most restaurants now post their calorie counts on their websites and even right in their stores. Instead of hiding their nutrition, chains from Boston Market to California Pizza Kitchen are introducing healthier options and letting us make informed choices about the most important choice of all—what we put into our bodies. Here's how it all happened:

December 2007

Eat This, Not That! is released. Dave Zinczenko and coauthor Matt Goulding say it all in their dedication, calling out Applebee's, Olive Garden, Outback, Red Lobster, and T.G.I. Friday's: "We hope this book plays some part, small or large, in compelling you to provide what every diner in America deserves: full disclosure." Shortly thereafter, we publish a Restaurant Report Card on the home page of Yahoo!, grading every major restaurant chain in America and providing phone numbers and email addresses of those that refuse to release their nutrition information. Soon after, Red Lobster and Olive Garden both go public with their info. (Today, each and every one provides full nutrition information for all of their offerings.)

December 2007

Nestle sends a cease-and-desist letter. We are not impressed. Kraft protests our accusation that Capri Sun is nothing more than sugar water. A few months later, they announce they're dropping the sugar content of their entire Capri Sun line by 25 percent.

April 2008

An *Eat This, Not That!* blog entitled "The Worst Drink on the Planet" exposes Baskin-Robbins for producing a 2,310-calorie Heath Bar milk shake. The company later scraps the drink as well as its entire line of "premium" milk shakes.

May 2008

Eat This, Not That! names Jamba Juice's Chocolate Moo'd Power Smoothie the Worst Drink in America. The company removes the Power size from the menu and, in a letter to *Eat This, Not That!*, company spokesman Tom Suiter declares the company is setting out

to become "the healthiest restaurant chain in America."

December 2008

Eat This, Not That! Supermarket Survival Guide is released. The book runs a series of Label Decoders to expose misleading label claims. A year later, the FDA sends a flurry of warning letters to food processors to crack down on inflated label claims.

April 2009

VitaminWater, which had previously protested our naming it The Worst "Healthy" Drink in America, launches VitaminWater Zero. It quickly becomes a bestseller; VitaminWater thanks us for the inspiration.

June 2009

Eat This, Not That! exposes Jack in the Box's Bacon Cheddar Potato Wedges as the "Trans-fattiest Food in America." The company responds by replacing its fryer oil with trans-fat-free oil.

June 2009

Jamba Juice unveils its new line of preservative-free, no-HFCS drinks. CEO James White writes, "*Eat This, Not That!* has always been an industry leader in providing healthy eating/healthy living advice to diners."

October 2009

Applebee's and Outback Steakhouse go public with their nutrition information; both release new lines of low-calorie offerings.

November 2009

After castigating Romano's Macaroni Grill for being one of America's unhealthiest restaurants, Dave Zinczenko appears on the *Today* show to praise the company's CEO Brad Blum's healthy reimagining of more than half the chain's menu.

December 2009

Zinczenko and Goulding release *Cook This, Not That: Kitchen Survival Guide*, giving readers a home oasis away from the craziness of contemporary restaurant calorie counts. *Grill This, Not That!* and two more *Cook This, Not That!* books follow.

December 2009

Gatorade removes HFCS from its products; Hunt's Ketchup follows suit a few months later. HFCS consumption begins to drop for the first time in 30 years.

February 2010

New York City becomes the largest municipality to enact a law requiring restaurant chains to display calorie counts.

March 2010

The Affordable Care Act is signed, and with it comes a stipulation that all chain restaurants with 20 or more outlets nationwide must post nutritional information on their menus. This goes fully into effect four years later.

August 2010

IHOP posts its nutritional information for the first time. Dairy Queen starts selling 7-ounce Mini Blizzards after repeated attacks from *Eat This, Not That!* about the caloric loads of their larger cups.

January 2011

Carl's Jr. and Hardee's, whose CEO had previously declared "healthy eating" to be a manufactured media concept, go national with their new *Eat This, Not That!* line of turkey burgers, all under 500 calories.

March 2012

After an *Eat This, Not That!* story calls out the restaurant chains that fudge their serving sizes to make their calorie counts appear lower, both P.F. Chang's and Uno Chicago Grill straighten up and fly right, adjusting their calorie counts to more accurately reflect their portions.

August 2014

The new EatThis.com launches, and with it comes more bad news for fried-food purveyors everywhere. *The Wall Street Journal* reports on the decline in growth for fast-food companies like Burger King and McDonald's. "Customers in their 20s and 30s are defecting to competitors.... Increasingly, younger diners are seeking out fresher, healthier foods...."

September 2014

Four years after the release of *Drink This, Not That!* spurred a flurry of legislative initiatives—including a proposed ban on supersized sodas in New York and a tax on sugary drinks in San Francisco—the big three soda makers (Coca-Cola, PepsiCo and Dr Pepper Snapple Group) pledge to work together to cut beverage calories in the American diet 20 percent by the year 2025.

November 2014

The FDA announces sweeping changes: By late 2015, calorie counts must be displayed at all sit down restaurants, takeout joints, bakeries, ice cream parlors, pizza chains, amusement parks and movie theaters, if the establishment has more than 20 outlets—and on vending machines, too.

5 DAILY HABITS THAT BLAST BELLY FAT

Double chin, spare tire, muffin top, cankles— we have more words for body fat than Eskimos have for snow. But the worst fat of all is belly fat. Belly fat (also called visceral fat) actually works to undermine your health—sending out inflammatory compounds that do everything from eroding muscle to increasing your risk of dementia. And to paraphrase the dean from *Animal House*, "Fat, weak, and demented is no way to go through life, son."

Fortunately, there are ways to fight back that don't involve running the gamut from aerobicizes to Zumba and living on only peanut butter or raw foods or whatever the diet trend of the moment is. All you need to jump-start your weight loss is to add these simple habits into your daily routine.

Swap Your Cup(s) o' Joe for Green Tea

Sipping on green tea throughout the morning has been proven to whittle your waist, but too much coffee has the opposite effect. What makes green tea so waist-friendly are compounds called catechins, belly-fat crusaders that blast adipose tissue by revving the metabolism, increasing the release of fat from fat cells (particularly in the belly), and then speeding up the liver's fat-burning capacity. In a recent study, participants who combined a daily habit of four to five cups of green tea each day with a 25-minute sweat session lost two more pounds than the non-tea-drinking exercisers. Meanwhile, a research team in Washington found that the same amount of coffee (5+ cups/day) doubled visceral fat.

Consult The Kernel

I'm not suggesting a movie theater binge, but without the butter and excess salt, popcorn can be an apple-shaped snacker's best friend. At only 30 calories, a cup of popped kernels provides more than 9 grams of whole grains—a dietary staple of people with the littlest middles. A Tufts University study found that participants who ate three or more servings of whole grains (oats, quinoa, brown rice, wheat) had 10 percent less belly fat than people who ate the same amount of calories from refined carbs (white stuff: bread, rice, pasta). Further research is required to figure out exactly why this is the case, but the hypothesis is that it has to do with the high fiber and slow-burn properties of whole grains. When it comes to diet, being unrefined is a good thing!

Try a Pepper Upper

Yes, you WOULD like pepper on that. Whenever the waiter cracks that pepper grinder, he releases piperine, a powerful compound found in black pepper that has been used for centuries in Eastern medicine to treat multiple health conditions, including inflammation and digestive troubles.

But recent animal studies have found that piperine may also have the profound ability to interfere with the formation of new fat cells—a reaction known as adipogenesis, resulting in a decrease in waist size, body fat, and cholesterol levels.

Eat from Your Palms

If you haven't yet graduated from coconut-oil suntanning to coconut-oil cooking, it's time to join the trend. Studies suggest that just two tablespoons of virgin coconut oil each day can have you ready for the tropical beaches in no time. What makes coconut oil superior to other fats is its medium-chain triglycerides. Unlike the long-chain fatty acids found in animal sources of

saturated fat, coconut oil doesn't seem to raise your cholesterol and is more likely to be burned as energy than stored as blubber. Its high smoke point makes it great for just about every dish, from eggs to stir-fries, and a perfect substitute for butter when baking (you could even try some on your popcorn for a double dose of belly-blasting goodness).

Indulge Your Darkest Desires

You've probably heard about the virtues of dark chocolate—a little preliminary research has been justifying late-night binges for years now. Research shows that the fiber in chocolate, especially when paired with fruit, feeds the healthy bacteria in your gut, leading to reduced overall

body fat and a shrinking waist. And in one study, mildly overweight women who ate a Mediterranean diet that included two servings of dark chocolate each day showed a significant reduction in waist size compared with when they were on a similar, cocoa-free meal plan. Researchers say it has to do with the flavonoids, heart-healthy compounds in chocolate that have important antioxidant and anti-inflammatory properties. But most of what's labeled "dark chocolate" is entirely ineffective. Buy a bar that says "70% cacao" or higher (cacao is the actual chocolate bean itself, minus the sugar and additives). And stay away from anything labeled "Dutch" or "alkalized," a process that destroys the majority of nutrients in the chocolate.

HOW TO LOSE WEIGHT WITH THIS BOOK

The basic belief has always been that, for adults, calculating your potential weight gain is simple. It takes about 3,500 calories' worth of food to build a pound of body fat, and 3,500 calories' worth of activity to burn that pound off: calories in minus calories out divided by 3,500 equals the number of pounds that a given meal or daily diet will help you to gain or lose.

Since early 2014, however, more and more researchers have looked at the increasingly robust American landscape and thought, "There's got to be more to it than this." And in fact there is. New research shows that too many calories, when combined with too little nutrition, can do more than just tip the scales of that weight-gain equation. When we overeat without giving our bodies the nutrients it needs—especially early in life—we trigger our fat genes to turn "on." Now our genetic propensity to gain weight is accelerated, and our bodies become much more efficient at converting incoming calories to fat. That's why some people seem to diet constantly but never lose weight—their fat genes are revving on high, and just reducing calories by cutting out certain food groups like all meat, or all carbs, or all foods that begin with the letter T, simply won't work.

Here's why that's good news: When we start swapping out egregiously bad foods and swapping in healthier versions, we can actually impact the behavior of our genes. While you can never fully turn them back "off," you can dim their powers. The better you eat, the more your fat genes deactivate. The more they deactivate, the more weight you lose—and it becomes a virtuous cycle. Weight loss leads to even greater weight loss.

But to start the process, you have to reduce calories in—without skipping meals or cutting out your favorite foods—while maintaining calories out. And that's what *Eat This, Not That!* is all about.

Understanding the Numbers

On the "calories out" side, we have your daily activities: cleaning house, standing in line at the post office, hauling groceries, and so on. Often, when people discover extra flab hanging around their midsections, they assume there's something wrong with this side of the equation. Maybe so, but more likely it's the front end of the equation—the "calories in" side—that's tipping the scale. That side keeps track of all the cookies, fried chicken, and piles of pasta you eat every day.

In order to maintain a healthy body weight, a moderately active female between the ages of 20 and 50 needs only about 1,800 calories per day, according to the Centers for Disease Control and Prevention. The average man fitting the same profile needs about 2,200 calories per day. Those numbers will fluctuate depending on whether you're taller or shorter than average, whether you run marathons or resist exercise like the plague, or whether you spend your days moving furniture, chasing a room full of toddlers, or just sitting in a cubicle. (For a more accurate assessment, use the calorie calculator at mayoclinic.com.)

The problem is, many of the foods that we consider "normal" servings are, in fact, so packed with calories that we can easily blow through that 1,800 to 2,200 figure in just one sitting. For example, let's say you and your love have date night at Outback. You romantically split a Bloomin' Onion, enjoy a healthy-looking Aussie Chicken Cobb Salad with Crispy Chicken and Thousand Island Dressing, and then—because you ordered the salad—you split one of those yummy Chocolate Thunder from Down Under desserts. All you ate was a salad, and you split the appetizer and dessert. Healthy meal? In fact, you've just downed **3,050 calories.** That means each of you is 1/3 of the way to an extra pound of fat today—and you haven't even figured in breakfast or lunch yet.

But if you'd come armed with *Eat This, Not That!*, you might have made different choices. If you'd ordered the Shrimp on the Barbie (no need to share, eat the whole thing), an Asian Sesame Salad with Seared Ahi and Sesame Viniagrette, and then shared a Classic Cheesecake, you'd have each cut your calorie total to 969—a respectable dinner that's less than a third of what you might have eaten. Even if you only have date night once a week, that's enough for each of you to lose 31 pounds a year!

Here's the math: 3,050 minus 969 equals 2,081 calories you just saved. Once a week means 2,081 times 52, which equals 108,212 calories in a year. And since it takes 3,500 calories to produce a pound of body weight, simple division leads you to 30.91 pounds.

That's the magic of *Eat This, Not That!* Within these pages are literally hundreds of simple food swaps that will save you from 10 to

THE MATH

3,050	calories in the big meal
- 969	calories in meal swap
2,081	calories saved with swap

2,081	calories saved in swap
x 52	once a week for a year
108,212	calories saved per year

108,212	calories saved per year
÷ 3,500	calories per pound of fat
30.91	**pounds saved per year!**

1,000 calories apiece. The more often you choose the "Eat This" foods over the "Not That" options, the quicker you'll notice layers of fat melting away from your body. Check this out:

A cup of Apple Cinnamon Cheerios contains 160 calories. A cup of Cinnamon Burst Cheerios contains 110 calories. Alter your breakfast every morning and **SAVE 5 POUNDS THIS YEAR!**

Two tablespoons of Kraft Roka Blue Cheese dressing will cost you 120 calories. Bolthouse Farms Yogurt Dressing Chunky Blue Cheese is just 35 calories. It's only 85 calories, what's the difference? But making one swap like this at home every day will help you LOSE 9 POUNDS THIS YEAR.

WHAT'S HEALTHIER: The Premium Grilled Chicken Ranch BLT Sandwich at McDonald's, or their Premium Crispy Chicken Ranch BLT Salad? Choose wrong and you've cost yourself 160 calories. (Hint: It's the sandwich!) Make the right choice every day and **DROP NEARLY 17 POUNDS IN A YEAR!**

A turkey sandwich from Panera Bread sounds like a reasonable lunch. But pass on the Sierra Turkey on Asiago Cheese Focaccia and opt instead for the Smoked Turkey Breast on Country. Pretty much the same meal? Not when you're saving 380 calories by making the swap. A move like this at lunch five times a week **SAVES YOU MORE THAN 39 POUNDS THIS YEAR!**

AND THE BEST NEWS IS: These swaps aren't isolated calorie savers. In these pages we'll show you how to save calories on everything from soups to salads, from Ruby Tuesday to T.G.I. Fridays, and every day in between.

TOP SWAPS
THE EAT THIS, NOT THAT!
HALL of FAME

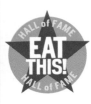

Nobody ever became an NBA star the first time they dribbled a ball, or a tour headliner the first time they picked up a guitar. Whether it's in Canton or Cleveland or Cooperstown, getting to the Hall of Fame means taking a million little steps that look, to the outside world, like one great leap. The same is true for weight loss. *Eat This, Not That!* was founded in 2007 on the idea that simple food swaps every day add up to big results over time. Slice just 100 calories from your daily intake and you shed 10 pounds in a year. It's not about draconian measures. It's about small changes and smart choices. Here, we present the 10 Hall of Fame of Swaps that have given people the power to change their lives.

BURGER

Steak 'n Shake Double Steakburger with Cheese

440 calories
25 g fat
(11 g saturated,
1 g trans)
590 mg sodium

EAT THIS!
HALL of FAME

NOT THAT!
HALL of SHAME

Five Guys Little Cheeseburger
with Lettuce, Tomato, Onions, and Mayo

673 calories
43 g fat
(17 g saturated)
767 mg sodium

*Save 233 calories and
18 grams of fat!*

In the battle between two of America's fastest-growing burger chains, the East Coast titan gets trounced by the scrappy Midwestern patty shack. Five Guys' smallest, relatively restrained cheeseburger packs more calories than a Big Mac and 233 calories more than a bilevel cheeseburger from Steak 'n Shake. From a sheer flavor standpoint, it's hard to argue that both places aren't putting out burgers superior to the hamburger heavyweights (after all, they're cooking fresh ground beef on flattops to order), but Five Guys proves fresh and healthy often have very little to do with each other.

BREAKFAST BURRITO

Burger King
Sausage Breakfast Burrito

290 calories

17 g fat
(6 g saturated)

810 mg sodium

Save 210 calories and 11 grams of fat!

Chick-fil-A
Sausage Breakfast Burrito

500 calories

28 g fat
(11 g saturated)

910 mg sodium

When it comes to dependably low-calorie fast-food chicken sandwiches, Chick-fil-A has the market cornered, but if you're on the hunt for sausage and egg wrapped in a warm tortilla, keep on driving. The chicken purveyor's breakfast burrito has as much fat as seven Chargrilled Chicken Sandwiches, not to mention unwholesome injections of hydrogenated soybean oil and various unpronounceable chemicals. Burger King's burrito, on the other hand, is surprisingly balanced, relying on just enough sausage to add flavor without excess fat.

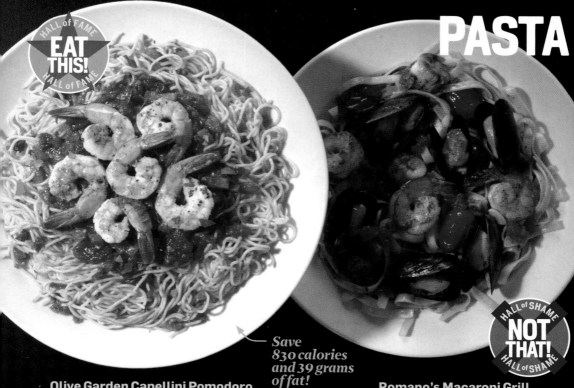

EAT THIS!
HALL of FAME
HALL of FAME

Save 830 calories and 39 grams of fat!

NOT THAT!
HALL of SHAME
HALL of SHAME

Olive Garden Capellini Pomodoro with Grilled Shrimp

480 calories
10.5g fat, (1g sat fat)
1530 mg sodium

Romano's Macaroni Grill Pasta di Mare

1,310 calories
57 g fat, (16 g saturated)
1,900 mg sodium

At Romano's Macaroni Grill, the much-vaunted Mediterranean diet takes a real beating. While in Italian, *di mare* means "of the sea," here it means "of the starch"—in fact, this dish contains 11 times more carbohydrates than protein. Olive Garden's shrimp dish, on the other hand, packs an impressive 41 grams of protein for a solid one-to-two ratio of protein to carbs. The difference is striking: Both dishes feature pasta, shellfish, olive oil, wine, garlic, and tomatoes, yet somehow Romano's comes out with twice the calories and an inexplicable glut of saturated fat.

27

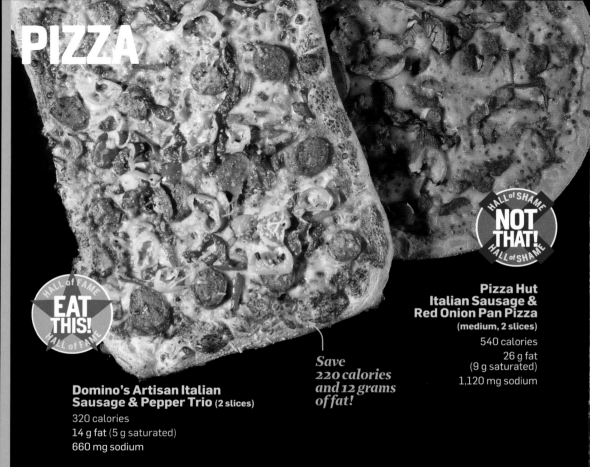

PIZZA

**Pizza Hut
Italian Sausage &
Red Onion Pan Pizza**
(medium, 2 slices)

540 calories
26 g fat
(9 g saturated)
1,120 mg sodium

*Save
220 calories
and 12 grams
of fat!*

**Domino's Artisan Italian
Sausage & Pepper Trio** (2 slices)

320 calories
14 g fat (5 g saturated)
660 mg sodium

Pizza Hut's pie represents pizza's two great pitfalls: oversized crust and fatty meat. That pushes carbs and fat to the forefront and relegates protein to a supporting role— bad strategy if you like to eat pizza regularly (who doesn't?). Domino's exceptional Artisan line relies on relatively thin crusts and lean toppings, and with this particular pizza, the trio of flavor-dense peppers prevents the heavier sausage from overrunning the pie. The result is one of the best pizzas in America, decadent enough to satisfy a serious pizza craving, lean enough to eat on a regular basis.

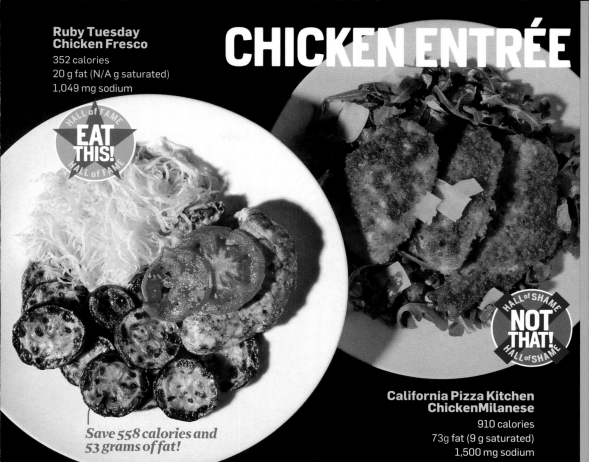

CHICKEN ENTRÉE

**Ruby Tuesday
Chicken Fresco**

352 calories
20 g fat (N/A g saturated)
1,049 mg sodium

EAT
THIS!
HALL of FAME

*Save 558 calories and
53 grams of fat!*

NOT
THAT!
HALL of SHAME

**California Pizza Kitchen
ChickenMilanese**

910 calories
73g fat (9 g saturated)
1,500 mg sodium

The difference between these two meals can be only partly explained by the fact that Ruby Tuesday grills its chicken instead of frying it. California Pizza Kitchen's dish looks like an inverted salad, after all. Where could all that fat come from? The chain doesn't provide the data we'd need to explain it, but CPK somehow greases up its bird with 73 grams of fat—roughly four times what you'll find in Ruby Tuesday's dish. Make this swap twice a week and you'll save 20 pounds within a year.

29

SALAD

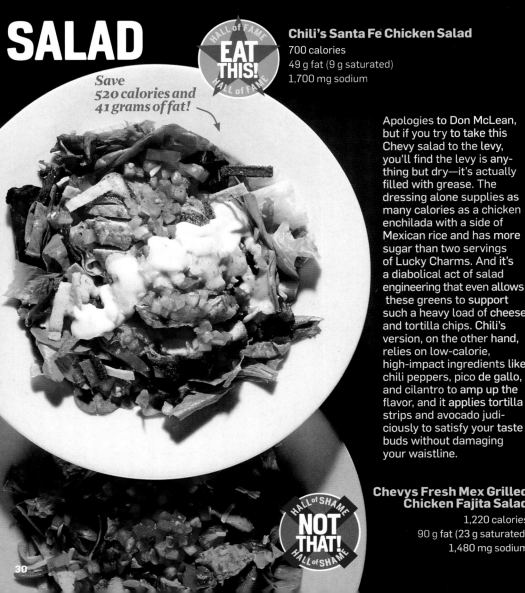

Save
520 calories and
41 grams of fat!

Chili's Santa Fe Chicken Salad

700 calories
49 g fat (9 g saturated)
1,700 mg sodium

Apologies to Don McLean, but if you try to take this Chevy salad to the levy, you'll find the levy is anything but dry—it's actually filled with grease. The dressing alone supplies as many calories as a chicken enchilada with a side of Mexican rice and has more sugar than two servings of Lucky Charms. And it's a diabolical act of salad engineering that even allows these greens to support such a heavy load of cheese and tortilla chips. Chili's version, on the other hand, relies on low-calorie, high-impact ingredients like chili peppers, pico de gallo, and cilantro to amp up the flavor, and it applies tortilla strips and avocado judiciously to satisfy your taste buds without damaging your waistline.

Chevys Fresh Mex Grilled Chicken Fajita Salad

1,220 calories
90 g fat (23 g saturated)
1,480 mg sodium

30

HALL of FAME
EAT THIS!
HALL of FAME

Ruby Tuesday Classic Barbecue Baby-Back Ribs
(half rack)

470 calories
24 g fat (N/A g saturated)
365 mg sodium

HALL of SHAME
NOT THAT!
HALL of SHAME

Chili's Memphis Dry Rub Baby Back Ribs
(half rack)

960 calories
49g fat (14g sat fat)
2,800 mg sodium

Save 490 calories and 2,435 milligrams of sodium

Chili's must have a side business manufacturing textiles. How else can you explain its dedication to making us wear larger and larger clothes? Their ribs are a perfect example: In a normal world, Memphis dry rub is the lower-calorie alternative to ribs with barbecue sauce. But at Chili's a full order racks up 1,920 calories. Order a side of Texas Cheese Fries and you've got a meal that's nearly 3,700 calories.

SUB

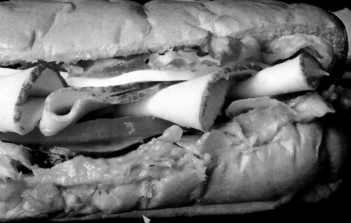

Subway Turkey & Bacon Avocado Sub (6")

390 calories
13 g fat
(3.5 g saturated)
860 mg sodium

Save 550 calories and 38 grams of fat!

Quiznos Turkey Bacon Guacamole Sub (regular)

940 calories
51 g fat
(15 g saturated, 0.5 g trans)
2,820 mg sodium

On the nutritional battlefield, Subway's subs win nearly every time, and this is no exception. Quiznos's liberal condiment policy allows for two calorie-dense spreads on this sandwich—guacamole and ranch—which combine to sabotage any shot at a light lunch. Subway's version balances indulgence (bacon, avocado) with refreshing simplicity (no excess condiments, all of the fresh vegetables you want). Plus your heart will thank you. Subway slashed sodium from every sandwich a few years ago, minimizing the salty strain on your cardiovascular system.

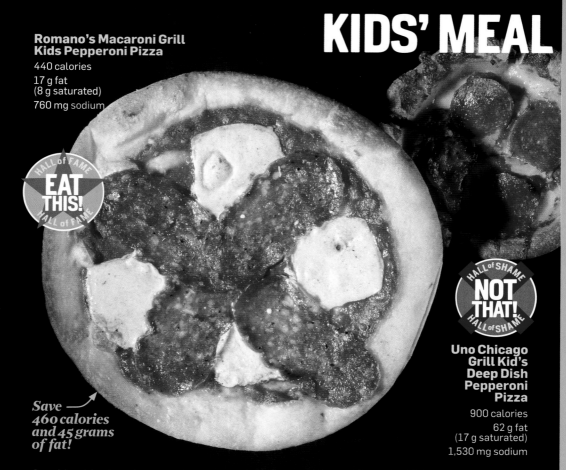

Romano's Macaroni Grill Kids Pepperoni Pizza

440 calories

17 g fat
(8 g saturated)

760 mg sodium

HALL of FAME
EAT THIS!
HALL of FAME

HALL of SHAME
NOT THAT!
HALL of SHAME

Uno Chicago Grill Kid's Deep Dish Pepperoni Pizza

900 calories

62 g fat
(17 g saturated)

1,530 mg sodium

Save 460 calories and 45 grams of fat!

Consider this: America's obesity rate is nearly three times that of Italy's. If that doesn't convince you to aim for authentic Italian pizzas (or to move to Tuscany), nothing will. Although Uno's Kid's pizza is a vast improvement over the chain's adult individual deep dish, it still packs more than 90 calories per ounce, making it more calorie dense than many fast-food shakes. Mac Grill approaches its pie as an Italian would, stretching the crust thin, allowing it to puff up, and then applying just the right amount of pepperoni and cheese.

SMOOTHIES

Jamba Juice Light Strawberries Wild Smoothie
(28 fl oz)

280 calories
0g fat
54g sugar

Save 317 calories and 87 grams of sugar!

Smoothie King Lemon Twist Strawberry
(32 fl oz)

597 calories
0g fat
141g sugar

The American Heart Association recommends that an adult male eat no more than 38 grams of added sugars a day. Each of these smoothies breaks through that barrier, but the Smoothie King manages to blow through four days' worth of added sugar. Plus, liquid calories are absorbed more quickly than solid calories, because the digestion process is quicker. That's a sugar rush that will send you flying!

DESSERT

Jack in the Box Chocolate Overload Cake

300 calories
7 g fat
(1.5 g saturated)
57 g carbohydrates

EAT THIS!
HALL of FAME

Applebee's TripleChocolate Meltdown

960 calories
52 g fat
(34 g saturated)
122 g carbohydrates

NOT THAT!
HALL of SHAME

Save 660 calories and 45 grams of fat!

It's not often we suggest that people turn to Jack in the Box for nutritional refuge, but in a minor miracle the West Coast behemoth has managed to produce one of the lowest-calorie chocolate treats we've ever come across. Skip the medium fries and order this instead and you'll take in fewer carbs and a third fewer calories. The scariest thing about Applebee's Chocolate Meltdown is that despite sharing the same general makeup as the Chocolate Overload cake (look at it!), it somehow packs 15 times the saturated fat. This is what a good swap is all about: Eating the healthiest possible versions of the foods you really want to eat (burgers! pizza! chocolate cake!)

Chapter 1

FOOD RIGHT NOW

The food world moves fast. If you blinked, you might have missed these major developments in our restaurants and supermarkets

Forty years ago, there were no disposable plastic water bottles littering America's landscape. Now there are billions of them. Twenty years ago, no one had really heard of gluten intolerance. Today, everyone and their uncle is suffering from it. Ten years ago, chia seeds were what you used to grow little fuzzy plant pets—who knew you could eat them? Now they're the superfood of the moment, and scientists in Kentucky have even discovered how to cultivate these previously tropical plants in the U.S.

The food landscape moves fast. Seemingly ground-shaking trends, like low-fat eating, rise and recede like waves. Small movements, like foraging, slowly evolve from a couple of hippies traipsing around Central Park to a strategy that fuels some of the best restaurants in the world. And technologies—from the re-invention of sous-vide (plastic pouch cooking) to the rise of Instagram—can change the way we consume food in an instant. Here are some of the most interesting developments of the last year.

GMOs Get Called Out!

In 2014, Vermont became the first state to pass a law that would require the labeling of GMOs. "We believe we have a right to know what's in the food we buy," said Governor Peter Shumlin as he signed the bill. The law is scheduled to go into effect in July 2016, although we can already see the dollar signs lighting up as the food industry gets ready to pour money into challenging the movement. In November of 2014, big food producers went head-to-head with consumer advocates in both Oregon and Colorado over proposed GMO labeling laws. According to the *Wall Street Journal,* big food outspent consumer groups by about $27M in anti-labeling campaign ads. Surprise, surprise: In both states, the ballot measures were defeated. Maine and Connecticut have passed GMO-labeling laws, but they won't go into effect until another state successfully launches its own labeling program. Look for Orwellian-sounding advocacy groups like the Biotechnology Industry Organization to continue campaigning mightily on behalf of food companies who'd like us to know as little as possible about what we're putting in our bodies.

#conspiracytheory

The FDA Steps In

After 21 years, the FDA has finally proposed an overhaul of the Nutrition Facts label that appears on packaged foods, putting calorie counts in larger type. More important, the new labels would update serving sizes to recognize what people actually eat and drink, making it harder for food packagers to claims that, for example, a serving of Snapple Peach Tea is 80 calories when a bottle actually contains twice that. Just as important, the administration has established new rules requiring any business with more than 20 outlets nationwide that sell prepared foods to eat on premises—including restaurants, amusement parks and even movie theaters—to post calorie counts.

#itsabouttime

Even 7-Eleven Gets Healthy

Half the time we go to 7-Eleven, it's because our designated driver had to stop for gas. The chain is the ultimate tank-topping spot for late-night munchies and, as such, a terrible place to be making healthy food choices. So kudos to the chain for partnering with P90X creator Tony Horton to create products like spicy quinoa salad and cold-pressed juices including celery, apple, cucumber, spinach, kale, and even exotics like wheatgrass and clover sprouts. They also unveiled a line of under-400-calorie sandwiches, salads, and wraps made by a company called Fresh Grill Santa Ana. Time will tell whether this is enough to save them from the eternal damnation wrought by their near-simultaneous introduction of Doritos Loaded—a mozzarella-stick/Doritos chip hybrid with half a day's sodium in one 4-piece container and 60 percent of its calories from fat.

#munchieattack

McDonald's Hits a Wall

The world's largest restaurant chain reported its sharpest decline in global sales in more than a decade. According to the *Wall Street Journal,* traditional fast-food joints are struggling both in the U.S. and across the globe, especially among millennials, who are as likely to meet up with friends at Chipotle or Panera Bread, as they are one of the big three burger chains. Part of the issue: A lot of "fast casual" chains like Chipotle or even Starbucks make a big show of social responsibility and ethically raised foods, which resonates with younger people who were raised in the era of *Food, Inc.* and *Supersize Me.*

#fallenarches

The Big Three Make a Pledge

In September 2014, Coca-Cola Co. and PepsiCo, Inc. joined with Dr. Pepper Snapple Group (NOT the name of a '70s funk band) and pledged to cut calories in soda by 20 percent by 2025. A former executive for the one of the companies told us that as beverage makers were feeling the heat of legislative initiatives, health advocacy groups and, yes, *Eat This, Not That!,* the race was on to find alternatives to sugar, high-fructose corn syrup, and the chemical additives in diet soda that would give soft drinks a healthier halo. The pledge is meant to stall further action—like the soda tax enacted by voters in Berkeley, California, in November of 2014—until manufacturers can find a solution.

#sweetrelief

Everything Is Coming to Your Front Door

You've heard of Pea Pod and Fresh Direct? Now everyone from Amazon to Walmart to Google (yes, Google) is trying to muscle in on the grocery delivery business. Some companies are experimenting with the standard warehousing model, while others are trying a grocery-shopping version of Uber, where you place your order via app and, if there's a freelance shopper in the area, they pop into a local supermarket, buy your groceries, and drop them off at your house. New York and San Francisco are the hotbeds of this new trend, but home delivery will likely be coming to your hometown in the near future.

#neverleavethecouch

Your Gut Is the New Hot Zone

Ever since Jamie Lee Curtis started pitching yogurt to baby boomers, concerns about gut health have started to percolate up. In 2014, belly bacteria was second only to Ebola as America's top health obsession. "Increasingly, scientists, physicians, and the public are recognizing that the gut microbiota, the microbes that live within our intestines, shape our health and wellbeing in innumerable ways," reported the Harvard School of Public Health. And in *The 21-Day Belly Fix,* one of nearly a dozen books on the subject released in 2014, Tasneem Bhatia, M.D., reported that 9 out of 10 patients she sees are suffering from some health effects of imbalanced gut bacteria. The culprits: too much stress, too many medications (including antibiotics, nonsteroidal anti-inflammatories like Advil, and antidepressants), and not enough bacteria-feeding fiber. Dr. Bhatia and others recommend a regimen that includes a daily dose of apple cider vinegar to promote healthier buggers. #goingbuggy

We're Getting Hip to "Natural"

In 2014, Trader Joe's paid out $3.4M to customers upset that many products labeled "all-natural" actually contained synthetic ingredients. Whole Foods is facing a similar lawsuit. And it's not the first time consumers have kicked back against this meaningless term: In 2011, Frito-Lay was sued by consumers over the "all-natural" label on its Tostitos and Sun Chips. As a result, the industry is wisely backing away from "natural" claims: in 2013, 22 percent of new products contained the "natural" label, down from 30 percent in 2011 and 2012. #wontgetfooledagain

Food Is Saving the World

A decade ago, films like *Food Inc.* got a lot of people thinking about corporate animal agriculture, but most of us thought of it as like the weather: Everybody talks about it, but what can you do? Until recently, that is, when companies like Beyond Meat and Hampton Creek started to create vegan versions of meat and eggs with the stated purpose of disrupting our food supply chain and altering the very way in which our food is raised. In 2014 they hit the mainstream, with coverage on NPR and in the *New York Times,* and distribution in places like Whole Foods. Instead of faking the taste of meat with soy or fungus-based materials like Quorn, for example, these companies break down the molecular composition of meat and then rebuild it using non-animal products, with the stated mission of reducing global warming and industrial animal farming. #steppingup

EAT THIS, NOT THAT! AWARDS

AWARD
EAT THIS!
WINNER

At Eat This, Not That!, we spend a lot of time bashing restaurant chains, food manufacturers, and general ne'er-do-wells of the industrial agricultural complex for their lack of transparency, duplicitous labeling practices, and insistence in shoving as much fat, salt, and chemicals into our bodies as they can. Sometimes, we feel like Alexander and the Terrible, Horrible, No-Good, Very Bad Food.

So we thought it made sense to stop and celebrate some of the good guys out there—the food companies, small and large, who are stocking our shelves, menus, and bodies with foods that are wholesome, nutritious and just plain good. According to the 2014 Health & Wellness Survey by the Grocery Manufacturers Association (GMA), more than 10,000 new "healthier" products have been introduced into supermarkets in just the last four years. Here then are the recipients of the Eat This, Not That! Awards.

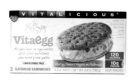

VITALICIOUS
VitaEgg Flatbread Sandwiches

Low-calorie, high in fiber and protein, and, most interesting, boasts 160 mg of omega-3 DHA fatty acids, on par with what you'd get from a couple of ounces of canned tuna.

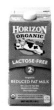

HORIZON
Organic Lactose-Free Milk

For the lactose intolerant, a welcome new option, organic lactose-free milk.

SMART BALANCE
Buttery Spread

One of the top national brands in alternative spreads made the leap this year to produce all of its products with 100% non-GMO sourced ingredients.

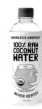

HARMLESS HARVEST
Raw Coconut Water

For purists, this is as close as you can get to cracking open a coconut yourself. Harmless Harvest uses high-pressure processing to bottle organically grown coconut water.

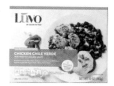

LUVO
Frozen Foods

The concept is "restaurant-quality" frozen meals using nutritious ingredients, no artificial sweeteners or artificial flavors, with no more than 500 calories per meal and less than 500 mg sodium. Luvo has attracted partnerships with everyone from diet author Mark Hyman, M.D., to Derek Jeter.

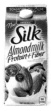

SILK
Protein+Fiber Almond Milk

Traditional almond milk is low in calories and high in calcium, but often has none of the protein or fiber that almonds provide. Silk found a way to capture the good stuff and help keep us feeling full and satisfied.

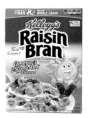

KELLOGG'S
Raisin Bran Omega-3 with Flaxseed

Parents love it when food manufacturers help them sneak nutrition into the lives of their unsuspecting children. Here, Kellogg's adds whole flaxseed and soluble corn fiber to its standard whole-wheat cereal, resulting in a cereal with 5 grams of fiber per cup. (Now if it could just create a version with a little less sugar coating the raisins.)

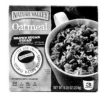

NATURE VALLEY
Oatmeal for the Keurig

Better living through technology! The perfect way to avoid the temptation of the office snack machine: You can keep these Keurig cups of oatmeal in your desk and brew yourself a cup of oatmeal in no time.

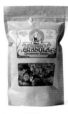

MICHELE'S
Apple Quinoa Granola

Formerly sold only at farmers markets, this product is now available online. This granola uses organic products and includes everyone's favorite new superfood, quinoa. Michelesgranola.com

DEEBEE'S
Organic TeaPops

Tea and fruit in a frozen pop sounds like an awesome idea. DeeBee's takes it all the way with a frozen treat that's (deep breath): certified non-GMO, organic, kosher, vegan, gluten-free, dairy-free, nut-and-soy free, and with no refined sugars. Phew!

HARVEST SOUL
Green Fusion and Tropical Fusion

Harvest Soul uses a high-pressure processing technology that protects its juices' natural levels of antioxidants. These "chewable juices" include a blend of fruits and vegetables mixed with crunchy and chewable seeds, nuts and berries, which give them an unusual boost of protein and fiber.

AWARD
EAT THIS!
WINNER

OCEAN SPRAY
PACt water

We've had enough of "nutritional" waters that are not much more than high-fructose corn syrup, a concoction of chemicals, and a splash of vitamin C. Ocean Spray has stepped up with a product that sports only 10 calories per bottle, and 80 milligrams of cranberry PACs. PACs, or proanthocyanidins, are natural elements found in some plant foods including cranberries, tea, dark chocolate, apples and grapes. Among their main role in the human body is to protect collagen and elastin—basically, the connective tissue proteins that help you resist aging. We'll take it!

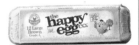

HAPPY EGG COMPANY

Thanks to confusing labeling rules, "cage-free" or "free-range" doesn't necessarily mean the eggs come from free-roaming chickens. Cage-free simply means no cages, but doesn't guarantee the hens ever get outside; free-range means they have access to the outdoors, but not that they will be encouraged (or understand how) to get out-side. Happy Egg promises to sell only little protein bomb-lets dropped from truly free-range chickens who roam the equivalent of 4 football fields of space every day.

JAMBA
All-Natural Fruit & Veggies Smoothie– Green Fusion

Not everything at your local Jamba Juice is exactly a health food (a 22-ounce Surf Rider can pack 450 calories and nearly 100 grams of sugar). But this smoothie kit contains whole pieces of frozen fruit and vegetable blocks that, when blended with one cup of apple juice, makes two, 8-ounce smooth-ies. Contains green apple, mango, pineapple, kiwi, banana, broccoli, spinach and spirulina, with just 120 calories.

VITALICIOUS
VitaPizza

It's almost unfair to your belly fat. The newly reformulated VitaPizzas contain up to 14 grams of belly-filling protein, another 14 grams of heart-healthy fiber, and no more than 5 grams of fat per serving, for a caloric load that's about half of what your average frozen pizza offers. At just 220 calories, this might be the best late-night snack in the universe.

COMING TO A NEIGHBORHOOD NEAR YOU
These emerging restaurant chains are cooking up something unique

Zoë's Kitchen

Mediterranean-inspired food, where grilling is the predominant method of cooking and the cuisine is focused on vegetables, olive oil, and lean protein. There are no fryers or microwaves.

LOCATIONS: 132 locations across 13 states in the South and Southwest, as well as New Jersey and Pennsylvania.

Bareburger

One of a number of small chains (including BRGR and Tallgrass) offering exclusively grass-fed beef in their burgers. Almost everything in Bareburger restaurants are built from sustainable materials, including tabletops made from trees felled in storms and booths made from recycled vinyl. Even its take-out containers are biodegradable.

LOCATIONS: New York, Pennsylvania, Connecticut, New Jersey, Ohio

Pizzeria Locale

It's not a chain yet, but Pizzeria Locale is backed by Chipotle, and it's not exactly shy about growing quickly. The Colorado-based pizza shop uses artisanal recipes and a 1,000-degree oven to create traditional pizzas designed by James Beard—award-winning chefs Lachlan MacKinnon-Patterson and Bobby Stuckey. Wait for it...

LOCATIONS: Boulder and Denver, Colorado

True Food Kitchen

A selection of vegan, vegetarian, and gluten-free superfoods like acai, kale, quinoa, and seabuckthorn. Developed in partnership with Dr. Andrew Weill, True Food's motto is "feel better, live longer, and make your mouth happy."

LOCATIONS: Arizona, California, Texas, Colorado, Georgia, Virginia

Elevation Burger

100% organic, grass-fed, free-range, ground-on-site beef burgers and french fries cooked in olive oil. The restaurants are built from renewable materials such as bamboo.

LOCATIONS: 30 locations in Texas, Michigan, Indiana, and along the East Coast.

LYFE Kitchen

An increasingly national chain that serves locally sourced food. Everything on the menu is less than 600 calories.

LOCATIONS: California, Colorado, Illinois, Nevada, New York, Texas

FOOD ABOMINATIONS
The Worst New Foods

Every year, in the minefield that is the American food scene, there are new and utterly inventive booby traps laid. And this year, the new calorie bombs are among the most dangerous we've ever seen.

Major food companies actually save their most horrible inventions for overseas audiences, like McDonalds' Arabia Mega Mac (four patties for a whopping 736 calories). The real insanity in the U.S.A. comes from local sources, like PYT Burger of Philadelphia's D'oh Nut burger, a doughnut stuffed with a bacon cheeseburger, or the 8-pound Hugo Boss burger available at Charlotte Hornets home games.

But you don't have to go to the Middle East—or even the Eastern Conference—to suffer the slings and arrows of our harrowing hash slingers. This year, a lot of very bad ideas have come to restaurants and grocery stores right near you.

NABISCO CHIPS AHOY! CHEWY BIRTHDAY FROSTING FILLED

A cookie stuffed with sugary frosting, and 7 different artificial food dyes to make it look like a birthday cake. There's nothing to celebrate here, and you won't need a pinch to grow an inch—or two.

150 calories, 7 g fat, 13 g sugars, 1 g protein

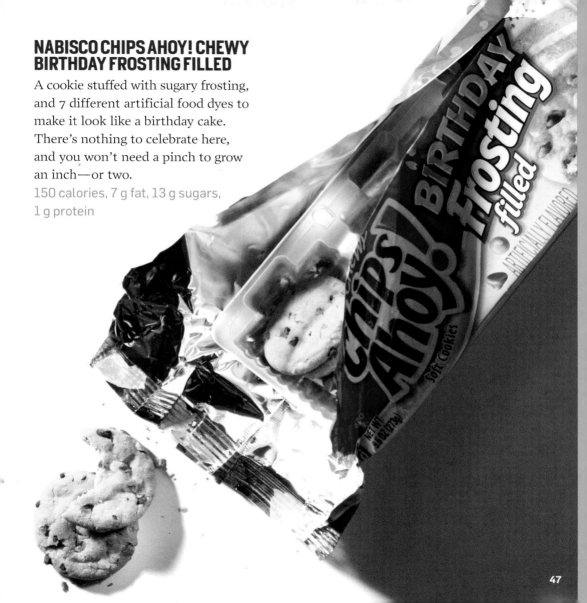

EGGO BITES PANCAKES CHOCOLATEY CHIP

The giveaway word here is "chocolatey," which means there's not enough actual cocoa in the food to legally call itself chocolate. No fiber, either. There are, however, 10 grams of sugar in these little diskettes of white flour and vegetable oil.

140 calories, 3.5 g fat, 10 g sugars

CRACKER JACK'D ENERGY TRAIL MIXES

The prize at the bottom is a much larger belt. Despite the nuts and fruits on the package, the second, third, and fourth ingredients are sugar, vegetable oil, and graham cracker crumbs. Looks like it's our wallets that got jacked.

140 calories, 7g fat, 7g sugars

TACO BELL A.M. SAUSAGE CRUNCHWRAP

There's nothing we can add to the words "sausage crunchwrap." Don't skip breakfast—except this one.

710 calories, 46 g fat (14 g saturated fat), 3 g sugars

JACK IN THE BOX CHICK-N-TATER MELT MUNCHIE MEAL

Fried chicken, bacon, hash browns, and three cheeses stuffed into a buttery croissant. But wait—the meal also comes with a couple of tacos, fries, and a soda. Your terrible total:

1,756 calories, 109 g fat (28 g saturated fat), 10 g sugars.

COFFEE-MATE NESTLE TOLL HOUSE CHOCOLATE CHIP COOKIE CREAMER

The idea of a "nondairy creamer" almost sounds healthy, doesn't it? But Coffee-mate is made with water, sugar, and partially hydrogenated oils—you know them as trans fats. This new version of an already awful product at least brings a little honesty to the table with its name. You're not drinking coffee. You're drinking junk food.

35 calories, 1.5 g fat, 5 g sugars

WONKA PEEL-A-POP

Made to look like a healthy banana, it's actually a push pop surrounded by a taffy-like "peel" that uses ingredients like propylene glycol mono-stearate—a de-greasing agent that was deployed to help clean up the Deepwater Horizon spill. This makes that chewing gum that turned Violet Beauregarde into a blueberry look harmless by comparison.

65 calories, 2 g fat, 12 g sugars

SONIC GRAPE WITH NERDS CANDY REAL ICE CREAM SLUSH, LARGE

Imagine the sugar equivalent of 59 Twizzler sticks. Now imagine drinking those Twizzler sticks through a straw.

1,640 calories, 52 g fat
(37 g saturated fat), 282 g sugars

CHUCK E. CHEESE'S YOGURT SQUEEZES

Advertised as a snack that "balances health with fun," each pop contains only 2 grams of protein and 10 grams of sugar, along with a lot of artificial food coloring. So really, health and fun are balanced—you get very little of either.

70 calories, 0.5 g fat, 10 g sugars

PAPA JOHN'S FRITOS CHILI PIZZA

Papa John's seasonal concoction of pizza, beef chili, and yes, Fritos is an insult to almost every cuisine known to man. By our estimates, a whole pie would come salted up with nearly 6,000 mg of sodium.

Per 2 slices: 720 calories, 30 g fat, 12g saturated, 1,400 mg sodium

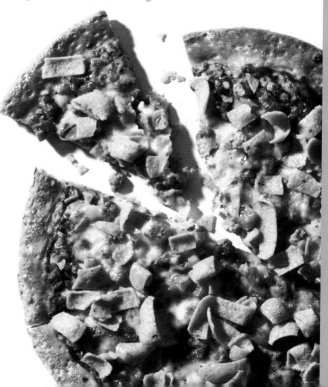

Chapter 2

THE TRUTH ABOUT YOUR FOOD

The advertisements make every cheesy, gooey, greasy meal seem so naturally delicious. The reality is something less enticing.

Wouldn't it be refreshing if, just once, a cable news anchor came on and said, "In today's top story, everything we told you in yesterday's top story was wrong"? Wouldn't it be great if the people who are paid to keep us informed about everything acknowledged that they don't always get everything right?

Nowhere are the nattering nabobs of news less sure of themselves than in the realm of nutrition. For decades, we've been slapped with wave after wave of food hype, promoted by the media, by celebrities, by big food and agriculture companies, even by the U.S. government (remember how we were all supposed to give up fat and eat nothing but carbs back in the 1990s?). We've pounded pomegranate juice, guzzled green smoothies, acceded to acai, duked it out with Dukan. And yet we just keep getting fatter and sicker.

The reason: Much of what we believe about food is really just hearsay, a game of nutritional telephone handed down from science journals to newspapers to television to your Aunt Phoebe to your mom and then to you, with marketers in between, messing with the message. As a result, we swing wildly back and forth with our weight battles, chasing one nutritional hobgoblin after another. (Don't eat beef, eat seafood! But only if it doesn't have mercury! Or if it's line caught! Or if it's grass fed—no wait, that's the beef! Eat that!)

The entire mission of *Eat This, Not That!* is to make your nutritional life simpler. As trends teeter-totter and research reaches and redacts, one thing stays the same: We like the food we eat. We like pizza, burgers, pies, even the occasional salad. We just want to be able to eat them and know we're doing the right thing. So enjoy the food you love, just eat the best possible versions of them. And while you're at it, ignore these nutrition myths—they're only confusing you.

You Must Force Yourself to Eat Kale

The superpowers of kale, like the dangers of the Bermuda Triangle, have been highly exaggerated. A 2014 study at William Paterson University ranked fruits and vegetables by their nutrient density, based on their levels of 17 different nutrients that have been linked to improved cardiovascular health. Not surprisingly, the top 16 were all leafy greens, which pack the most nutrition per calorie. (Coming in at #17 was red bell peppers.) But kale didn't even make the top 10. In fact, simple spinach and even Romaine lettuce beat the alleged supergreen, as did parsley and chives. Even stuff you normally throw away—the greens atop beets—pack more nutrition.

Sugar Is Healthier than High-Fructose Corn Syrup

Sugar is the master of disguise. Maltodextrin, brown rice syrup, dextrose, sucrose—it's got more alter egos than the Avengers. But it's most well-known costume is high-fructose corn syrup. Whether HFCS is worse than plain ol' table sugar has long been a contentious issue. Here's what you need to know: In a 2014 review of five studies comparing the effects of sugar and HFCS, there was no difference found in changes in blood glucose levels, lipid levels, or appetite between table sugar consumption and HFCS consumption. In other words, your body can't tell one from the other—they're both just sugar. HFCS's real sin is that it's super cheap, and as a result, it's added to everything from cereal to ketchup to salad dressing. Is it a good idea to minimize the HFCS in your diet? Absolutely. But sugar's role as a more "natural" alternative has been exaggerated.

Sea Salt Is a Healthier Version of Regular Salt

Everyday table salt comes from a mine and contains roughly 2,300 milligrams of sodium per teaspoon. Sea salt comes from evaporated seawater, and it also contains roughly 2,300 milligrams of sodium. That makes them, well, roughly identical. Advocates point to the fact that sea salt also contains other compounds like magnesium and iron, but in truth, these minerals exist in trace amounts. To obtain a meaningful dose, you'd have to take in extremely high and potentially dangerous levels of sodium. What's more, traditional table salt is regularly fortified with iodine, which plays an important role in regulating the hormones in your body. Sea salt, on the other hand, gives you virtually zero iodine. The bottom line is this: If switching from table salt to sea salt causes you to consume even one extra granule, then you've just completely snuffed out whatever elusive health boon you hope to receive. Plus you've wasted a few bucks.

Energy Drinks Are Better for You than Soda

Energy drinks like Red Bull, Monster, and Full Throttle attempt to boost your energy with a cache of B vitamins, herbal extracts, and amino acids. But what your body's going to remember most (especially around your waistline) is the sugar in these concoctions; a 16-ounce can delivers as much as 280 calories of pure sugar, which is about 80 calories more than you'd find in a 16-ounce cup of Pepsi. What's more, a University of Maryland study found energy drinks to be 11 percent more corrosive to your teeth than regular soda. So here's the secret that energy drink companies don't want you to know: The only proven, significant energy boost comes from caffeine. If you want an energy boost, save yourself the sugar spike and drink a cup of coffee. (A cup of black joe: 5 calories.

Make this swap once a day and lose nearly 29 pounds this year!)

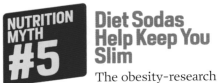

NUTRITION MYTH #5 Diet Sodas Help Keep You Slim

The obesity-research community is becoming increasingly aware that the artificial sweeteners used in diet soda—aspartame and sucralose, for instance—lead to hard-to-control food urges later in the day. One Purdue study discovered that rats took in more calories if they'd been fed artificial sweeteners prior to mealtime, and a University of Texas study found that people who consume just three diet sodas per week were more than 40 percent more likely to be obese. Try weaning yourself off by switching to carbonated water and flavoring with lemon, cucumber, and fresh herbs.

A study in the *American Journal of Public Health* found that more obese adults drink diet soda than healthy-weight adults and that, among the overweight and obese adults studied, those who drank diet soda ate more calories than those who consumed sweetened/regular soda. Researchers have also linked regular diet soda consumption with decreased response to artificial sweeteners and a decreased link between sweet tastes and energy value, meaning their bodies may grow to disassociate sweetness with satiety cues, making it easier to overeat and, therefore, gain weight.

NUTRITION MYTH #6 Yogurt Is Good for the Bacteria in Your Belly

Sure, some yogurts contain beneficial bacteria that can send reinforcements to your gut when you need them. Lactobacillus acidophilus is the bacteria you want to look for, with yogurts that say "live active cultures." But most yogurts are so high in sugar that they do more to promote unhealthy gut bacteria than anything else. (Unhealthy bacteria feed on sugar in your belly the same way they do around your teeth.)

Low-Fat Foods Are Better for You

As it applies to food marketing, the term "low fat" is synonymous with "loaded with salt and cheap carbohydrates." For instance, look at Smucker's Reduced Fat Peanut Butter. To replace the fat it skimmed out, Smucker's added a fast-digesting carbohydrate called maltodextrin. That's not going to help you lose weight. A study in the *New England Journal of Medicine* found that over a two-year span, people on low-carb diets lost 62 percent more body weight than those trying to cut fat. (Plus, the fat in peanut butter is heart-healthy monounsaturated fat—you'd be better off eating more of it, not less!)

"Trans-Fat Free" Food Is Actually Trans-Fat Free

The FDA's guidelines allow companies to claim 0 grams of trans fat—even broadcast it on the front of their packages—as long as the food in question contains no more than 0.5 grams of trans fat per serving. But here's the deal: Due to trans fat's inextricable link to heart disease, the World Health Organization advises people to keep their intake as low as possible, maxing out at about 1 gram per 2,000 calories consumed. If your cupboard's full of foods with almost half a gram per serving, you might be blowing past that number every single day. The *American Journal of Health Promotion* recently published an article urging the FDA to rethink its lax regulations, but until that happens, you should avoid all foods with "partially hydrogenated oil" (meaning trans fats) on their ingredients statements.

Foods Labeled "Natural" Are Healthier

The FDA makes no serious effort to control the use of the word "natural" on nutrition labels. Case in point: 7UP boasts that it's made with "100% Natural Flavors" when, in fact, the soda is sweetened with a decidedly unnatural dose of high-fructose corn syrup. "Corn" is natural, but "high-fructose corn syrup" is produced using a centrifuge and a series of chemical reactions. Other "natural" abusers include Natural Cheetos, which are made with maltodextrin and disodium phosphate, and "natural advantage" Post Raisin Bran, which bathes its raisins in both sugar and corn syrup. The worst part is, you're likely paying a premium price for common junk food.

 Egg Substitutes Are a Smart Way to Lower Cholesterol

NUTRITION MYTH #10

Egg yolks contain dietary cholesterol; this much is true. But research has proven that dietary cholesterol has almost nothing to do with serum cholesterol, the stuff in your blood. Wake Forest University researchers reviewed more than 30 egg studies and found no link between egg consumption and heart disease, and a study in Saint Louis found that eating eggs for breakfast could decrease your calorie intake for the remainder of the day.

 Eating Junk Food Helps Battle Stress

NUTRITION MYTH #11

You've been there: Stressed out and sprawled across your sofa with one arm elbow-deep in a bag of cheese puffs. In the moment, it can be comforting, but a study published in the *British Journal of Psychiatry* found that people who consumed the most highly processed foods were 58 percent more likely to be depressed than those who ate the least.

 Dark Chocolate Is Good for You

NUTRITION MYTH #12

It would be great if all you had to do to eat healthy was look for chocolate bars that were darker than Kristen Stewart's mascara.

Unfortunately, the secret to unlocking the health benefits of chocolate are a bit more complicated than that. Plenty of studies have shown that polyphenols—nutrients found in darkly colored plant foods like chocolate—can do everything from lowering blood pressure to raising our ability to burn fat. A 2013 study in the journal *Diabetic Medicine* even found that eating dark chocolate lessened the effects of high blood sugar in diabetic patients. Unfortunately, the more chocolate is processed, the more of the polyphenols are lost. Creating "Dutch" chocolate, in which an alkalizing agent is added to the cocoa to reduce acidity, destroys up to 77 percent of the nutrients in the cocoa. To get the health benefits that have been touted since the time of Montezeuma, look for a dark chocolate that says 70% cacao (or higher) on the label. The rest? It's just candy.

it's just oatmeal that you made from scratch, and then sweetened yourself with a little fruit. But most of what's sold as oatmeal today is more like a package of Kool-Aid mix. Consider Instant Quaker Oatmeal Strawberries & Cream, which features delicious sounding "flavored and colored fruit pieces." What does that mean, exactly? What they've done is taken dried apples and/or figs and injected them with corn syrup solids, corn starch, and trans fats, and mixed it in something called a "creaming agent." Or check out the Fruit & Maple Oatmeal offering at McDonald's. It's a breakfast cereal with 32 grams of sugar—the equivalent of nearly 13 cups of Kix cereal!

NUTRITION MYTH #14
Bananas Are the Best Source of Potassium

Your body uses potassium to keep your nerves and muscles firing efficiently, and an adequate intake can blunt sodium's effect on blood pressure. One 2009 study found that

NUTRITION MYTH #13
Oatmeal Is Good for You

Okay, oatmeal really is good for you, if

a 2:1 ratio of potassium to sodium could halve your risk of heart disease, and since the average American consumes about 3,400 milligrams of sodium each day, your goal should be 6,800 milligrams of daily potassium. You're extremely unlikely to ever reach that mark—and never with bananas alone. One medium banana has 422 milligrams and 105 calories. Here are the sources that earn you roughly the same amount of potassium in fewer calories:

POTATO / half a medium spud / 80 calories

APRICOTS / 5 whole fruit / 80 calories

CANTALOUPE / 1 cup cubes / 54 calories

BROCCOLI / 1 full stalk / 50 calories

SUN-DRIED TOMATOES / a quarter cup / 35 calories

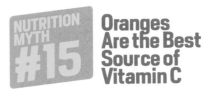

Oranges Are the Best Source of Vitamin C

Far more than a simple immune booster, vitamin C is an antioxidant that plays a host of important roles in your body. It strengthens skin by helping to build collagen, improves mood by increasing the flow of norepinephrine, and bolsters metabolic efficiency by helping transport fat cells into the body's energy-burning mitochondria. But since your body can neither store nor create the wonder vitamin, you need to provide a constant supply. An orange is the most famous vitamin-C food, and although it's a good source, it's by no means the best. For 70 calories, one orange gives you about 70 micrograms of vitamin C. Here are five sources with just as much vitamin C and even fewer calories:

PAPAYA / ¾ cup / 50 calories

BRUSSELS SPROUTS / 1 cup / 40 calories

STRAWBERRIES / 7 large fruit / 40 calories

BROCCOLI / ½ stalk / 25 calories

RED BELL PEPPER / ½ medium pepper / 20 calories

Peanut Butter Is a Health Food

In its best form, peanut butter actually is

a health food. That's because peanuts are packed with monounsaturated fats, the heart-healthy fat that actually helps you lose weight. Here's how the ingredients of a healthy jar of peanut butter should read:

Peanuts.

But most peanut butter doesn't look like that. Here's what the label of Jif Reduced Fat Creamy Peanut Butter Spread reads like:

Peanuts, corn syrup solids, sugar, pea protein, salt, fully hydrogenated vegetable oils, mono and diglycerides, molasses, magnesium oxide, niacinamide, ferric orthophosphate, zinc oxide, copper sulfate, folic acid, pyridoxine hydrochloride.

Now, we know your kids constantly beg you for seconds of pyridoxine hydrochloride, but is that something they need? Most peanut butters are highly processed and loaded with sugars and trans-fatty oils, and contain less of the healthy monounsaturated fats that you truly need. "Peanut butter spread" is even worse.

The word "spread" indicates that it's at least 10 percent additives. Look for "natural" peanut butter (Smucker's and Justin's both make great versions) and don't be fooled by any low-fat promises.

Comfort Food Chases Away the Blues

A bowl of tomato soup and a grilled-cheese sandwich on a cold winter's day. A big spoonful of mac & cheese when you're down on your luck. Comfort food just makes you feel better, doesn't it?

Actually, it doesn't. In a 2014 study aptly titled "The Myth of Comfort Food," researchers showed participants depressing films to "induce a negative effect." Then they gave them either comfort food, foods that weren't considered comfort foods, or no food at all. Result: The subjects got over their bad moods in equal time, regardless of whether or not they ate. Is feeling bad a good excuse for eating bad? Turns out, it's not.

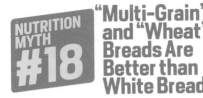

NUTRITION MYTH #18: "Multi-Grain" and "Wheat" Breads Are Better than White Bread

Wait a minute—isn't "multi-grain" one of the biggest buzzwords in nutrition? And haven't we been trained to pick the wheat bread over the white at every turn? Yes, but unfortunately those labels are about as credible as your local congressman's campaign promises. "Wheat bread" is generally white bread with caramel or molasses added to make it look dark and healthy. "Multi-grain" just means that different kinds of junky refined grains may have been used. Always look for the words "100% whole wheat" or "100% whole grain" on the package.

NUTRITION MYTH #19: Wraps Are Healthier than Regular Sandwiches

Those skinny little wraps are so flimsy, so delicate, so fusion-cuisine-friendly. How can they not be better than the average lump of bread? Well, consider Subway's wrap, for one. It packs 310 calories—before you even add the first whiff of meat or sauce. The reason is that, in order for the tortilla to wrap around like that, it needs added fat, often in the form of soybean oil and hydrogenated oils. (In fact, when ordering Mexican food, you're usually better off with a hard taco than a soft, for the same reason.)

NUTRITION MYTH #20: Potatoes Are Empty Carbs

Once the proud spud stud of the American dinner plate, potatoes have been downgraded in recent years to a lowly status not seen since the Irish blight. But unlike the commentators on cable news, the common taters in your kitchen actually have something worth chewing on. A USDA study of potatoes recently found levels of phytochemicals such as flavonoids and kukoamines that rival the amounts found in broccoli, spinach, and Brussels sprouts. Wait a minute:

Kukoamines? You haven't heard of them because they were previously believed to exist only in Chinese medicinal plants, but they have been shown to lower blood pressure by decreasing free-radical damage and inflammation, and getting more of them into your daily diet makes a lot of sense. If you have a craving for fries, try a batch of crispy oven-baked spuds: Cut a medium Russet potato into 8 wedges, toss with olive oil, salt and black pepper (add some paprika if you want to get fancy), and roast in a 400-degree oven until browned on the outside and tender all the way through.

Nutrition Bars Are Actually Nutritious

In a world where we really called it as it is, nutrition bars would be known by another name: calorie bars. Most of them are so polluted with additives that their ingredients list looks like Charlie Sheen's blood test results. For example, PowerBar Vanilla Crisp touts itself as "fuel for optimum performance," but unless you're talking about a performance by the Chemical Brothers, we're not sure exactly what it means. With four different types of sugar, it packs more of the white stuff than an adult woman should eat in an entire day. If you like the idea of a snackable bar that packs in the nutrition, read the ingredients carefully: Brands like KIND, Larabar, and Clif have plenty of smart offerings. But most of what's out there is just candy.

SECRETS THE DIET INDUSTRY DOESN'T WANT YOU TO KNOW

Much like our political scene, the American food scene has splintered into wildly divergent interest groups, all of whom follow their own unshakeable belief systems and are pretty much sure that everybody else who doesn't think like them is nuts. G-freers, Cavemen, Juicers, Vegans—the local grocery store looks like a tribal caravan on its way to Burning Man.

But while each of these movements has plenty to recommend it— lowering white flour, upping protein, vitamins and minerals—none is the cure-all its marketers want you to believe. Here's a skeptical tour through some of the more questionable aspects of the new diet movements.

The Diet Industry Doesn't Want You to Know...
TRANS FATS ARE VEGAN

What do Little Debbies, Doritos Spicy Sweet Chili Tortilla Chips, Oreos, Red Bull, Hershey's Syrup, and Sour Patch Kids all have in common?

They're all endorsed by PETA as part of a vegan diet. And none of them belong in your kitchen.

Veganism—the complete eschewing of any animal-based food, including dairy, eggs, and even honey—used to be the sole domain of yurt-dwellers, yoga enthusiasts, and Moby. No longer. Notorious Big-Mac lover Bill Clinton went vegan a few years back. Jay-Z and Beyoncé bestowed their golden touch on veganism by going without animal products for 22 days to jump-start their 2014. In fact, one in 50 Americans now consider themselves vegan, according to a 2012 Gallup poll.

On the surface, veganism would seem to be the most unassailable of all diet trends. How can one frown on the idea of eating more plants, maximizing fiber and micronutrients, and cutting down on the saturated fats in red meat and dairy—not to mention reducing your carbon footprint, striking out against slaughterhouses, protecting Bambi, and otherwise saving the planet? A 2012 study found that people who eat meat-free have significantly lower levels of LDL "bad" cholesterol, and another found that they had a 32 percent lower risk of hospitalization or death from heart disease. But the peeps from PETA have a small secret: Sugar, salt, high-fructose corn syrup, chemical food dyes, and trans fats are all vegan, and they're hidden in the special sauce of a lot of animal-free products.

Take Amy's Kitchen Thai Pad Thai, a vegan frozen meal that somehow contains 22 grams of sugar. Panera Bread's

Classic Salad has 12 grams of sugar. Add the White Balsamic Apple Vinaigrette and you're up to 23 grams of sugar; you'd get less if you ate a couple of Krispy Kreme doughnuts for dinner. Or check out Stonyfield's O'Soy Raspberry Yogurt with 27 grams of sugar—the equivalent of a Snicker's bar. And the quest for animal-free shortening products often leads to partially hydrogenated oils—you know them as artery-clogging trans fats. A PETA-endorsed margarine like Fleischmann's Light contains partially hydrogenated corn oil, plus something called propylene glycol, which is also used as a plastic resin and to de-ice airplanes. (Fleischmann's claims "og trans fat," but check out the nutrition label: a tablespoon contains 4.5 grams of fat, but

Fleischmann's then lists 1 g monounsaturated fat, 2 grams polyunsaturated fat, and .5 grams of saturated fat. We're not math geniuses, but that adds up to 3.5. Something's missing.)

Another unfortunate side effect of meat-free living can be high-sodium living. Two Morningstar Farms Veggie Dogs may give you only 100 calories, but you're also getting 860 mg of sodium—about the same as in three servings of Cheetos Cheese Curls—and more than 40 ingredients, half a dozen of them being forms of MSG.

Several studies have shown that vegans are prone to deficiencies in vitamins B12, A, and D, as well as calcium, iron, zinc, and long-chain fatty acids, all of which are found primarily in animal proteins. And part of that problem is

that our modern food world isn't particularly friendly to vegans, forcing many to resort to packaged foods and the kind of junk that PETA recommends we eat. When we make animal welfare a priority, we lose sight of the other health issues involved. Studies show that the more processed foods you eat, the more you weigh—regardless of how many calories you consume. Swapping out processed foods for more colorful vegetables, especially leafy greens, will help reduce your risk of most of these deficiencies.

BOTTOM LINE:
A vegan diet is no different from any other diet: It should be focused on whole foods that you can control. On a vegan diet, no animals should suffer harm. Most of all, you.

INDUSTRY SECRET:
Vegan Foods Can Be Cruel, Too!

Just two pancakes made from Bisquick give you half a day's allotment of trans fats, the artery-clogging, manmade alternative to animal fats that's found in margarine, shortenings, and some cooking oils. But are you going to eat just two? Even if you use almond milk to make it vegan, Bisquick sticks not to your ribs but to your heart.

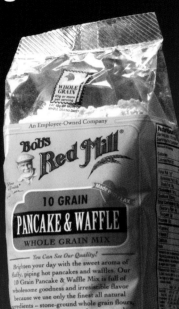

EAT THIS INSTEAD
Bob's Red Mill Organic 7 Grain Pancake & Waffle Mix (⅓ cup)

190 calories

1 g fat
(0g saturated fat, 0g trans fat)

6 g fiber

2 g sugars

7g protein

WORST VEGAN FOOD
Betty Crocker Bisquick Original Pancake and Baking Mix (⅓ cup)

150 calories

4 g fat (1 g saturated fat, 1 g trans fat)

0 g fiber

1 g sugar

3 g protein

The Diet Industry Doesn't Want You to Know...
YOUR JUICING SYSTEM IS "CLEANSING" YOU WITH SUGAR

We Americans live in a world of extremes. We work more hours than any other country, but we spend the most on leisure activities. We exercise more than any other culture on the planet, but we're also the fattest folks on the face of the Earth.

And that extremism is reflected in how we eat—and drink. If junk-food junkiedom is one end of the spectrum, the opposite pole is our new-found obsession with juice cleansing. BluePrint juices are expected to reach sales of $100M after a full roll-out at Whole Foods at the end of 2014. In New York and Los Angeles you can't throw an apple without hitting a trendy juice bar.

But while the idea of cleansing your body with green, healthy juice sounds great, these cleansing agents are often no more than spoonfuls of sugar. BluePrint's P.A.M. juice, a mixture of pineapple, apple and mint (hence PAM) is included in two of its three cleansing systems. But by condensing two high-sugar fruits, PAM isn't much healthier than SPAM: Each drink packs 45 grams of sugar, more than you'd find in a can of Coca-Cola. That makes BluePrint's $65-a-day program a sweet deal— too sweet.

Along for the juicing joyride are brands that have snuck so-called healthy smoothies onto produce aisle shelves.

A 15-ounce bottle of Bolthouse Farms' Green Goodness has nearly 60 grams of sugar, the equivalent of 12 Chips Ahoy cookies.

And because juicing strips these foods of their fiber, those sugar calories are absorbed like a bullet to the belly. That means your healthy juice can cause an insulin spike—which leads directly to calories being stored in fat cells. One major 2014 study found sugar plays a role in chronic disease independent of weight gain. "Too much sugar doesn't just make us fat," one doctor wrote. "It can also make us sick."

BOTTOM LINE:
Cleanse or not, a juice should have fewer than 20 g of sugar, and in most cases even less. Using sugar to "cleanse" your body of toxins is like using a toilet brush to rid your coffee cup of mold.

INDUSTRY SECRET:
Green Isn't Always Lean

If you were trying to cleanse your body of toxins, would you stick two and a half Kit Kat bars in a blender and then drink them down? That's the sugar equivalent of what you're getting when you ride the Naked Green Machine.

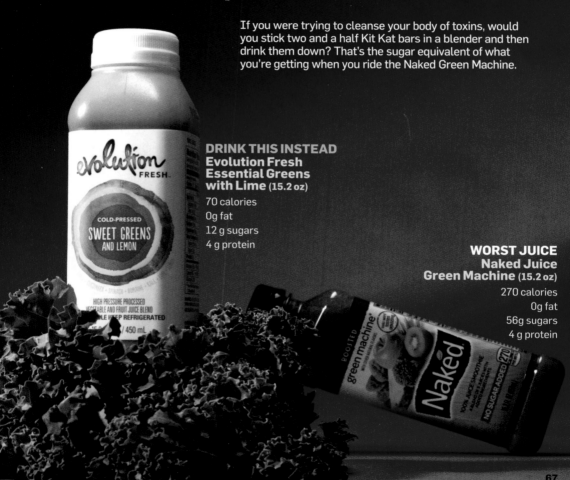

DRINK THIS INSTEAD
Evolution Fresh
Essential Greens
with Lime (15.2 oz)

70 calories

0g fat

12 g sugars

4 g protein

WORST JUICE
Naked Juice
Green Machine (15.2 oz)

270 calories

0g fat

56g sugars

4 g protein

67

GLUTEN-FREE OFTEN MEANS NUTRITION-FREE

When tennis star Novak Djokovic was devouring opponents in 2011 on his way to a 41-match winning streak, everyone wanted to know, What's this guy on? According to Djokovic's own diet book, *Serve to Win*, the streak was powered by what he wasn't on: gluten.

It's not like the industry needed another celebrity endorsement. Miley Cyrus, Drew Brees and Gwyneth Paltrow are just a few of the big-name disciples of the gluten-free gospel. According to a 2013 poll, a third of Americans are trying to restrict gluten. As a result, what was a $935 million industry in 2006 is estimated to top sales of $15 billion by 2016.

It used to be that living sans gluten was relegated to the roughly 1 percent of Americans with celiac disease. But now the gluten-free gurus preach the diet for everyone, claiming it increases energy and helps people lose weight. Here's the problem: Eliminating wheat—especially products like cereals and whole-grain bread—means we're also taking out important nutrients. Scandinavian researchers found that a significant percentage of people following a gluten-free diet suffered from deficiencies of folate, vitamin B12, phosphorus, zinc and calcium. The *British Journal of Nutrition* reported in 2009 that gluten-free living led to a reduction in beneficial gut bacteria needed for a healthy immune system. And maybe most disturbing, the dietary trend has been shown to increase plasma levels of something called homocysteine, which is a risk factor for cardiovascular disease.

Part of the problem is that gluten-free baked goods and pastas tend to be made of nutrition-free materials like refined corn or rice, or potato or tapioca starch, and often make up for missing gluten by adding fat and sugar. Oh, and in a nice bit of irony, those empty calories cost an average of 242 percent more than basic wheat products.

BOTTOM LINE:
Going gluten-free is fine as long as you double down on fiber-based nutrients like beans, lentils, brown rice and quinoa, and avoid expensive gluten-free products that go right to your glutes.

INDUSTRY SECRET:
All that's Gluten-Free Isn't Gold!

At first glance, Udi's seems like that rare exception: a gluten-free cereal that's actually good for you. That's because the package lists 130 calories and just 5 g of sugar per serving. But look closer, and you see a serving is a mere ¼ cup—barely enough to cover the bottom of your cereal bowl. Four times that amount is what a typical cereal serving would be—and now you're eating almost as many calories as a Big Mac, before you pour on the milk.

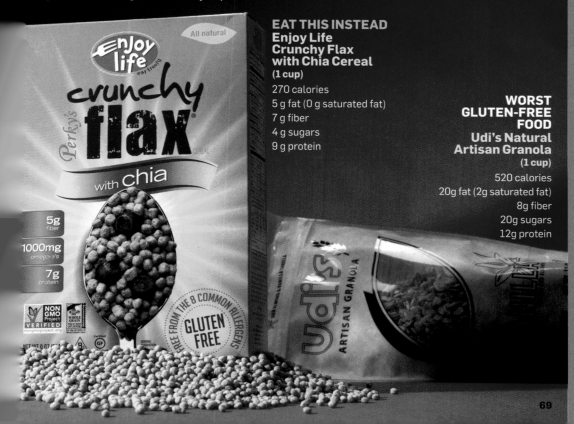

EAT THIS INSTEAD
Enjoy Life
Crunchy Flax
with Chia Cereal
(1 cup)

270 calories
5 g fat (0 g saturated fat)
7 g fiber
4 g sugars
9 g protein

WORST
GLUTEN-FREE
FOOD
Udi's Natural
Artisan Granola
(1 cup)

520 calories
20g fat (2g saturated fat)
8g fiber
20g sugars
12g protein

STICKING TO THE STONE AGE CAN MAKE YOUR BONES AGE

Americans have a bad case of stone-age nostalgia.

Beards are in. Barefoot running is all the rage. And the paleo diet is hot. It was the top health term searched for on Google in 2013.

The idea behind paleo is that many of today's chronic diseases are caused by eating foods that we haven't evolved properly to digest. Eliminate grains, dairy and beans, and we'll devolve our way out of the obesity crisis. Well, there's another reason why the ancients didn't suffer the indignities of modern middle age—because most of them got killed and eaten before they reached the age of wanting a Porsche.

When we imagine cavemen, we imagine them dragging a woolly mammoth back to the cave and having a barbecue. But real cavemen ate meat only rarely; mostly they ate berries, seeds, nuts, and greens. That's a lot different than stopping by Chipotle to order a double-steak, double-guacamole burrito bowl.

This stone-age swap can have serious drawbacks. Eliminating dairy cuts two top sources of calcium and vitamin D. Calcium helps facilitate muscle contractions. Without enough of the mineral to make those cells fire, the body steals calcium from the bones. Its dairy comrade, vitamin D, aids in calcium absorption. A deficiency in either is particularly alarming for women who are more susceptible to osteoporosis.

Even if you're munching on loads of vegetables, as many paleo experts suggest, you still risk falling short on fiber. Take spinach, a favored leafy green. We love its cancer-fighting powers, but consider that you'd have to eat 10 cups of the foliage to get as much fiber as two slices of whole-wheat bread.

BOTTOM LINE:
The life of a Paleolith was short and brutal, in part because nobody was waiting back at the cave to make him a sandwich. Eating more fruits and vegetables, more nuts and seeds, and more lean meats is a great food foundation. But there's no reason to cut out healthy foods like beans and whole grains just because they weren't on sale at the 10,000 BC 7-Eleven.

INDUSTRY SECRET:
Cavemen Didn't Live on Beef!

Once you eliminate beans, corn, wheat flour, and cheese from a Mexican restaurant meal, it's pretty hard to find anything to eat. Chipotle's Burrito Bowls let you skip the tortilla, and the beans, and go dairy free, but that leaves you with only a handful of food choices, most of which are packed with calories.

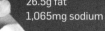

EAT THIS INSTEAD
Chipotle Salad with Chicken, Romaine, Guacamole, Veggies, and Salsa

430 calories
26.5g fat
1,065mg sodium

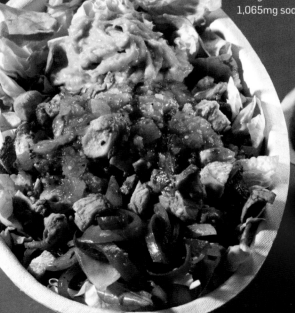

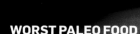

WORST PALEO FOOD
Chipotle Mexican Grill Double Steak, Double Guacamole, Veggies and Salsa Burrito Bowl

825 calories
52.5 g fat
1,970 mg sodium

THE WORST FOODS IN AMERICA

At *Eat This, Not That!*, we're cooking up a great idea for a television show. It's got all the elements of a huge hit—postapocalyptic zombie survival show meets cooking competition. We're calling it *The Walking Fed*.

And the great news is, it's a reality show. Because right now, the people cooking our meals in America's most popular restaurants seem utterly intent on turning us all into slow-moving, unthinking, ravenous creatures who wander from chain to chain, searching for our next disgusting meal.

If you don't think we're living through a food apocalypse, just take a look at how catastrophic our restaurant calorie counts have gotten. In a recent study in the *Journal of the American Medical Association,* researchers looked at 19 chain restaurants, studying the typical breakfast, lunch, and dinner. Their findings: The average restaurant meal contains:

- **1,128 calories, or about 56 percent of a person's daily calorie intake**
- **2,269 milligrams of sodium, or 95 percent of a person's daily recommended intake (In fact, researchers consider 600 milligrams or less a "healthy" meal, yet only 1 percent of all chain restaurant meals meet this standard.)**
- **58 grams of fat (89 percent of what we should eat in a day).**

As a result, the average American man now eats, every single day,

- **⅔ cup of sugar**
- **½ cup of fats and shortenings**
- **2 teaspoons of salt**
- **500 calories more than he burns off**

Now look at what this collusion of calories has wrought: We spend nearly $200 per year per person—man, woman and child—in America on prescription drugs to fight diabetes, high blood pressure, and elevated cholesterol. It's time for us to put an end to the horror show. The list on the following pages presents the 20 most cunning villains in a world studded with shadowy characters. Next time one of these nutrition nightmares comes knocking at your door, double-bolt it and turn off the lights.

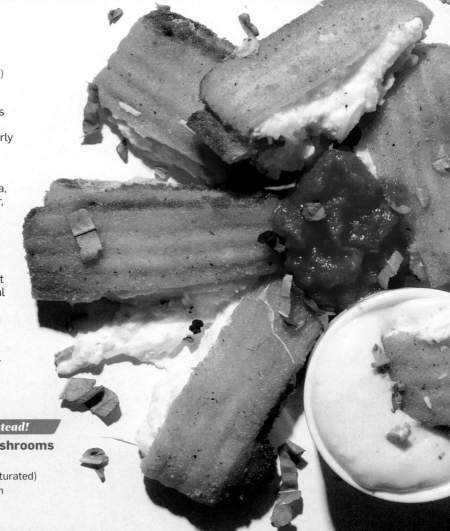

20 WORST FRANKENFOOD

Olive Garden's Lasagna Fritta

1,070 calories
71 g fat (29 g saturated)
1,650 mg sodium

This appetizer sounds like a fantasy food dreamed up in the early morning hours at a college frat house: "Dude, imagine if you took hunks of lasagna, dipped them in batter, and tossed them in the deep fryer." Unfortunately, Olive Garden's crazy pasta creation is the real deal, and so is its cost to your health. A meal starter with half a day's calories and a day's saturated fat? That's one fantasy we'd rather not fulfill.

Eat This Instead!
Stuffed Mushrooms

380 calories
30 g fat (8 g saturated)
860 mg sodium

**Cinnabon
Caramel Pecanbon**

1,080 calories
50 g fat (20 g saturated)
76 g sugars

The cinnamon bun is an inherently unscrupulous pastry—there's just no way to slather big blobs of dough with butter and frosting and end up with a sensible treat—but this caramel catastrophe from Cinnabon is just plain inexcusable. Here, Cinnabon, that peddler of so much dietary mischief, takes its classic bun—which already packs an astounding 880 calories—and defiles it with a dousing of caramel syrup and a pile of pecans. This type of shameless excess results in a day's saturated fat, half a day's calories, and nearly 20 teaspoons of sugar. Save your own buns and indulge elsewhere.

 Eat This Instead!

Classic Bites (4)

420 calories
17 g fat (7 g saturated)
25 g sugars

18 WORST FRIES

Steak 'n Shake
Chili Cheese Fries
(large)

1,170 calories
67 g fat (22 g saturated, 3.5 g trans)
2,150 mg sodium

Here's the most distressing dietary fact we know: French fries are the most consumed "vegetable" in America. They also happen to be one of the most dubious caloric investments in the nutrition world. They're bad enough on their own, but when doused with trans-fatty processed cheese and loaded with greasy ground beef, they become a side dish so twisted it'll make a burger blush. In fact, you could scarf three Steakburgers with cheese and still take in fewer calories than you would with these spuds. Our advice: Skip fries altogether and order another burger.

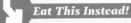

Eat This Instead!
Bacon Cheese Fries
(small)

360 calories
20 g fat (6 g saturated, 1.5 g trans)
710 mg sodium

76

IHOP
Crispy Chicken
& Spinach Salad

1,280 calories
81 g fat
(24 g saturated, 1.5 g trans)
2,440 mg sodium

The poor spinach never saw it coming. The simple menu description screams wholesome and healthy, but nothing could be further from the truth. With this bowl of mischief, IHOP debases one of the most nutritious greens on the planet by suffocating it with deep-fried chicken, bacon, and one too many handfuls of Cheddar cheese. You could order the chain's worst burger—the Monster Bacon'N Beef Cheeseburger made with Bacon Patties—and a side of fries—and still not reach the calorie load of this health-food fraud. Unfortunately, other than the basic Simple & Fit House Salad and the Side Caesar Salad, none of the pancake purveyor's salads come with fewer than 700 calories.

 Eat This Instead!

Honey-Lime
Chicken Salad

410 calories
21 g fat (4 g saturated)
1,160 mg sodium

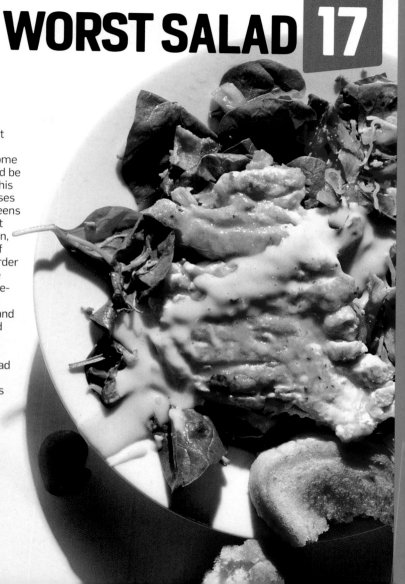

16 WORST FAST-FOOD BURGER

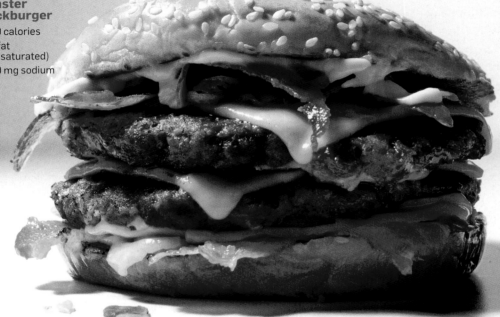

Hardee's Monster Thickburger

1,330 calories
95 g fat
(35 g saturated)
2,820 mg sodium

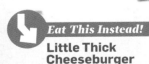

Eat This Instead!

Little Thick Cheeseburger

430 calories
23 g fat (9 g saturated)
1,150 mg sodium

"Monster" is right. This burger beast comes at your diet full force, saddling your gut with four strips of bacon, three slices of processed cheese, and two ⅓-pound slabs of greasy ground beef. Coincidentally, ⅓ of a pound is exactly how much flab you'll add to your middle if you inhale one of these bad boys. At Hardee's, consider "little" a relative term. The Little Thick Cheeseburger is one of the only ways to leave the chain's drive-thru window with your waistline intact.

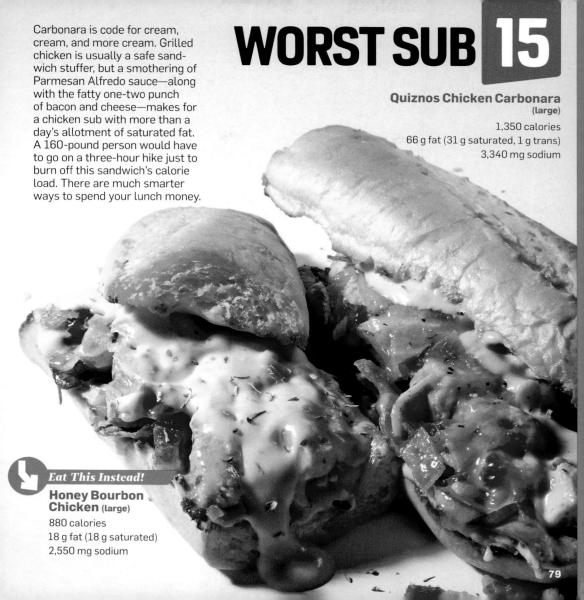

Carbonara is code for cream, cream, and more cream. Grilled chicken is usually a safe sandwich stuffer, but a smothering of Parmesan Alfredo sauce—along with the fatty one-two punch of bacon and cheese—makes for a chicken sub with more than a day's allotment of saturated fat. A 160-pound person would have to go on a three-hour hike just to burn off this sandwich's calorie load. There are much smarter ways to spend your lunch money.

WORST SUB 15

Quiznos Chicken Carbonara
(large)

1,350 calories
66 g fat (31 g saturated, 1 g trans)
3,340 mg sodium

Eat This Instead!

Honey Bourbon Chicken (large)

880 calories
18 g fat (18 g saturated)
2,550 mg sodium

14 WORST HEALTH-FOOD FRAUD

The folks at the Cheesecake Factory aren't exactly forthcoming about what goes on behind their culinary curtain, so we're honestly not sure how they managed to take grilled chicken and avocado—two of the healthiest foods on the planet—and turn them into a sandwich with more calories than their worst burger. The bacon, cheese, and mayo certainly don't help matters, but the Factory must be hiding a secret ingredient that magically turns any reasonable food into a nutritionist's nightmare. We may never know the truth, but all you need to know is this: Stay away from this sandwich.

Cheesecake Factory Grilled Chicken and Avocado Club

1,400 calories
N/A g fat (23 g saturated)
2,100 mg sodium

Eat This Instead!

Factory Burger

740 calories
N/A g fat (16 g saturated)
1,020 mg sodium

WORST EGGS 13

Perkins
Southern Fried Chicken Biscuit Platter

1,490 calories
83 g fat
(44 g saturated)
4,580 mg sodium

Unless you're stocking up to hibernate for the winter, there's no reason to ever order a menu item that contains the word "platter." Your cholesterol could shoot up just reading the menu description: fried chicken, biscuits, fried eggs, cheese, gravy, bacon, and hash browns. The collective impact translates into two days' worth of sodium and saturated fat, and a calorie count fit for three breakfasts. We can't think of a worse way to start your day.

 Eat This Instead!

Classic Eggs
and Smoked Bacon with Toast and Fresh Fruit

670 calories
40 g fat (12 g saturated)
1,100 mg sodium

12 WORST SIT-DOWN BURGER

Chili's Southern Smokehouse Bacon Burger

1,550 calories
90 g fat
(27 g saturated)
4,130 mg sodium

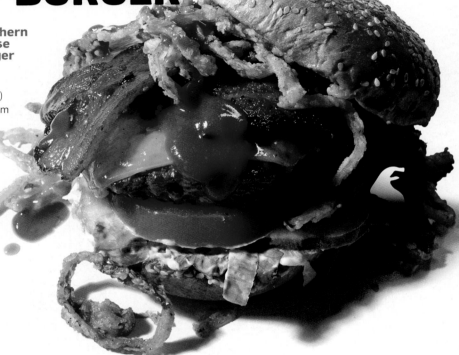

Eat This Instead!

Custom Combinations Classic Sirloin (10 oz)

440 calories
24 g fat (8 g saturated)
1,330 mg sodium

A typical burger at Chili's will cost you a cool 1,400 calories—without fries!—and with this ground-beef bomb, the chain pulls out all the gut-busting stops: cheese, bacon, fried onions, barbecue sauce, and mayo. This blatant display of excess translates into a sandwich with nearly as many calories as three Big Macs and nearly double your recommended daily allotment of salt. There's only one way to safely get your meat fix at Chili's: Order a steak and pair it with respectable sides.

WORST DESSERT

The word "Thunder" is a pretty clear indicator that you're about to do some serious damage to your diet, but this sundae's nutrition stats are impressively heinous. The calorie culprits: a brick of a brownie, a hefty scoop of vanilla ice cream, a crown of whipped cream, and a deluge of chocolate sauce. Even if you split this dessert with three friends, you'll still take in a meal's worth of calories and a day's saturated fat. When you consider that the Classic Cheesecake is one of the great caloric bargains in America, there's no excuse to throw away 1,200 calories.

Outback Steakhouse Chocolate Thunder from Down Under

1,558 calories

106 g fat (56 g saturated)

140 g carbohydrates

Eat This Instead!

Classic Cheesecake

334 calories

24 g fat (16 g saturated)

23 g carbohydrates

83

10 WORST CHIPS & DIP

Chili's Skillet Queso with Chips

1,590 calories
97 g fat
(35 g saturated)
3,920 mg sodium

Eat This Instead!

Fried Cheese with Marinara Sauce

720 calories
41 g fat (17 g saturated)
2,140 mg sodium

Cheese dips are bad news to begin with—their fluid consistency can fool you into downing more calories than you realize—and the addition of fatty ground beef makes Chili's version the most hazardous chip sauce in America. Order this little cheese pot and you risk scooping up almost two days' worth of saturated fat and nearly a day's calories. Those would be some sad stats for an entrée, but for an appetizer, they're downright deplorable. Other than its rib and burger plates, this is the most offensive item Chili's has to offer.

WORST MILK SHAKE

9

Baskin-Robbins Chocolate Chip Cookie Dough Milkshake
(large)

1,600 calories
72 g fat
(46 g saturated,
2 g trans)
181 g sugars

We're thankful that Baskin ditched the 2,310-calorie Heath Bar Shake that used to haunt our every waking moment, but there are still more than a few nutritional nightmares to be found on its menu. Even an average small shake at the chain houses 16 teaspoons of sugar! Order a large cookie dough and you'll gulp down more than two days' worth of saturated fat, 56 Chips Ahoy! cookies' worth of sugar, and enough calories to add half a pound to your gut. A word of caution: When you can drink your dessert, you're asking for trouble.

Eat This Instead!

Chocolate Chip Cookie Dough Ice Cream
(1 large scoop, 4 oz)

280 calories
15 g fat (10 g saturated)
24 g sugars

85

8 WORST BURRITO

Baja Fresh Enchilado Style Nacho Burrito

1,670 calories
82 g fat (36 g saturated)
4,650 mg sodium

The trouble with burritos? It takes a whole lot of food to fill out those big tortillas. And when chains opt for particularly fattening fillers—which, let's be honest, is often the case—it's a recipe for a full-scale caloric assault. Case in point: This Baja burrito bomb is stuffed with creamy salsa, cheese sauce, and shredded Jack and Cheddar cheeses. As if that weren't bad enough, the chain offers patrons the option to order their burrito "Enchilado" style, which translates to a smearing of cheese and salsa, a pile of deep-fried chips, and a glob of sour cream. *Ay caramba!*

Eat This Instead!

Chicken Americano Soft Tacos (2)

460 calories
20 g fat (9 g saturated)
1,180 mg sodium

WORST FISH 7

Applebee's New England Fish & Chips

1,690 calories
126 g fat (22 g saturated, 1.5 g trans)
2,840 mg sodium

Attack of the beige! Whenever your dinner is monochromatic (in this case, the off-brown hue of deep-fried junk), you know you're in trouble. Don't blame the fish—seafood is packed with lean, muscle-building protein and heart-healthy fats. No, the trouble here lies with a massively unbalanced fish-to-fat ratio. A coating of crispy batter and a heaping pile of deep-fried potatoes is no way to treat the golden child of nutrition. Plus, trans fats? Really? That's so 2005! When it comes to seafood, always abandon ship on fried fish and opt for grilled instead.

Eat This Instead!

Blackened Tilapia
(with Fried Red Potatoes and Seasonal Vegetables)

470 calories
18 g fat (5 g saturated)
1,370 mg sodium

87

6 WORST BREAKFAST

**The Cheesecake Factory
French Toast Napoleon**

1,700 calories
N/A g fat (51 g saturated)
1,270 mg sodium
160 g carbohydrates

We give Cheesecake Factory props for rolling out some lighter options as of late, but its menu is still home to the most caloric fare in the country. What's worse, the Factory insists on keeping its nutrition info under lock and key. And we can't say we blame them. True to its namesake, this breakfast plate attempts to make up for its nutritional shortcomings by enticing diners with indulgent ingredients like cream-drenched bread, piles of pecans, and a snowstorm of powdered sugar. The result: You're starting your morning with the carbohydrate equivalent of a half dozen hot dog buns and more saturated fat than 20 slices of CPK's BBQ Chicken Pizza.

Eat This Instead!
Energy Breakfast

640 calories
3 g saturated
1,260 mg sodium

5

Friendly's Create Your Own Munchie Mania: Kickin Buffalo Strips + Fries + Buffalo Wings (6)

1,800 calories
134 g fat (22 g saturated)
4,880 mg sodium

It takes guts to name your restaurant Friendly's and then dish out this type of vicious waistline attack. Any food that's been smothered in batter and dunked in the deep fryer is a nutritional loser by default, but the added blow of oily, sugary sauces makes this poultry plate a particularly fattening failure. Order this combo and you'll wolf down nearly a day's calories and more sugar than you'd find in 150 Honey Teddy Grahams. Doesn't get much more unfriendly than that.

Eat This Instead!

Grilled Chicken Breast on a Wheat Roll
with Monterey Jack & Chedder Blend

590 calories
26 g fat (12 g saturated)
1,620 mg sodium

4 WORST APPETIZER

**Outback Steakhouse
Bloomin' Onion**

1,953 calories

116 g fat
(48 g saturated,
4 g trans)

3,700 mg sodium

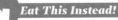

Eat This Instead!

**Grilled Shrimp
on the Barbie**

312 calories
20 g fat (4.6 g saturated)
587 mg sodium

According to Outback's website, its signature starter is "hand-carved by a dedicated bloomologist." We have no idea what that means, but consider bloomology the science of diet destruction. This bouquet of batter-dipped produce is the caloric equivalent of eating an entire medium Pizza Hut pepperoni pizza—before your dinner! What's more, it also delivers two days' worth of cholesterol-boosting trans fats and enough sodium to keep your cardiologist up at night.

WORST GRILLED ENTRÉE 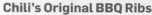 3

Chili's Original BBQ Ribs
(full rack) with Cinnamon Apples
and Homestyle Fries

2,290 calories
112 g fat (34 g saturated)
4,585 mg sodium

Tasty as they are, ribs are among the fattiest cuts on the pig, so when they get the big-chain treatment (monster portions, excess sauce, and lackluster sides), they're pure nutritional mayhem. The heart-rattling stats here: more than a day's calories and more than two days' saturated fat. And, as if that's not enough, if you order this ridiculous rib plate, you'll also take in four times the recommended daily dose of sodium. Consider this dish cardiac kryptonite. If you want ribs, try our baby backs in *Grill This, Not That!* (they'll save you nearly 2,000 calories). Otherwise, stick with grilled chicken or steak.

 Eat This Instead!

Margarita Grilled Chicken

610 calories
16 g fat (3 g saturated)
2,450 mg sodium

2 WORST PASTA DISH

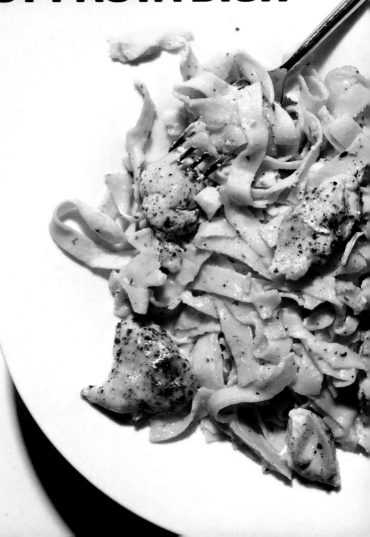

**The Cheesecake Factory
Fettuccini Alfredo
with Chicken**

2,300 calories
N/A g fat (103 g saturated)
1,297 mg sodium

Aside from the Atkins craze, Alfredo sauce is the worst thing to ever happen to pasta. You'd be better off bathing the noodles in a bowl of butter (seriously—this dish has more fat than a full stick of butter!). Thankfully, the Cheesecake Factory recently took a break from destroying the hearts and guts of the American public to unveil its lower-calorie SkinnyLicious menu. We're not crazy about the name (though it's an improvement on the denigratory name of its old low-cal menu, the Weight Management Menu), but we love its nutrition stats: The pasta plate swap on this page will save you 1,760 (!) calories.

 Eat This Instead!

**SkinnyLicious
Pasta**

540 calories
N/A g fat
(1 g saturated)
660 mg sodium

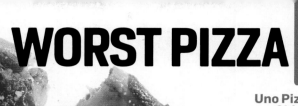

WORST PIZZA 1

**Uno Pizzeria & Grill
Chicago Classic
Individual Pizza**

2,300 calories

164 g fat
(53 g saturated,
1 g trans)

4,910 mg sodium

Uno changed its name
in 2014, but hasn't lifted
a finger to change its
atrociously caloric menu.
We're running out of ways
to express its nutritional
transgressions, so we'll
break it down like this:
If you ate just one of these
"individual" pies each
week, you'd take in enough
calories to gain 34 pounds
in a year. There's not a
single Uno pizza option we
can recommend; the best
we can do is hold our nose
and point to the flatbreads.

Eat This Instead!

**Roasted Eggplant,
Spinach & Feta Flatbread**

880 calories

32 g fat (11 g saturated)

1,500 mg sodium

Chapter 3

THE
EAT THIS, NOT THAT!
MENU DECODER

From juice bars to yogurt shops, your guide to modern food trends

If the gang from *Friends* were transported into today, they'd have an awful hard time recognizing their favorite coffee shop hangout. Central Perk would probably have closed, forced out by a chain like Starbucks or Gregory's. Instead of a shock of Eminem-style hair, the baristas would all have tattoos and beards. And the cushy couches would now be hard-backed chairs, where driven digital entrepreneurs were pounding away at their latest app idea. Phoebe and her six-string wouldn't fly in today's caffeinated commerce palaces.

In fact, the way we consume food has changed immeasurably since the 1990s. The *Seinfeld* Soup Nazi trend came and went, only to be replaced by Juice Nazis, and the diners that served "damned good cherry pie" in *Twin Peaks* have all turned into yogurt shops. But the biggest change of all might be the health halos that have been bestowed on many of the newest dining trends, from the above-mentioned juice and yogurt spots to the outcropping of "authentic" Mexican cantinas and the growth of vegan restaurants. And the truth is, you can find healthier fare at some of these places more easily than you might have found it in the old greasy spoons.

But eating and drinking well at the new joint that opened up where The Halfmoon Diner used to stand isn't a given. Use these guides to help you cruise through the new foodie landscape.

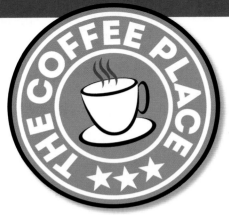

THE COFFEE PLACE

Long ago, coffee shops were the environs of folks like Bob Dylan and Allen Ginsburg who wrote poetry and smoked clove cigarettes and argued about Miles Davis over cups of espresso. Then came the internet, the Great Recession, and Pumpkin Spice Lattes.

Nowadays, the men and women sitting next to you at your local Starbucks are as likely to be working on a Kickstarter campaign to fund their next app launch as they are on finding the perfect word to rhyme with "Daddy-O."

That means a trip to the coffee shop can be an all-day affair, especially for those of us who have been laid off, downsized, furloughed, disengaged, or our new favorite corporate copout, "job-separated." So finding the right spot to set up shop—and picking the best, healthiest coffee and snacks to fuel your financial future—makes a lot of sense.

Egg & Cheese It

An egg-and-cheese sandwich usually comes in under 400 calories no matter where you go, as long as it's not on a bagel. Plus, the protein hit helps temper your appetite as the day wears on.

Listen For The Grind

The closer you grind to brew time, the better. Coffee is most Americans' number one source of polyphenols—the micronutrients that make the Mediterranean diet so effective. But it's flavor, and health benefits, begin to erode rapidly once the beans are broken up and exposed to air.

Espresso Yourself

Darker, more concentrated espresso is much higher in polyphenols than regular brew, says Barry Sears, Ph.D., author of *The Mediterranean Zone.* If you prefer a longer, milder drink, ask for an Americano, which is basically an espresso mixed with water. It tastes similar to a regular cup of coffee, but with even greater health benefits.

Go Cold Brewed

When regular brewed coffee is chilled and stored, two things happen. First, it begins to lose whatever nuance of taste it once possessed. Second, it starts losing the polyphenols that give coffee its health benefits. The best iced coffee is cold brewed; it takes more time to make so it will be more expensive, but you'll taste the difference.

Never Roam Near Styrofoam

Styrofoam cups can leach styrene, a neurotoxin that can cause depression and a loss of concentration. Highly acidic or hot beverages— in other words, coffee—draw the plastic compound out more effectively than, say, cold water would. Look for a regular joint that serves coffee in paper, or bring your own.

Leave the Scone Alone

The great, rich, flaky taste that makes a scone so appealing comes from gobs of butter, flour and sugar. With up to 500 calories a pop, this pastry is better left behind the glass.

Ban Bran Muffins

One of the great health food imposters, bran muffins are simply excuses to get you to eat cupcakes for breakfast. Each can deliver about 440 calories, with nearly a quarter of them coming from fat.

Embrace The Noise

It's not just the coffee that makes a

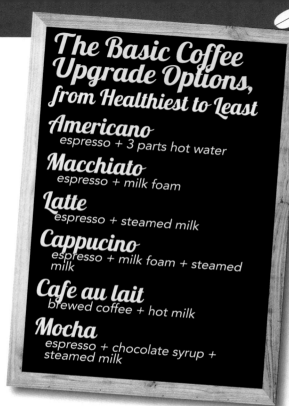

The Basic Coffee Upgrade Options, from Healthiest to Least

Americano
espresso + 3 parts hot water

Macchiato
espresso + milk foam

Latte
espresso + steamed milk

Cappucino
espresso + milk foam + steamed milk

Cafe au lait
brewed coffee + hot milk

Mocha
espresso + chocolate syrup + steamed milk

coffee shop great to work in: A study in the Journal of Consumer Research found that a little ambient noise actually increases creativity. They report that moderate (70 dB) versus low (50 dB) level of ambient noise enhances performance on creative tasks and increases the buying likelihood of innovative products.

MEXICAN CANTINA

Mexican food is a cuisine on the cusp. In 2014, *Eat This, Not That!* surveyed the 10 fattiest foods in chain restaurants. Three of the top 10 were from Mexican restaurants: On the Border's Firecracker Stuffed Jalapenos with Salsa Ranch (138 g of fat, 1,900 calories); Dos XX Fish Tacos (155 g of fat, 2,240 calories); and Chili's Bacon Ranch Beef Quesadilla (135 g fat, 1,800 calories). Add to that the ongoing insult to Mexican culture that is Taco Bell—inventors of the Waffle Taco—and it's clear that we need some culinary reform, stat. *Dios Mio!*

Yet at the same time, Chipotle—the anti-Taco Bell—is the fastest-growing chain in America. Its super-customizable menu (more than 65,000 possible combinations) and focus on naturally raised meats has hit the millennial market right in the wallet. And it's shown Mexican food made healthy is a winner, which means more and more restaurants will be following suit.

So skip the tired old chains and check out your local cantina. And by the way, want to cut 200 calories or more out of every Mexican meal? El Pass-o on the tortilla chips. They do nothing but make you thirsty and get you to order more beer. The guacamole is just as healthy and delicious if you eat it with a fork.

Guacamole
Avocados are high in fat, but its the monounsaturated kind, so (like olive oil) it's good for your heart. Also contains vitamin E, a disease-fighting antioxidant.

Bean Burrito
Ask about the type of beans. If they're whole, this could be the healthiest thing on the menu. (The fiber in beans lowers cholesterol and helps make you feel full.) If they're refried (mashed and cooked in lard), you're better off with the chicken burrito.

Mojado
It means "wet" in Spanish, and normally denotes a burrito that is shrouded in melted cheese and then drowned in a rich, salty tomato- and chili-based sauce.

Chicken Fajitas
A heap of onions and peppers is a plus, but to keep this sizzling skillet from breaking the caloric bank, skip the cheese and the sour cream—it will save you 300 calories and 15 grams of fat. To slice additional calories, ask for just one tortilla and stuff it full.

Our Traditional Specials

GUACAMOLE
with homemade corn tortillas.

BURRITOS
A meal in itself that starts with a large flour tortilla and your choice of any meat, then we add rice, beans and cheese all wrapped inside. Frijoles de la olla by request.

BURRITO MOJADO
A flour tortilla filled with your choice of meat and beans topped with lettuce, tomato, cheese, and your choice of red or green salsa.

BURRITO AMERICANO
Grilled steak or chicken, smothered with Glazed Onions and garnished with Lettuce, Tomatoes, Cheese, Sliced Avocados & Felipe's sauce, all wrapped in a Tortilla.

FAJITAS POLLO
Combination of chicken, bell peppers, tomatoes and onions grilled to order

TOSTADAS
A crisp corn tortilla spread with beans, your choice of entree, topped with fresh lettuce, guacamole sauce and cheese.

NACHOS
First we start with a layer of beans, add a good portion of fresh chips, add more beans, your favorite meat and cover it with melted cheese and guacamole

QUESADILLAS
Your choice of meat and melted cheese in between two flour tortillas

TAQUITOS & FLAUTAS
Our homemade taquitos are made with corn tortillas and our flautas are made with flour tortillas, topped with guacamole & lettuce.

CHILE RELLENO
A Chile Poblano stuffed with cheese and topped with special sauce.

TACOS
All tacos are served on a soft flour tortilla with cheese and lettuce. Hard shell or corn tortilla by request.

TACO SALAD
Lettuce, rice, beans, jack and cheddar cheese, fresh salsa, guacamole, sour cream served with or without crisp shell

ENCHILADAS
A soft corn tortilla, stuffed with cheese or meat, and smothered with enchilada sauce or tomatillo sauce then topped with melted cheese and lettuce.

MOLE
Mexico's national mole dish. A blend of ancho chiles, almonds, peanuts and filberts. Served with chicken.

MEXICAN RICE
A fresh batch made everyday

Soft Taco
Real Mexican tacos are served on soft corn tortillas, and you should embrace the authenticity; made with just whole grains (i.e. corn) and water, they'll save you 100 calories per taco over the flour variety.

Taco Salad
It's a huge fried tortilla shell with ground beef, cheese, sour cream, and a few token shreds of iceberg lettuce. The result: 900 calories, 55 grams of fat, and perhaps the most liberal use of the word "salad" ever.

Enchiladas
Tortillas dipped in fat, stuffed, rolled, covered with cheese, and baked. Topped with sour cream, two of them carry 748 calories, 55 percent of which is from fat.

Mole
A vast improvement on melted cheese and sour cream.

Rice
Skip it. Fried in oil in many Mexican restaurants, it packs 380 calories and nearly 11 grams of fat in about 1 cup.

House of Sushi

A little over a decade ago, Anthony Bourdain shocked foodies with a big secret from his Kitchen Confidential: Never order seafood on a Monday, because fish markets are closed on Sunday, so Monday's fish is probably a couple of days old. But whichever day you do find yourself in the local sushi joint, keep this little cheat sheet handy.

Soy Sauce Japanese sushi purists scoff when they see Westerners drowning their fish in puddles of soy muddied with a mound of wasabi. They should: A single tablespoon of soy sauce has over 1,000 mg of sodium. At a reputable sushi spot, the chef will serve the fish exactly as it's intended to be eaten, which means hands off the soy.

Spanish Mackerel Oft-overlooked for more glamorous fish like salmon and tuna, the humble mackerel has twice the amount of heart-healthy, inflammation-reducing, cancer-fighting omega-3 fatty acids as salmon, making it one of the healthiest fish in the sea.

Tobiko The Japanese word for flying fish eggs. A tablespoon of the neon-colored stuff has about 20 percent of your daily cholesterol in it. Limit yourself to one tobiko-strewn item per sushi session.

Nigiri-Sushi
One serving consists of two pieces

Alaska King Crab
Amaebi *sweet shrimp*
Blue Fin Tuna
Ebi *boiled shrimp*
Escolar *seared fatty white tuna*
Hamachi *yellowtail*
Hirame *fluke*
Hotategai *scallop*
Hokkigai *surf clam*
Ika *squid*
Ikura *salmon roe*
Kanikama *crab stick*
Kanpachi *wild yellowtail*
Masago *crab roe*
Saba *spanish mackeral*
Shake *fresh salmon*
Shake *smoked salmon*
Spicy Tuna *original or jalapeno*
Spicy scallop *original or jalapeno*
Suzuki *bass*
Tai *red snapper*
Tako *boiled octopus*
Tarako *cod roe*
Tobiko *flying fish roe*
Tamago *layered chicken eggs*
Unagi *fresh water eel*
Uni *sea urchin*
Wakame *seaweed*
Quail egg

Maki-Sushi

One serving consists of 6 pieces

Alaska Roll *smoked salmon, cream cheese & masago*

California Roll *(crab stick & cucumber)*

Crab Salad Roll

Futomaki *(crab stick, shrimp, tamago, pickle & cucumber)*

Gobo Maki *(pickled burdock)*

Ikura Maki *(salmon roe)*

Kampo Maki *(oriental squash)*

Kappa Maki

Mexican Roll *boiled shrimp & avocado*

Negi Hamachi Maki *yellowtail & scallions*

Natto Maki *fermented soybeans*

Philadelphia Roll *smoked salmon, cream cheese & masago*

Sake Kawa Maki *smoked salmon skin & cucumber*

Shrimp Tempura Maki *shrimp tempura, cucumber & crab roe*

Spicy Scallop Maki *original or jalapeno*

Spicy Tekka Maki *spicy tuna original or jalapeno*

Spider Maki *soft shell crab roll & masago*

Takuwan Maki *pickled radish*

Tekka Maki *tuna roll*

Unagi Maki *fresh water eel*

Ume Maki 2 pcs *plum paste & oba leaf*

Maki Sushi "Maki" refers to sushi that's rolled on a piece of seaweed. The seaweed allows for additional ingredients to be added—not all of them wise.

California Roll The most popular menu item is also one of the most healthy. Just 300 calories for eight pieces, plus a dose of healthy fat from the avocado.

Spicy Tuna Roll The "spicy" comes from a fattening dab of Asian chili sauce mixed with mayo. Want something fiery? Ask for chili sauce on the side, or extra wasabi.

Edamame

High in protein and fiber and very low in calories, steamed soybeans make a good start to a meal. Ask them to serve your edamame salt-less, and apply it carefully yourself.

House Salad

Sounds healthy, right? The iceberg it's served on offers very little nutritionally, and 2 tablespoons of the oily ginger dressing can have up to 200 calories and 10 grams of fat. Branch out and try the seaweed salad, one of nature's most potent multivitamins, instead.

Yakitori

Skewers of lean meat and vegetables give you maximum nutrition for minimum calories. Couldn't be a better start to a meal: protein- and nutrientpacked and grilled over an open flame.

GRANDE TAPAS RESTAURANT

To bridge the long gap between lunch and dinner, the Spanish invented tapas, small bites to nosh on, often while standing at a bar and yelling obscenities at enemy fútbol teams. If you've ever had half a dozen chicken wings with a beer before heading home to dinner, you've had the American version of tapas. Served on small plates, tapas come with their own portion control. It takes about 20 minutes between the time your belly is full and your brain gets "full tank" signal. Tapas allows for that signal to get through in time to keep you satisfied, not stuffed. Order a few, and then, if you're hungry, order more.

ALMONDS AND OLIVES Along with a glass of vino, this is a traditional start to a Spanish meal. And it's a good one: All three of the beloved Spanish staples help fight off cardiovascular disease. No wonder Spaniards live longer than nearly everyone else on the planet.

PATATAS BRAVAS Cubed, fried potatoes covered with garlic mayo and hot sauce. Muy mal! Want heat? Go with roasted piquillo peppers instead.

TORTILLA ESPAÑOLA Ubiquitous staple of the tapas menu, this Spanish-style omelet gives paella a run for its money as the national dish. Made simply of egg, onion, and potato, it's a safe haven for confused and calorie-conscious diners alike.

VEGETABLES & CHEESES

ACEITUNAS Y ALMENDRAS
Assorted Marinated Olives & Marcona almonds

QUESO MAHÓN FRITO CON SALSA DE TOMATE
Fried Mahon Cheese with Spicy Tomato Sauce

PATATAS BRAVAS
Deep fried potatoes in a spicy sauce

BERENJENA FRITA AL SALMOREJO
Fried Eggplant with Salmorejo Sauce with Serrano Ham

TORTILLA ESPAÑOLA
The Classic Potato and Onion Omelette from Spain

PIMIENTOS DEL PIQUILLO AL AJILLO
Sauteed strips of roasted Piquillo Peppers with toasted Garlic slivers

PATATAS ALI-OLI
Fried Baby Red Potatoes with an unabashed Garlic Ali-oli

PIMIENTOS ASADOS

PAELLA Order the "mariscos" version whenever possible. It's traditional along the coast of Spain and includes a variety of clams, mussels, squid, and shrimp, much better than the chorizo and chicken thigh version that's also common.

GAMBAS AL AJILLO Shrimp with a ton of garlic. A single order of these crustaceans might be sautéed in up to ¼ cup of olive oil, which is good for your heart, but ultimately packs nearly 500 calories on its own.

CROQUETAS Breadcrumbs are wrapped around a filling made from a mix of flour, milk, butter, and cheese or ham, and then the whole package is deep-fried. Think: fat bomb.

MUSSELS & CLAMS A good rule of thumb is to gravitate toward the shellfish. Whether steamed with white wine and herbs or served with a chunky tomato sauce, the protein fills you up while the shell negotiating slows you down. A portion won't cost you more than 300 calories.

MEAT & CHEESE PLATE A common option in Spanish restaurants. Meats are sliced super thin, so order wisely and this can be a solid beginning to a meal. Pick lean lomo and jamón serrano over fat-speckled chorizo.

OUR SPECIAL
FISH & SEAFOOD PLATES

PAELLA DE MARISCOS
Prawns, mussels, squid, peppers, peas and onions served in a rich saffron rice.

PEZ EN ADOBO
Fresh Mahi-Mahi, cubed and marinated in the style of Cadiz, battered and perfectly fried

GAMBAS AL AJILLO
Sauteed Shrimp with sliced Garlic and Pequin Chile Flake served sizzling hot in a Cazuela

CALAMARES FRITOS CON DOS SALSAS
Flash fried Baby Calamari with Spicy Tomato Sauce and Roast Garlic Caper Alioli

VIEIRAS AL VINO BLANCO CON JAMÓN SERRANO
Sauteed Scallops with White Wine and Serrano Ham

CROQUETAS DE JAMÓN
Serrano Croquettes with Roast Garlic-Caper Alioli and Baby Greens

MEJILLONES AL VINO CON TOMATE
Steamed cultured Mediterranean Black Mussels with herbed White Wine and Tomato Broth

BOQUERONES EN ESCABECHE
Fresh white A___

MEAT & POULTRY

JAMÓN SERRANO
The famous mountain cured Ham of Spain, shaved to order

PINCHOS MORUNOS
Spicy marinated grilled Brochettes Lamb or Chicken

SPANISH MEAT & CHEESE PLATE
Chef's Selection of Spanish Cured Meats, Chorizo & Spanish Cheese

CHORIZO A LA PARRILLA CON PESTO
___ Parsley and Pine Nut Pesto

the yogurt place

Franchises like Pinkberry, Red Mango, and Yogurtland have created glowing, neon hubs of fermented dairy happiness, where moms park their strollers and indulge themselves and their children in harmless yogurt treats that are so much healthier than ice cream. They are healthier, right?

Pack your pith helmet, kids. We're taking a trip up denial.

While fro-yo is a little lower in fat than regular ice cream, that's not always a guarantee that you're getting a healthier treat than you'd find at Mr. Softee's truck. One half cup of Pinkberry's Peanut Butter, for example, is 140 calories—pretty good for a frozen treat. But wait—you haven't added the toppings yet. Nothing too sugary, just some roasted hazelnuts, some mochi, a little of that Nutella. Now your ½ cup is 340 calories—or almost exactly what you'd get from two scoops of Baskin-Robbins Cookie 'N Cream in a cake cone. And thanks to the "pump it 'til you're full" approach that yogurt shops encourage, it's hard to know exactly what you're eating. Some places, like Yogurtland, for example, list their calories by the ounce—that's great, if you're pouring the stuff into a shotglass. A real serving may be closer to 10 ounces once you've finally peeled your eager palms off the handle.

Choose Your Sugar

To keep your sugar intake in check, choose either a tart (i.e. low sugar) yogurt with candy toppings or a sugary yogurt without any candy on top. That will ensure you get a sweet dessert without going overboard.

Non-Fat

Beware of non-fat yogurt; the fat is usually replaced with a lot of sugar. In the battle between two evils, sugar is the nastier of the two.

Sugar-Free

Sugar-free yogurt rarely means unsweetened. Find out what type of sugar replacement they use. Studies continue to link artificial sweeteners to weight gain.

Sweet Toppings

Bin after bin of candy, cereal, syrup and nut toppings is hard to resist. Treat yourself by picking one favorite candy and limit yourself to one scoop. Use the most of your topping real estate on fresh fruit.

Fruit

Apples
Bananas
Blackberries
Blueberries
Cantaloupe
Honeydew
Kiwi
Mango
Peaches
Pineapple
Raspberries
Strawberries

Candy

Butterfinger
Chocolate Malt Balls
Chocolate Sprinkles
Gummi Worms
Gummi Bears
Heath English Toffee Bits
Hershey's Chocolate Chips
Kit Kat bars
M&Ms
Milk Caramel Turtles
Nerds

Nuts

Oreos
Cashews
Hazelnuts
Peanuts
Pecans
Pistachios
Walnuts
Almonds

Fruit Toppings

Is the fruit fresh cut or swimming in syrup? You want fresh cut fruit, not the sugary canned stuff.

The Cup

Considering you pay by the weight, yogurt shops want you to fill up with as much yogurt as possible. Use the smallest cup size, and don't go above the brim.

Syrups and Sauces

Cool it with those self-serve syrup or sauce pumps. Each pump distributes ½ ounce, which can easily run you 50 calories per pump.

Nuts

All nuts are healthy, but walnuts are especially so for their high levels of brain-healthy omega-3 fatty acids.

Free Samples

Free in money terms is not the same as free in calorie terms. Those sample cups hold about 20 calories of yogurt. If you're going to try half the flavors in the store, you're going to have both very annoyed counter folks and maybe an extra 100 calories on top of your dessert.

Bowls made of Food

Waffle bowls are like ice cream cones; they just increase the empty calories.

Taste of Thai

For a lot of us, Thai seems like the healthier, lighter alternative to Chinese food. And many of the dishes you'll find here fill that role—the summer rolls are like spring rolls, without the long hot-oil bath. Spicy peanut sauce is a healthier choice by far than some of the heavy Chinese sauces. And soups like tom yum rely much less on sodium than egg drops do, and much more on healthy spices like lemongrass and cilantro.

But there are plenty of boobie traps on the Thai menu as well. The word "Pla," for example, should make you say "Blah!" It basically means "deep-fried." And keep an eye on fancy versions of rice (sweet coconut) or iced tea—they generally carry serious doses of sugar.

ROLLS (spring and summer)

Spring=deep-fried. Summer=not deep-fried. Now choose accordingly.

SATAY

Lean grilled meat on a stick slathered in a spicy peanut sauce. Seriously satisfying, low-fat food.

VEGETABLES

Laced with ginger, garlic, and chilies, Thai-style vegetables pack huge flavor for few calories. Try splitting an entrée with a companion and sharing a side of sizzling vegetables to round out the meal.

FRIED RICE

Nearly as oil-soaked as its Chinese counterpart.

APPETIZERS

Crispy Spring Rolls
(vegetables)
Steamed Dumpling
(chicken or vegetables)
Potstickers w
(chicken or vegetables)
Chicken Sate
Vietnamese Spring Rolls
(shrimp or tofu)
Fried Shrimp Rolls

VEGETABLES & TOFU

Sauteed Spinach
Szechwan String Beans
Garlic Eggplant
Orange Tofu
Red Curry Vegetables
Steamed Vegetable Plate
Vegetable Deluxe
(sauteed asparagus, snow peas, baby bok choy, and broccoli)

RICE

Thai Fried Rice
Spicy Basil Fried Rice
(choice of chicken, beef, tofu, or vegetables)
Special Brown Rice
(stir fried brown & wild rice with vegetables, and eggs)
Seafood Fried Rice
(shrimp, scallops, crab)

HOUSE SPECIALTIES

Thai BBQ Chicken

BBQ Pork Ribs

PadThai
(our most popular noodle dish)

Terry's Special
(sauteed bok choy, broccoli, and chicken with steamed brown & wild rice)

Mongolian BBQ beef

Garlic Scallops

Fish
(with black bean sauce)

Green Curry
(our popular curry dish from Bangkok)

Thai Chilli
(fish lightly fried and topped with thai chilli sauce)

Fillet of Sole
(lightly fried and topped with house curry sauce)

Steamed Fillet of Sole
(with house ginger and steamed vegetables)

Pla Lard Prik
(crispy snapper with chili, garlic and tamarind)

BEVERAGES

Our Special Thai Iced Tea or Coffee
(with non- dairy creamer)

PAD THAI

An average portion of this popular noodle entrée can be 600 calories, but it's usually very low in saturated fat, making it a pretty good option.

PLA LARD PRIK

The crispy whole snapper's "crispy" part comes from its bath in a wok of hot, bubbling oil. Eat the whole thing with rice and the meal tops out around 900 calories.

GREEN CURRY

Thai curries, regardless of color, are based around coconut milk. While high in saturated fat, most of that comes from lauric acid, which has been shown in more than 60 studies to decrease your risk of cardiovascular disease. Pick a lean protein like shrimp or chicken, and this makes for a healthier option than many of the noodle-based dishes.

TOFU

Acts like a soybean sponge, sucking up anything it comes into contact with. When it's fried, that often translates into a heavy dose of oil and little else. Ask for it sauteed, or stick to vegetables.

THAI ICED TEA

Any potential benefits of the brute-strength black tea are hopelessly diluted by the addition of sweetened condensed milk and a few fistfuls of sugar. Sip this and your blood sugar levels will soar, which signals your body to start storing fat.

MARRAKECH
MIDDLE EASTERN CUISINE

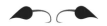

Perfect for the three V's (vegans, vegetarians, and people from Vermont), Middle Eastern restaurants are great go-tos for times when you want a healthy meal that's low on the meat and packed with veggies.

The success of Halal Guys—a food cart in New York City that attracted lines of people not seen since the last One Direction tour—has sparked a rush of interest in Middle Eastern cuisine. The Guys are opening a chain of 100 stores across the U.S. over the next few years, while Just Falafel, a United Arab Emirates franchise, is opening across the U.S. and Canada as well. Here's how you can find nutritional peace in the Middle East.

Pita & Hummus: Hummus has become one of the hot health foods of the last few years, and for good reason. Made from chickpeas and ground sesame seeds, plus olive oil (although most commercial brands use cheaper canola oil), hummus is packed with fiber, protein, and healthy fats. But a large pita can run you 165 calories, and just because it feels foreign doesn't make it anything more than plain empty carbs.

Babaganoush: A tasty, creamy eggplant dip that looks like it contains mayo, but actually is made from eggplants, tahini and olive oil.

Tahini sauce: Tahini is a paste made from ground sesame seeds, but the tahini sauce that is liberally spread on falafel sandwiches is made of tahini, olive oil and spices/seasoning. Ask for tahini on the side so you can control the amount that goes on your sandwich.

Tabouleh: A super-healthy choice, tabouleh is made of chopped parsley (an unsung superstar with more nutritional punch, ounce per ounce, than kale), plus tomatoes and bulgur with a dash of olive oil and lemon juice. Bulgur is a grain that contains 8 g of fiber per cooked cup.

Falafel: Have a falafel, you'll never feel awful. Just don't have too many: A falafel is a ball of ground chickpeas and/or fava beans that's then deep fried. Still, a 2-inch falafel ball is only about 60 calories and 3 grams of fat.

Traditional Favorites

HUMMUS BI TAHINI
Puree of chickpeas, tahini, lemon and garlic served as a dip

SPICY HUMMUS
Our delicious hummus with a spicy flare

BABAGHANOUSH
Charcoal-grilled eggplant, tahini, olive oil, lemon juice, & garlic

TABOULEH
Our traditional Lebanese Tabouleh Salad

GARLIC DIP
Our homemade garlic dip

KIBBEE NAYE TARTARE
Raw kibbee mixed with wheat wheat and our special seasoning

KIBBEE NAYE MHAMASA
Raw kibbee served with fried meat on the side

KIBBEE KRASS
Stuffed oval shaped nuggets of ground lamb and burghul

FALAFEL
Fried chick pea and coriander patties with tahini sauce

SHAWARMA
A platter of the tenderest cuts of meat from the gyro

GRILLED CHEESE
Grilled goat's milk cheese

Specialty Sandwiches

SPINACH PIES
Dough filled with seasoned spinach, onions, walnuts, and pine nuts

GYRO PITA
Toasted pita filled with Spicy tender meat from the gyro.

CHEESE RIKAKAT
Filo pastry filled with halloumi cheese, deep fried

LAHME BI AJIN
Minced meat baked over our homemade thin crust

After Dinner!

OUR HOMEMADE DESSERTS   TURKISH COFFEE

Kibbeh: Usually made from beef or lamb and bulgur, these balls are fried just like falafel, so eat with caution.

Shawarma: Spiced, marinated meat (usually lamb, but sometimes beef, veal or chicken), that is molded around a rotating spit and slowly roasted. They shave slices of the meat and serve it in a pita. Because fattier cuts are typically used to form the mold, and then further marinated in more fat, shawarmas typically run in the 600-calorie neighborhood, once you've added in the pita and sauces.

Gyro/Laffa/Pita Sandwiches: These beef, lamb or chicken sandwiches contain a liberal amount of carbs (the wrap or pita) as well as substantial amounts of sauces like hummus or tahini. You are better off ordering a platter which contains all the same ingredients but allow you to control how much you eat.

Dessert: Many desserts in Middle Eastern restaurants contain heavy amounts of honey, nuts and butter.

Turkish Coffee: Turkish coffee is usually served with sugar already mixed in, so you don't have any control over how sweet it is. Consider it a dessert.

THE VEGAN PLACE

Ignorance is bliss. And once you've read a bit about how cows, pigs and chickens are raised, it's hard to feel particularly blissful while eating a bacon cheeseburger. The more we know about how our food is treated before it gets turn into food, the more of us are turning to veganism.

Unfortunately, most cuisines of the world—especially traditional American cuisine—are built around meat products. With the exception of some Chinese restaurants, most places that seem like they'd be safe for vegans—from cheesy Italian joints to eggy coffee shops—rely on beasts to carry their nutritional burdens. That's one reason why vegan restaurants are popping up around the country.

If there's one rule of happy veganism, however, it's this: Don't ever pretend you're eating meat. No matter how much you manipulate tofu or wheat gluten, it will never taste like meat. Stick with a veggie-based dish and a grain, the staples of any vegan diet; you might find yourself discovering veg and grain combos you never knew existed.

TOFU: a block of soybean curd. Soy is high in naturally occurring chemicals called phytoestrogens, which have the opposite effect of testosterone, and can influence our hormonal balance and lead to weight gain.

TEMPEH: made from fermented soybeans, but unlike tofu, it uses whole soybeans so it is more dense. This density makes it a better protein source with 18 grams of protein compared to 9 for the same amount of tofu (100 grams).

SEITAN: made from wheat gluten, it does a great job of looking like beef, so you will find it in a lot of vegan stir fry.

Our Specials

Black Bean & Quinoa Veggie Burgers
Our house specialty! The most tender and juicy Quinoa burger you've ever tasted!

Norimaki Delight Teriyaki Tofu
Roasted red peppers, cucumber, marinated kale, seasoned brown rice, and parsley-almond pesto.

Live Zucchini Enchiladas
With cashew cheese, crunchy sprouts, guacamole, cashew sour cream, toasted pumpkin seeds, cucumber-jicama salsa, chipotle sauce

Spiced Chickpea Cake
Sautéed kale, broccoli, onions & jalapeños, red pepper-coconut curry sauce, date-apricot-ginger chutney, toasted almonds

Chipotle-Grilled Tempeh
Roasted shallots, sweet potatoes, brussels sprouts, pumpkin seeds, fennel & leek purée

Pumpkinseed-Crusted Seitan
With quinoa-corn pilaf, sautéed lobster mushrooms, broccoli, leeks, & a smoky tomato-chipotle sauce with radish salad

Fresh from the Oven
ANGEL'S SOURDOUGH
Rustic, whole grain square served with miso-tahini spread, rich & smooth!

QUINOA: While not technically a meat replacement, it is a good non-meat source of protein that has gained a lot of recent popularity. One cup contains 8 grams.

BREAD: The bread at a vegan restaurant is every bit as bad for you as the loaves at the Italian joint next door. Replacing protein and fat with empty carbs is a lousy trade too many vegans make, so limit yourself to one small piece with your meal.

DESSERT: Don't fall into the trap thinking that vegan sweets are healthier. Milk and eggs may be off the table, but sugar is still fair game, as are a host of other sweeteners like agave and honey. Some vegan desserts may end up with more sugar than regular desserts, to make up for the lack of animal fats.

DRINKS: A soda sweetened with organic agave or cane sugar is just as much of a waste of calories as a Pepsi. Stick with water, or unsweetened ice tea.

Chapter 4

AT YOUR FAVORITE RESTAURANTS

Simple ways to eat all your favorite foods— and dodge the calorie bombs

Here's a number you should keep in mind: 43. That's the percentage of calories you're going to eat this year that will come from restaurants, catering companies and other folks who, unlike you and your mom, don't really care very much about your health. So you'd better plan to be extra vigilant yourself.

And that's hard to do at a restaurant. Researchers call it the "special occasion mentality," and it sets in whenever we eat out at the local Applebee's or Arby's. Restaurants are where we celebrate our victories and drown our defeats—so it's worth it to splurge, right?

Unfortunately, the majority of Americans eat at restaurants every day or two. In fact, in our recent poll, one out of every three respondents said they'd eaten from a restaurant within the last 24 hours. That makes dining out about as "special" as taking a shower.

In this chapter, you'll discover exactly how not-so-special some of your restaurant favorites really are, and some smart ways to ensure that the terrific spread at the buffet doesn't turn into a terrific spread at your waistline. And along the way, you'll discover swaps that will save you hundreds, even thousands of calories in a single meal.

A&W

A&W's Canadian outlets have ditched the trans-fatty frying oil, so why do the American stores continue to soak its rings, fries, and chicken strips in this hazardous liquid? Beyond the trans fat issues, A&W offers little refuge for the health-conscious eater. The menu is long on old-time classics (burgers, fries, shakes) with new-age nutritionals (a 760-calorie burger, a 900-calorie milk shake). Despite its full menu, A&W is still a root-beer float shop at heart.

SURVIVAL STRATEGY

The best item on the entire menu is the Grilled Chicken Sandwich. Start with that or a small burger, skip the sides and the regular root beer, and finish (if you must have something sweet) with a small sundae or a vanilla cone.

Eat This
Original Bacon Cheeseburger

530 calories
30 g fat (10 g saturated, 0.5 g trans)
1,160 mg sodium

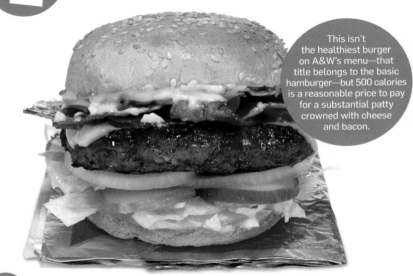

This isn't the healthiest burger on A&W's menu—that title belongs to the basic hamburger—but 500 calories is a reasonable price to pay for a substantial patty crowned with cheese and bacon.

Other Picks

Grilled Chicken Sandwich

400 calories
15 g fat
(3 g saturated)
820 mg sodium

Corn Dog Nuggets
(regular)

280 calories
13 g fat
(3 g saturated, 0.5 g trans)
830 mg sodium

Hot Fudge Sundae

350 calories
11 g fat
(6 g saturated)
15 g sugars

690 calories
39 g fat (14 g saturated, 1 g trans)
1,350 mg sodium

Not That!
Papa Burger

1,140
CALORIE BOMB
CheeseCurds
(large)

80 g fat
(42 g saturated,
2.5 g trans)
2,440 mg sodium

We can't say we're surprised that deep-fried cheese blobs aren't the health food of the year, but half a day's calories, nearly 3 days' worth of saturated fat, and 2.5 grams of dangerous trans fats in a single side dish is preposterous, even by junk-food standards.

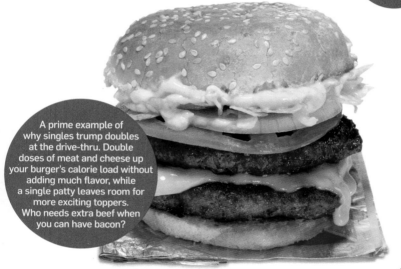

A prime example of why singles trump doubles at the drive-thru. Double doses of meat and cheese up your burger's calorie load without adding much flavor, while a single patty leaves room for more exciting toppers. Who needs extra beef when you can have bacon?

Other Passes

Reese's Polar Swirl
740 calories
31 g fat
(14 g saturated, 0.5 g trans)
85 g sugars

Chili Cheese Fries
410 calories
17 g fat
(5 g saturated, 3.5 g trans)
990 mg sodium

Chicken Strips
with Ranch Dipping Sauce
660 calories
46 g fat
(7.5 g saturated, 2 g trans)
1,290 mg sodium

ICE CREAM
STACKUP

Signature Soft Serve Cone
200 calories
22 g sugars

Root Beer Float
(medium)
350 calories
64 g sugars

Vanilla Shake
(medium)
900 calories
71 g sugars

APPLEBEE'S

It's easy to see why it took Applebee's so many years to release it's nutritional information. The 1,330-calorie Riblets Basket, the 1,390-calorie Oriental Chicken Salad, and the 2,370-calorie Appetizer Sampler are just a few of the little nightmares lurking on the menu. The bright spots on the menu include the steaks and the ever-expanding "Have It All" menu (despite some serious sodium issues).

SURVIVAL STRATEGY

Skip the meal-wrecking appetizers, pastas, and fajitas, and be very careful with salads, too; more than half of them top 1,000 calories. Concentrate on the excellent line of lean steak entrées, or anything from the fantastic 550-calorie-or-less "Have It All" menu.

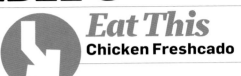

Eat This
Chicken Freshcado

440 calories
10 g fat (2 g saturated)
1,250 mg sodium

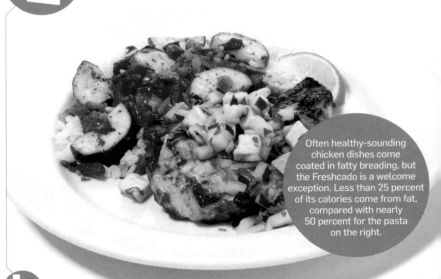

Often healthy-sounding chicken dishes come coated in fatty breading, but the Freshcado is a welcome exception. Less than 25 percent of its calories come from fat, compared with nearly 50 percent for the pasta on the right.

Other Picks

Roma Pepper Steak

510 calories
27 g fat
(12 g saturated)
1,860 mg sodium

Classic Turkey Breast Sandwich
with side of fruit

650 calories
29 g fat
(4.5 g saturated)
910 mg sodium

Garlic Mashed Potatoes

250 calories
14 g fat
(2.5 g saturated)
600 mg sodium

1,120 calories
55 g fat (30 g saturated)
2,620 mg sodium

Not That!
Chicken Broccoli Pasta Alfredo

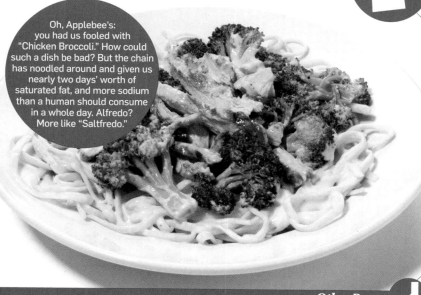

Oh, Applebee's: you had us fooled with "Chicken Broccoli." How could such a dish be bad? But the chain has noodled around and given us nearly two days' worth of saturated fat, and more sodium than a human should consume in a whole day. Alfredo? More like "Saltfredo."

HEALTH-FOOD FRAUD

Oriental Chicken Salad

1390 calories
98 g fat
(15 g saturated, 1.5 g trans)
1,610 mg sodium

How can chicken on a bed of greens do this much damage? At first we assumed it was the fried chicken, but ordering it grilled only saves you 100 calories. The collision of crispy noodles and oily dressing in this Oriental salad leaves us totally disoriented!

Guilty Pleasure

Garlic Mashed Potatoes

250 calories
14 g fat (2.5 g saturated)
600 mg sodium

Mashed potatoes at sit-down chains are usually loaded with cream and butter, but Applebee's managed to make its version with fewer calories and fat grams than a baked potato or small Caesar salad.

Other Passes

Loaded Mashed Potatoes

460 calories
31 g fat
(12 g saturated)
970 mg sodium

Boneless Wings
with Honey BBQ Sauce

1,250 calories
55 g fat
(11 g saturated, 0.5 g trans)
3,060 mg sodium

Steak Sizzling Skillet Fajitas

1,330 calories
48 g fat
(22 g saturated, 1 g trans)
5,240 mg sodium

ARBY'S

Just a few years ago, you could pull up to the Arby's window, order a grilled chicken sandwich, and be pretty sure you were keeping lunch under 500 calories. But the chain took a step backwards by eliminating its roast chicken line. Credit Arby's for nixing the trans fat from its frying oil years ago, but the restaurant doesn't offer a single side that hasn't had a long soak in a bath of hot oil.

SURVIVAL STRATEGY

You're not doing yourself any favors by ordering off the Market Fresh menu; that head-fake leads to dead ends like an 800-calorie Roast Turkey Ranch & Bacon Sandwich. A regular roast beef or Melt Sandwich will save you an average of nearly 300 calories over a Market Fresh sandwich or wrap.

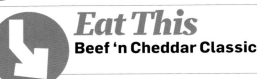

Eat This
Beef 'n Cheddar Classic

450 calories
20 g fat
(6 g saturated)
1,310 mg sodium

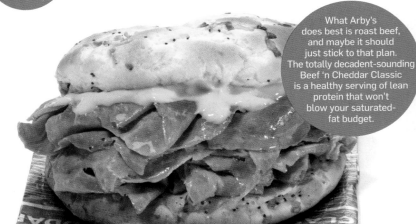

What Arby's does best is roast beef, and maybe it should just stick to that plan. The totally decadent-sounding Beef 'n Cheddar Classic is a healthy serving of lean protein that won't blow your saturated-fat budget.

Other Picks

Grand Turkey Club
480 calories
24 g fat (8 g saturated)
1,610 mg sodium

Roast Turkey Chopped Farmhouse Salad with Balsamic Vinaigrette
360 calories
25 g fat (9 g saturated)
1,250 mg sodium

Potato Cakes (small)
230 calories
14 g fat (2 g saturated)
460 mg sodium

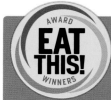

800 calories
35 g fat (9 g saturated, 0.5 g trans)
2,250 mg sodium

Not That!
Market Fresh Roast Turkey, Ranch & Bacon Sandwich

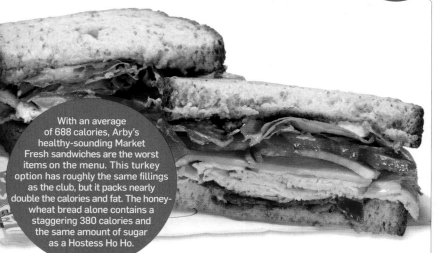

With an average of 688 calories, Arby's healthy-sounding Market Fresh sandwiches are the worst items on the menu. This turkey option has roughly the same fillings as the club, but it packs nearly double the calories and fat. The honey-wheat bread alone contains a staggering 380 calories and the same amount of sugar as a Hostess Ho Ho.

Ham & Swiss Melt

300 calories
9 g fat (3.5 g saturated)
1,030 mg sodium

The best bang for your nutritional buck at Arby's. It not only is low in calories and fat, but also delivers 18 grams of protein to help keep hunger pangs at bay.

BEEF SANDWICH STACKUP

Jr Roast Beef
210 calories
8 g fat

Roast Beef Classic
360 calories
14 g fat

Bacon Beef 'n Cheddar
510 calories
23 g fat

French Dip and Swiss
540 calories
23 g fat

Beef 'n Cheddar Mid
560 calories
27 g fat

Other Passes

Steakhouse Onion Rings
410 calories
20 g fat (3 g saturated)
1,690 mg sodium

Crispy Chopped Farmhouse Salad
with Honey Mustard Dressing
600 calories
39 g fat (10 g saturated)
1,250 mg sodium

Angus Three Cheese & Bacon Sandwich
630 calories
30 g fat
(11 g saturated, 0.5 g trans)
2,220 mg sodium

AU BON PAIN

There are plenty of ways you could go wrong here, but Au Bon Pain couples an extensive inventory of healthy items with an unrivaled standard of nutritional transparency. Use the on-site nutritional kiosks to seek out one of dozens of paths to a sensible meal. Or simply opt for one of the excellent soups or salads, or pair two smaller items from the All Portions menu.

SURVIVAL STRATEGY

Banish bagels and baked goods from your breakfast routine and opt for eggs instead. As for lunch, soups are a great option and there are plenty of low-calorie options on the All Portions menu, but steer clear of the Mediterranean Power Pack. It sounds vaguely healthy, but what it's actually packing is a hefty 1,020 calories.

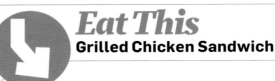
Eat This
Grilled Chicken Sandwich

480 calories
15 g fat (2 g saturated)
1,230 mg sodium

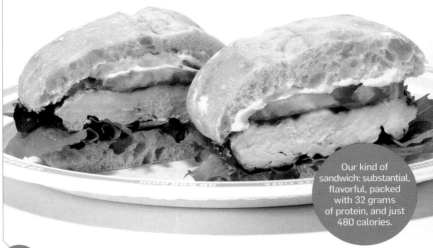

Our kind of sandwich: substantial, flavorful, packed with 32 grams of protein, and just 480 calories.

Other Picks

Classic Chicken Salad Sandwich

450 calories
12 g fat (2 g saturated)
990 mg sodium

Chicken Gumbo Soup (medium)

190 calories
9 g fat (1 g saturated)
930 mg sodium

Chocolate Dipped Cranberry Almond Macaroon

290 calories
16 g fat (13 g saturated)
25 g sugars

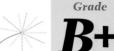

770 calories
34 g fat (14 g saturated)
1,790 mg sodium

Not That!
Newport Turkey Sandwich

You think white meat is healthier than red meat? Think again. When it comes to deli slices, turkey, ham, and roast beef all pack about the same amount of calories, fats, and protein per serving, which means when you're looking for the healthiest option, it all comes down to bread and condiments.

740 CALORIE BOMB
Pecan Roll

43 g fat
(18 g saturated)
48 g sugars

You could eat two Double Chocolate Cupcakes and still not reach the calorie load of this pecan-encrusted disaster. Unless you want to cultivate rolls of your own, avoid this pastry at all costs.

Other Passes

Double Chocolate Chunk Muffin
580 calories
24 g fat (7 g saturated)
49 g sugars

Chicken and Vegetable Stew
(medium)
340 calories
19 g fat (5 g saturated)
1,040 mg sodium

Black Angus Steak and Cheese Sandwich
840 calories
46 g fat (19 g saturated)
1,560 mg sodium

SIDE STACKUP

Chicken Noodle Soup
110 calories
2 g fat

Beef Chili
300 calories
13 g fat

Turkey Chili
380 calories
14 g fat

Lobster Bisque
410 calories
30 g fat

Macaroni & Cheese
560 calories
35 g fat

121

BAJA FRESH

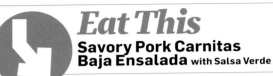

Baja Fresh is like communism or friends with benefits: In theory, it sounds great, but in practice, it fails miserably. It's nice that Baja makes all of its menu items fresh on-site, but why can't it make a simple chicken burrito with fewer than 600 calories? And what's up with all of the "naturally occurring" trans fats in their quesadillas and nachos? To minimize damage, turn to the tacos—then turn for the door.

SURVIVAL STRATEGY

Unless you're comfortable stuffing 54 grams of fat into your arteries before dinner, avoid the nachos at all costs. In fact, avoid almost everything on this menu except tacos, the torta, or a salad topped with salsa verde and served without the elephantine tortilla bowl.

Eat This

Savory Pork Carnitas Baja Ensalada with **Salsa Verde**

385 calories
18 g fat
(6 g saturated)
1,780 mg sodium

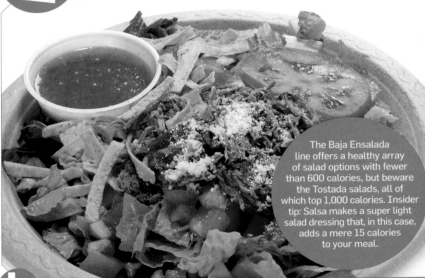

The Baja Ensalada line offers a healthy array of salad options with fewer than 600 calories, but beware the Tostada salads, all of which top 1,000 calories. Insider tip: Salsa makes a super light salad dressing that, in this case, adds a mere 15 calories to your meal.

Other Picks

Steak Original Baja Taco (2)

460 calories
16 g fat
(4 g saturated)
520 mg sodium

Shrimp Americano Soft Taco (2)

460 calories
20 g fat
(9 g saturated)
1,280 mg sodium

Side Salad

130 calories
6 g fat
(1.5 g saturated)
430 mg sodium

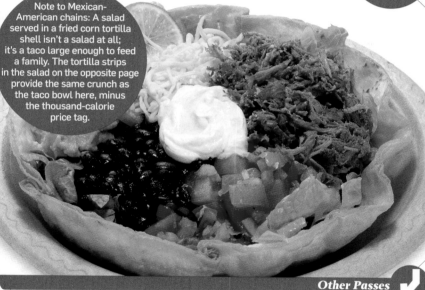

1,180 calories
62 g fat
(17 g saturated, 1 g trans)
2,520 mg sodium

Not That!
Savory Pork Carnitas Tostada Salad

Note to Mexican-American chains: A salad served in a fried corn tortilla shell isn't a salad at all; it's a taco large enough to feed a family. The tortilla strips in the salad on the opposite page provide the same crunch as the taco bowl here, minus the thousand-calorie price tag.

TORTILLA STACKUP

Chicken Original Baja Taco (2)
420 calories

Chicken Americano Soft Taco (2)
460 calories

Chicken Baja Burrito
790 calories

Charbroiled Chicken Nachos
1,010 calories

Charbroiled Chicken Quesadilla
1,330 calories

Other Passes

Chips and Salsa Baja

810 calories
37 g fat
(4 g saturated, 1.5 g trans)
1,140 mg sodium

Shrimp Fajitas with Flour Tortillas

1,120 calories
32 g fat
(10 g saturated)
3,410 mg sodium

Charbroiled Steak Quesadilla

1,430 calories
87 g fat
(41 g saturated, 3 g trans)
2,600 mg sodium

123

BASKIN-ROBBINS

Baskin-Robbins has a long tradition of carrying some of the worst frozen fare in the country. Sure, it shed its atrocious line of Premium Shakes, but it's going to take a lot more downsizing to earn a higher grade from us. The Premium Sundae line averages 1,055 calories, and even the average small Fruit Blast Smoothie contains 71 grams of sugars. If not for the frozen yogurt and sherbet, this grade would be even worse.

SURVIVAL STRATEGY

With choices like frozen yogurt, sherbet, and no-sugar-added ice cream, Baskin's lighter menu is the one bright spot in this otherwise dark world. Beyond that, look to the freezer for a Grab-N-Go treat. Stacked next to even a smoothie, these are great bets.

Eat This

Oreo Cookies 'n Cream Ice Cream in a Cake Cone (two 2.5-oz scoops)

345 calories
18 g fat
(10 g saturated)
24 g sugars

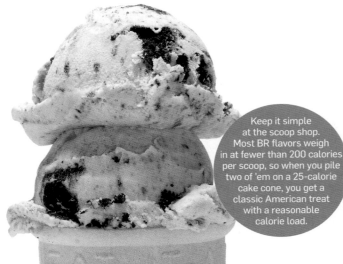

Keep it simple at the scoop shop. Most BR flavors weigh in at fewer than 200 calories per scoop, so when you pile two of 'em on a 25-calorie cake cone, you get a classic American treat with a reasonable calorie load.

Other Picks

Cappucino Blast Made with Soft Serve (small)

190 calories
6 g fat (4.5 g saturated)
26 g sugars

Chocolate Chip Cookie Dough Ice Cream (two 2.5-oz scoops in a cake cone)

385 calories
18 g fat (12 g saturated)
30 g sugars

Soft Serve Cookie Sandwich

180 calories
5 g fat (3 g saturated)
17 g sugars

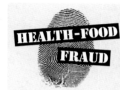

Grade

C−

1,330 calories
61 g fat
(31 g saturated, 1 g trans)
146 g sugars

Not That!
Oreo Layered Sundae

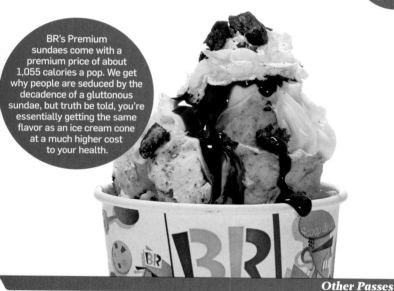

BR's Premium sundaes come with a premium price of about 1,055 calories a pop. We get why people are seduced by the decadence of a gluttonous sundae, but truth be told, you're essentially getting the same flavor as an ice cream cone at a much higher cost to your health.

HEALTH-FOOD FRAUD

Mango Banana Smoothie (large)

880 calories
3 g fat
192 g sugars

Smoothies have a sterling reputation in nutritional circles, but unless they're made without added sugars and served in small doses, they're really just dessert in disguise. Case in point: This mango monstrosity has more sugar than half a dozen Snickers bars.

Other Passes

Peanut Butter 'n Chocolate Ice Cream (two 2.5-oz scoops in a cake cone)

425 calories
26 g fat (12 g saturated)
32 g sugars

Chocolate Chip Cookie Dough Shake (medium)

980 calories
42 g fat
(27 g saturated)
114 g sugars

Turtle Cappuccino Blast (small)

510 calories
14 g fat
(8 g saturated)
70 g sugars

CONE STACKUP

Cake Cone
25 calories
0 g sugars

Sugar Cone
45 calories
3 g sugars

Waffle Cone
130 calories
11 g sugars

125

BEN & JERRY'S

What sets Ben & Jerry's apart from the competition amounts to more than just an affinity for jam bands and Hacky Sacks. The company remains committed to the quality of its ingredients. All dairy is hormone free and the chocolate, vanilla, and coffee ingredients are all Fair Trade Certified. From a strictly nutritional standpoint, though, it's still just an ice cream shop, and Ben & Jerry's average scoop is packed with more fat and sugar than most of its competitors.

SURVIVAL STRATEGY

With half of the calories of the ice cream, sorbet makes the healthiest choice on the menu. If you demand dairy, the frozen yogurt can still save you up to 100 calories per scoop.

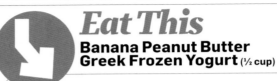

Eat This
Banana Peanut Butter Greek Frozen Yogurt (½ cup)

220 calories
10 g fat
(3 g saturated)
22 g sugars

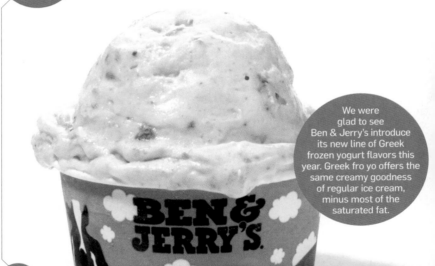

We were glad to see Ben & Jerry's introduce its new line of Greek frozen yogurt flavors this year. Greek fro yo offers the same creamy goodness of regular ice cream, minus most of the saturated fat.

Other Picks

Vanilla Toffee Bar Crunch Ice Cream (½ cup)

170 calories
4 g fat (2.5 g saturated)
20 g sugars

Super Pomegranate Smoothie (large)

190 calories
0 g fat
36 g sugars

Cherry Garcia Ice Cream (½ cup)

240 calories
13 g fat (9 g saturated)
23 g sugars

360 calories
24 g fat
(13 g saturated)
25 g sugars

Not That!
Peanut Butter Cup Ice Cream (½ cup)

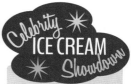

Celebrity
ICE CREAM
Showdown

Ben and/or Jerry managed to cram more than half a day's saturated fat into this peanut butter–chocolate bomb, making it the worst scoop on the menu, and one of the worst in America. The frozen yogurt on the opposite page is a much safer way to get your PB fix at B&J's.

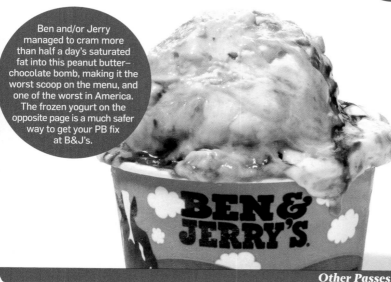

BEN & JERRY'S.

Liz Lemon Greek Frozen Yogurt

180 calories
4.5 g fat (2.5 g saturated)
21 g sugars

Stephen Colbert's Americone Dream

280 calories
16 g fat (10 g saturated)
28 g sugars

Phish Food

290 calories
14 g fat (9 g saturated)
32 g sugars

ALL THIS
- 1 small Sorbet Splash
- 1 small Berry Vanilla shake
- 1 scoop of Chunky Monkey ice cream

and
- an Ice Cream Float

OR THAT!
- 1 Banana Split

1,280 calories
67 g fat (41 g saturated)
118 g sugars

Other Passes

Chubby Hubby Ice Cream (½ cup)

340 calories
21 g fat (11 g saturated)
25 g sugars

Blueberry Cream Smoothie (large)

360 calories
8 g fat (2.5 g saturated)
55 g sugars

Coconut Seven Layer Bar Ice Cream (½ cup)

270 calories
17 g fat (10 g saturated)
21 g sugars

BLIMPIE

In the past, we admonished Blimpie for its love of trans fat. Since then, the chain has quietly removed all the dangerous oils from its menu and earned itself a place of honor in our book. But that doesn't mean the menu is free of danger. Blimpie likes to splash oil on just about everything containing deli meat, and there are a handful of sinful subs that top the 1,000-calorie mark.

SURVIVAL STRATEGY

A Bluffin makes a solid breakfast, and the Grilled Chicken Teriyaki Sandwich is one of the best in the business. But skip the wraps and most of the hot sandwiches. And no matter which sandwich you choose, swap out mayo and oil for mustard or light dressing.

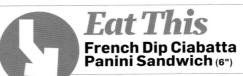

Eat This
French Dip Ciabatta Panini Sandwich (6")

430 calories
11 g fat
(4.5 g saturated)
1,820 mg sodium

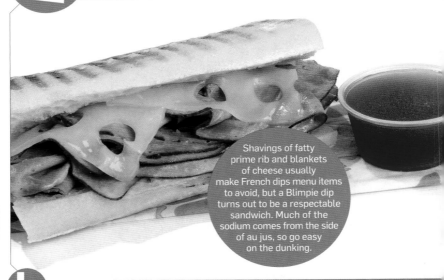

Shavings of fatty prime rib and blankets of cheese usually make French dips menu items to avoid, but a Blimpie dip turns out to be a respectable sandwich. Much of the sodium comes from the side of au jus, so go easy on the dunking.

Other Picks

Hot Pastrami Sandwich (6")

430 calories
16 g fat (7 g saturated)
1,390 mg sodium

Ham Egg & Cheese Bluffin

260 calories
9 g fat (4.5 g saturated)
930 mg sodium

Chocolate Chunk Cookie

180 calories
10 g fat (5 g saturated)
14 g sugars

590 calories
35 g fat
(11 g saturated)
1,410 mg sodium

Not That!
Philly Cheesesteak Sandwich (6")

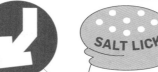

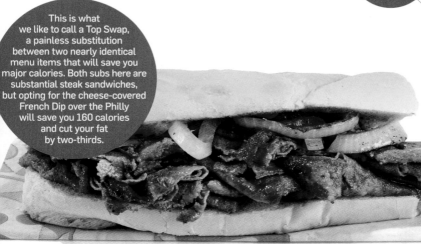

This is what we like to call a Top Swap, a painless substitution between two nearly identical menu items that will save you major calories. Both subs here are substantial steak sandwiches, but opting for the cheese-covered French Dip over the Philly will save you 160 calories and cut your fat by two-thirds.

SALT LICK

Meatball Parmigiana (12")

3,640 mg sodium
1,120 calories
58 g fat
(26 g saturated)

Blimpie loves the salt shaker, so anything Super Stacked will come at a cost to your blood pressure. This particular sub has more sodium than 227 Wheat Thin crackers.

Guilty Pleasure

Roast Beef & Provolone Sub (6")

430 calories
15 g fat (5 g saturated)
1,020 mg sodium

Roast beef gets a bad rap at the deli counter, but its calorie count and fat content are usually on par with turkey, ham, and other lean cold cuts. This sub has the same amount of saturated fat as Blimpie's Turkey & Provolone, but it feels a little more indulgent.

Other Passes

Sugar Cookie

320 calories
15 g fat (6 g saturated)
23 g sugars

Sausage Grilled Breakfast Sandwich

710 calories
45 g fat (19 g saturated)
1,920 mg sodium

Meatball Sandwich (6")

560 calories
29 g fat (13 g saturated)
1,820 mg sodium

BOB EVANS

No menu in America is more perplexing than Bob's. On one hand, the Ohio-based chain offers up an array of great entrées and side options, making it easy to cobble together a well-balanced meal. On the other, the menu is littered with land mines like 1,200-calorie multigrain pancakes and 1,000-calorie chicken salads. Until Mr. Evans shows us some consistency, we'll be showing him a lousy report card.

SURVIVAL STRATEGY

Breakfast should consist of staples like oatmeal, eggs, fruit, and yogurt (with maybe a slice or two of bacon); for lunch and dinner, stick with grilled chicken or fish paired with one of the non-fried vegetable sides. Or opt for one of Bob's perfectly portioned Savory Size entrées.

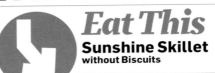

Eat This
Sunshine Skillet
without Biscuits

436 calories
24 g fat (10 g saturated)
1,410 mg sodium

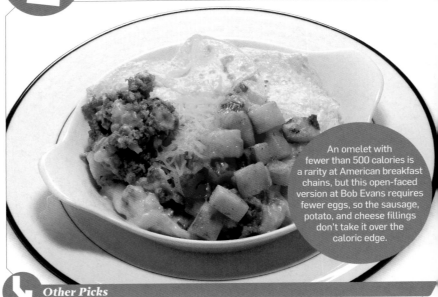

An omelet with fewer than 500 calories is a rarity at American breakfast chains, but this open-faced version at Bob Evans requires fewer eggs, so the sausage, potato, and cheese fillings don't take it over the caloric edge.

Other Picks

Meat Loaf
(with Mashed Potatoes and Green Beans)

575 calories
32 g fat
(15 g saturated)
2,225 mg sodium

The Farm Favorite Fried Chicken Sandwich

658 calories
26 g fat
(8 g saturated)
1,578 mg sodium

Fruit & Yogurt Plate and Cup of Oatmeal

439 calories
4 g fat
(0 g saturated)
78 mg sodium

884 calories
56 g fat (14 g saturated)
2,124 mg sodium

Not That!
2 Scrambled Eggs
with 3 Sausage Links and Hash Browns

Menu Magic

Ordering à la carte is usually your best strategy at big breakfast chains, but a couple of misguided choices can take your custom creation into dangerous territory. Switch the sausage to bacon and the hash browns to home fries, and you'll bring this meal down to a much more reasonable 418 calories.

Opting for mashed potatoes over french fries at Bob Evans will save you more than 300 calories and 12 g of fat. But be warned: This strategy won't work its magic everywhere. Many chains jack their mashed taters with copious amounts of cream and butter.

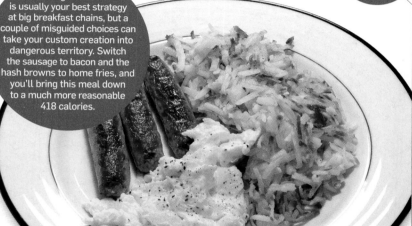

HIDDEN DANGER

Buttermilk Biscuit

Many of the breakfast items come with a side of two biscuits, which may feel like a bonus to hungry eaters, but the damage is often worse than the breakfast itself. Remember, it's these items—the bread basket, the chips and salsa, the "free" biscuits—that do the most damage to your waistline.

Other Passes

Fruit and Nut Multigrain Hotcakes (3) with Butter and Syrup

1,242 calories
25 g fat
(7 g saturated)
1,376 mg sodium

The Smokehouse Grilled Chicken Sandwich

890 calories
47 g fat
(17 g saturated)
2,642 mg sodium

Slow Roasted Chicken Pot Pie

862 calories
56 g fat
(22 g saturated)
2,623 mg sodium

476 calories
24 g fat
(14 g saturated)
1,570 mg sodium

BOSTON MARKET

Boston Market's menu remains a mixed bag of lean proteins and calorie-dense side dishes. Healthy combination platters can still be had, but tread lightly among its many nutritional land mines. What this menu really needs is less butter, less cheese, and makeovers of the Meatloaf, Pastry Top Chicken Pot Pie, and the entire line of Boston Carver sandwiches.

SURVIVAL STRATEGY

Pair roasted turkey, ham, white-meat chicken, or even beef brisket with a vegetable side or two, and you've got a solid dinner. But avoid calorie-laden dark-meat chicken, meat loaf, potpie, and almost anything served between two pieces of bread. And choose your sides carefully.

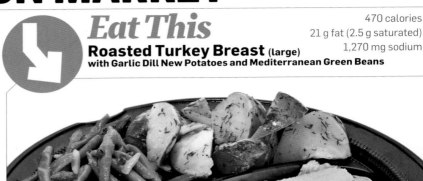

Eat This

Roasted Turkey Breast (large)
with Garlic Dill New Potatoes and Mediterranean Green Beans

470 calories
21 g fat (2.5 g saturated)
1,270 mg sodium

The piecemeal approach is still the best way to go at Boston Market, and there's no better place to start than with turkey breast. A 7-ounce piece contains 39 grams of protein, meaning that an astounding 83 percent of the turkey's 280 calories come from the metabolism-spiking macronutrient.

Other Picks

Rotisserie Chicken
¼ dark
(1 thigh, 1 drumstick)

310 calories
20 g fat
(6 g saturated)
670 mg sodium

Turkey Breast
(regular)

200 calories
9 g fat
(0 g saturated)
710 mg sodium

Cinnamon Apples

250 calories
3.5 g fat (0.5 g saturated)
720 mg sodium

1,040 calories
46 g fat (16.5 g saturated)
2,150 mg sodium

Not That!
Half Rotisserie Chicken
with Mashed Potatoes and Cornbread

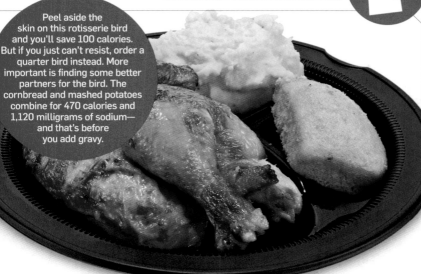

Peel aside the skin on this rotisserie bird and you'll save 100 calories. But if you just can't resist, order a quarter bird instead. More important is finding some better partners for the bird. The cornbread and mashed potatoes combine for 470 calories and 1,120 milligrams of sodium—and that's before you add gravy.

TEST TUBE FOODS

Meatloaf (large)

760 calories
44 g fat
(19 g saturated,
3.5 g trans)
1,340 mg sodium

Meatloaf might be comfort food, but the recipe for Boston Market's loaf boasts a 45-ingredient lineup of additives you won't find in your kitchen. That is, unless your mom's recipe calls for modified starch, maltodextrin, and xantham gum.

SIDE STACKUP

Fresh Steamed Vegetables
80 calories

Sweet Corn
120 calories

Mashed Potatoes
240 calories

Creamed Spinach
250 calories

Macaroni & Cheese
280 calories

Other Passes

Sweet Potato Casserole	Quarter White Rotisserie Chicken	St. Louis Style BBQ Ribs (½ rack)
430 calories	320 calories	1,180 calories
12 g fat (3.5 g saturated)	13 g fat (4 g saturated)	74 g fat (29 g saturated)
210 mg sodium	710 mg sodium	3,150 mg sodium

BURGER KING

BK invites you to "Take a Break from Boredom." You will definitely not be bored when you look down in panicked horror at the bathroom scale. The rule of thumb at Burger King is to be suspicious of anything that was invented after Taylor Swift was born: Newfangled options like 400-calorie wraps, sugar-loaded smoothies, and coffee drinks with nearly as many calories as a Whopper only make eating well more difficult. Thankfully, standbys like the Whopper Jr., basic hamburgers, and apple slices give you a way out.

SURVIVAL STRATEGY

Start your day with a Muffin Sandwich. For lunch, match the regular hamburger, the Whopper Jr., or the Tendergrill Sandwich with apple slices and water, and you'll escape for about 700 calories.

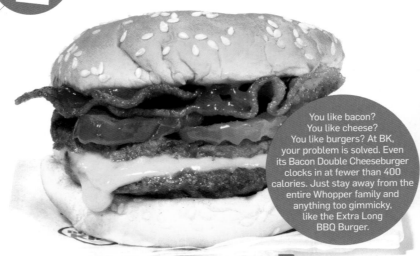

Eat This
Bacon Cheeseburger Deluxe

290 calories
14 g fat (6 g saturated, 0.5 g trans)
720 mg sodium

You like bacon? You like cheese? You like burgers? At BK, your problem is solved. Even its Bacon Double Cheeseburger clocks in at fewer than 400 calories. Just stay away from the entire Whopper family and anything too gimmicky, like the Extra Long BBQ Burger.

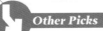

Other Picks

Tendergrill Chicken Sandwich

410 calories
16 g fat (2.5 g saturated)
830 mg sodium

Chicken Strips
(3 pieces)

340 calories
17 g fat (2.5 g saturated)
1,130 mg sodium

BK Breakfast Muffin Sandwich
(Sausage, Egg and Cheese)

430 calories
26 g fat (8 g saturated)
1,140 mg sodium

Not That!
A.1. Ultimate Bacon Cheeseburger

850 calories
51 g fat (22 g saturated, 3 g trans)
1,480 mg sodium

BK recently joined its Golden Arches rival in offering specialty burgers designed to imitate the more substantial burgers offered by sit-down chains. The problem? These pseudo-gourmet burgers translate into nothing more than bigger portions (aka bigger calorie loads). BK is not the place to go gourmet.

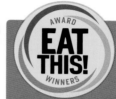

AWARD EAT THIS! WINNERS

Whopper Jr.
(without Mayo)

240 calories
10 g fat
(3.5 g saturated)
410 mg sodium

Sans mayo, the Whopper Jr. is a star beyond just the realm of Burger King. Order it solo for a solid snack or pair it with Chicken Tenders or a side garden salad for a satisfying meal.

ALL THIS
- **1 Hamburger**
- **Chicken Strips (3 pieces)**
- **Onion Rings (small)**
and
- **a Strawberry Sundae**

1,080 calories

OR THAT!
- **Triple Whopper with Cheese**

1,160 calories

Other Passes

Double Croissan'wich
(Sausage, Egg and Cheese)

790 calories
57 g fat
(21 g saturated, 1 g trans)
1,630 calories

Tendercrisp Chicken Sandwich

640 calories
36 g fat (6 g saturated)
1,270 mg sodium

Chicken Apple & Cranberry Garden Fresh Salad
with Tendercrisp Chicken and Dressing

680 calories
42 g fat (9 g saturated)
1,010 mg sodium

CALIFORNIA PIZZA KITCHEN

CPK's sneakiest trick is to make its "healthy" thin-crust pizzas somehow more caloric than its regular pies. A Five Cheese + Fresh Tomato Hand-Tossed will actually cost you nearly 200 calories per pie less than the Margherita Crispy Thin Crust. Oh, and if you order whole-wheat crust? Add another 140 calories. Salads range from 530 calories up to 1,500 for the Moroccan-Spiced Chicken—nearly what an adult woman should eat in a whole day.

SURVIVAL STRATEGY

Pair something from the nutrition-packed Lite Adventures menu with a cup of soup (Shrimp Scampi Zucchini Fettuccine with a cup of Dakota Smashed Pea + Barley brings you in at 640 calories), or split a Hawaiian pizza with your date.

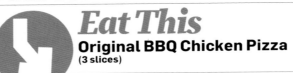

Eat This
Original BBQ Chicken Pizza
(3 slices)

535 calories
13.5 g fat
(7.5 g saturated)
1,445 mg sodium

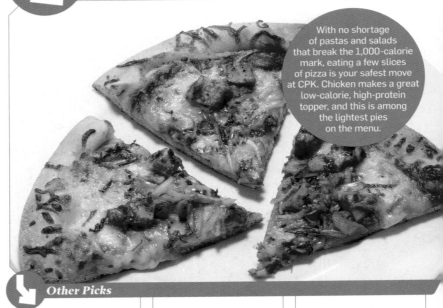

With no shortage of pastas and salads that break the 1,000-calorie mark, eating a few slices of pizza is your safest move at CPK. Chicken makes a great low-calorie, high-protein topper, and this is among the lightest pies on the menu.

Other Picks

Pepperoni Pizza
(3 slices)

560 calories
21 g fat
(10 g saturated)
1,380 mg sodium

Fire-Roasted Chile Relleno

420 calories
27 g fat
(11 g saturated)
870 mg sodium

Bianco Flatbread

380 calories
15 g fat
(9 g saturated)
740 mg sodium

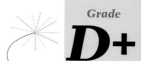

1,250 calories
81 g fat
(19 g saturated)
1,800 mg sodium

Not That!
The Original BBQ Chicken Chopped Salad (full), with Avocado

1,630 CALORIE BOMB
Chicken Piccata

78 g fat
(24 g saturated)
2,140 mg sodium

In the upside-down world of CPK, the healthier a dish sounds, the more caloric it probably is. That's the case with Chicken Piccata, which packs a full day's worth of sodium along with its 1,630 calories.

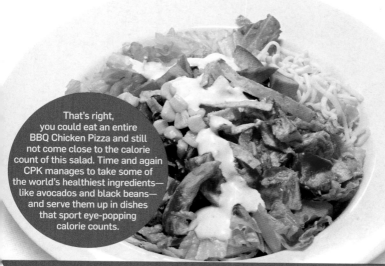

That's right, you could eat an entire BBQ Chicken Pizza and still not come close to the calorie count of this salad. Time and again CPK manages to take some of the world's healthiest ingredients—like avocados and black beans—and serve them up in dishes that sport eye-popping calorie counts.

Crust SELECTOR

Crispy Thin
570 calories
3 g fat (0 g saturated)
1,250 mg sodium

Hand-Tossed Original
580 calories
2.5 g fat (0 g saturated)
1,250 mg sodium

Hand-Tossed Wheat Whole Grain
720 calories
12 g fat (0 g saturated)
1,110 mg sodium

Other Passes

Tuscan Hummus
with Wheat Whole Grain Pita
970 calories
33 g fat
(0.5 g saturated)
1,520 mg sodium

Avocado Club Egg Rolls
1,190 calories
82 g fat
(20 g saturated)
2,280 mg sodium

The Meat Cravers Pizza (3 slices)
795 calories
38 g fat
(16 g saturated)
2,310 mg sodium

CARL'S JR.

Carl's Jr. may have the raciest ads in fast-food land, but some of its offerings are downright respectable, starting with its line of 500-calorie-or-less turkey burgers and Chicken Stars, the chain's version of nuggets that clock in at just over 40 calories apiece. Still, many of the burgers deliver twice the calories of a Big Mac, and almost everything on the breakfast menu makes for a bad morning.

SURVIVAL STRATEGY

Opt for any of the salads, but make sure you choose the low-fat balsamic dressing (35 calories) and not the blue cheese (320 calories). The Charbroiled BBQ Chicken Sandwich, or any of the turkey burgers make healthy options. Breakfast? Eat at home.

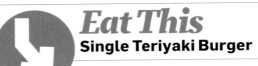

Eat This
Single Teriyaki Burger

630 calories
29 g fat (11 g saturated)
1,060 mg sodium

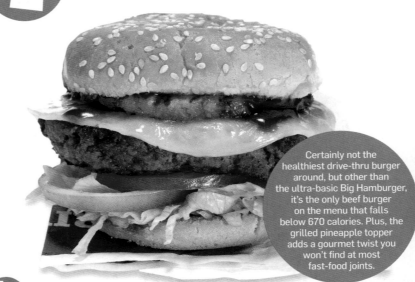

Certainly not the healthiest drive-thru burger around, but other than the ultra-basic Big Hamburger, it's the only beef burger on the menu that falls below 670 calories. Plus, the grilled pineapple topper adds a gourmet twist you won't find at most fast-food joints.

Other Picks

Guacamole Turkey Burger

480 calories
19 g fat
(6 g saturated)
1,000 mg sodium

Sourdough Breakfast Sandwich

470 calories
24 g fat
(12 g saturated)
1,340 mg sodium

Hand-Breaded Chicken Tenders (3)

260 calories
13 g fat
(2.5 g saturated)
770 mg sodium

930 calories
56 g fat (23 g saturated)
1,540 mg sodium

Not That!
Super Star with Cheese

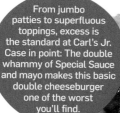

From jumbo patties to superfluous toppings, excess is the standard at Carl's Jr. Case in point: The double whammy of Special Sauce and mayo makes this basic double cheeseburger one of the worst you'll find.

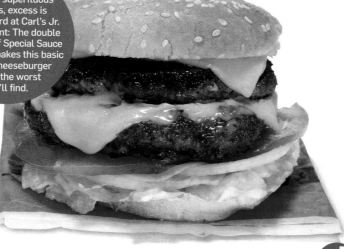

TEST TUBE FOODS

Breakfast Burger
800 calories
43 g fat
(18 g saturated, 1 g trans)
1,380 mg sodium

Smash a plate of eggs, bacon, and hash browns between two buns and you get a breakfast sandwich that's nearly three times the calories of an Egg McMuffin.

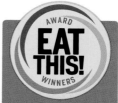

AWARD
EAT THIS!
WINNERS

Charbroiled Turkey Burgers (4 varieties)
480 to 500 calories
14 to 22 g fat
(4.5 to 6 g saturated)
960 to 1,150 mg sodium

In 2011, we worked with Carl's to design a line of lean, juicy turkey burgers with toppings like teriyaki and guacamole.

Other Passes

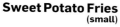

Sweet Potato Fries
(small)
360 calories
17 g fat
(3 g saturated)
590 mg sodium

Big Country Breakfast Burrito
720 calories
43 g fat
(18 g saturated)
1,380 mg sodium

Charbroiled Santa Fe Chicken Sandwich
560 calories
27 g fat
(7 g saturated)
1,290 mg sodium

THE CHEESECAKE FACTORY

The Cheesecake Factory stands nearly alone in its brazen refusal to reveal what's really in its food. And for good reason: In a recent survey of the most caloric restaurant foods in America, Cheesecake Factory scored 5 of the top 10! It made some progress when it introduced its SkinnyLicious menu, but most entrées still come with quadruple-digit calorie counts. Once again, the Cheesecake Factory retains the title of Worst Restaurant in America.

SURVIVAL STRATEGY

Your best survival strategy is to turn your car around and head home. Failing that, skip pasta, specialties, combos, and sandwiches at all costs. Split a pizza or a salad, or look to the SkinnyLicious menu.

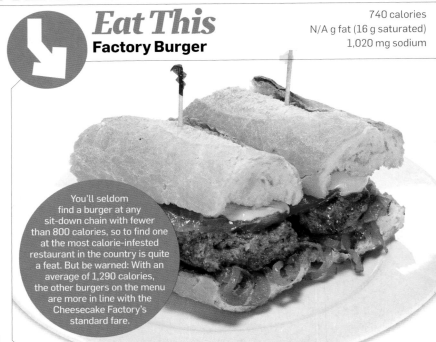

Eat This
Factory Burger

740 calories
N/A g fat (16 g saturated)
1,020 mg sodium

You'll seldom find a burger at any sit-down chain with fewer than 800 calories, so to find one at the most calorie-infested restaurant in the country is quite a feat. But be warned: With an average of 1,290 calories, the other burgers on the menu are more in line with the Cheesecake Factory's standard fare.

Other Picks

Grilled Mahi
470 calories
N/A g fat
(5 g saturated)
390 mg sodium

Vietnamese Shrimp Summer Rolls
660 calories
N/A g fat
(2 g saturated)
1,680 mg sodium

Giant Belgian Waffle (with Strawberries, Pecans, Cream)
740 calories
N/A g fat
(7 g saturated)
930 mg sodium

1,400 calories
N/A g fat (23 g saturated)
2,100 mg sodium

Not That!
Grilled Chicken and Avocado Club

> Only in the bizarro world of the Cheesecake Factory could a grilled chicken sandwich house nearly double the calories of a burger. We're consistently baffled by the chain's ability to cram staggering amounts of calories, fat, and salt into ordinary-sounding dishes. Add fries and you're looking at nearly 2,000 calories on a single plate.

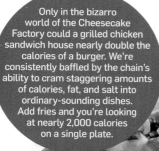

2,290
CALORIE BOMB
Bistro Shrimp Pasta

N/A g fat
(73 g saturated)
820 mg sodium

This is an unhealthy head fake if ever we've seen one. With more than an entire day's worth of calories, and more than three days' worth of saturated fat, the normally low-fat, low-cal shrimp is primed to turn you into a jumbo.

Other Passes

French Toast with Grilled Ham

1,570 calories
N/A g fat
(51 g saturated)
3,100 mg sodium

Thai Lettuce Wraps

1,030 calories
N/A g fat
(6 g saturated)
2,350 mg sodium

Miso Salmon

1,670 calories
N/A g fat
(39 g saturated)
2,420 mg sodium

PASTA STACKUP

Shrimp with Angel Hair
850 calories
2 g saturated fat

Pasta Marinara
1,210 calories
3 g saturated fat

Garlic Noodles
1,500 calories
22 g saturated fat

Pasta Carbonara
2,130 calories
81 g saturated fat

CHICK-FIL-A

Chick-fil-A ranks among the best of the country's major fast-food establishments, thanks to a line of low-calorie chicken sandwiches and an impressive roster of healthy sides like yogurt parfaits and various salads. But the menu does seem to be inching ever upward in the calorie and sodium departments. Any more movement and this A- becomes a B.

SURVIVAL STRATEGY

Instead of nuggets or strips, look to the grilled chicken sandwiches or the classic fried chicken sandwich. And sub in a healthy side—a salad or soup—for the standard fried fare. Just don't supplement your meal with a shake—none has fewer than 500 calories.

Eat This
Chick-fil-A Chicken Sandwich

440 calories
16 g fat
(3.5 g saturated)
1,400 mg sodium

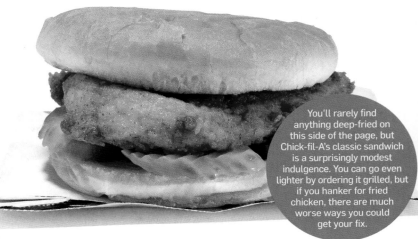

You'll rarely find anything deep-fried on this side of the page, but Chick-fil-A's classic sandwich is a surprisingly modest indulgence. You can go even lighter by ordering it grilled, but if you hanker for fried chicken, there are much worse ways you could get your fix.

Other Picks

Grilled Chicken Sandwich

320 calories
5 g fat
(1.5 g saturated)
800 mg sodium

Bacon, Egg, and Cheese Biscuit

450 calories
23 g fat
(11 g saturated)
1,040 mg sodium

Hearty Breast of Chicken Soup

130 calories
3 g fat
(1 g saturated)
790 mg sodium

740 calories
54 g fat
(12 g saturated)
1,890 mg sodium

Not That!
Cobb Salad
with Avocado Lime Ranch Dressing

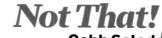

A prime example of how fast-food chains turn salads into junk food. High-fat toppings like fried chicken and shredded cheese make this salad one of the most caloric entrées on the menu.

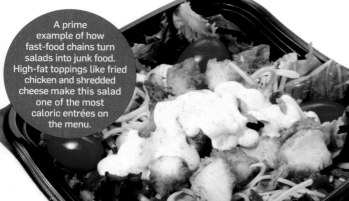

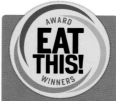

EAT THIS!
AWARD WINNERS

Grilled Market Salad

200 calories
5 g fat (2 g saturated)
570 mg sodium

A seriously healthy salad with berries, apples, red cabbage and carrots, all on top of a bed of mixed greens. The grilled chicken and a sprinkling of blue cheese loads you up with 23 grams of protein for a mere 5 grams of fat. We couldn't have designed a better muscle-up, slim-down food ourselves.

COOKIE STACKUP

Chocolate Chunk Cookie
330 calories
27 g sugars

Cookie Sundae
400 calories
52 g sugars

Cookies & Cream Milkshake (small)
520 calories
69 g sugars

Other Passes

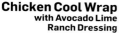

Chicken Cool Wrap
with Avocado Lime Ranch Dressing

650 calories
45 g fat
(10 g saturated)
1,420 mg sodium

Sausage, Egg, and Cheese Biscuit

670 calories
45 g fat
(19 g saturated)
1,340 mg sodium

Chicken Salad Sandwich

500 calories
20 g fat
(4 g saturated)
1,120 mg sodium

CHILI'S

Chili's serves up some of the country's saltiest, fattiest, most calorie-laden fare, from tacos and salads to baby back ribs. Worst among the offenders are the burgers, fajitas, and appetizers, including the 1,760-calorie Texas Cheese Fries. The Lighter Choices menu is Chili's attempt at healthier meals, but with only a handful of options and a sky-high average sodium count, nothing at Chili's will make you look particularly hot.

SURVIVAL STRATEGY

There's not too much to choose from after you eliminate the ribs, burgers, fajitas, and starters. Try a salad or the Make It a Combo section. Pair a Spicy Garlic and Lime Grilled Shrimp skewer with Margarita Chicken or sirloin and a side of black beans.

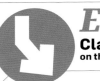

Eat This

Classic Sirloin (6 oz) with Sweet Corn on the Cob, Butter, and Steamed Broccoli

520 calories
19 g fat
(5.5 g saturated)
2,280 mg sodium

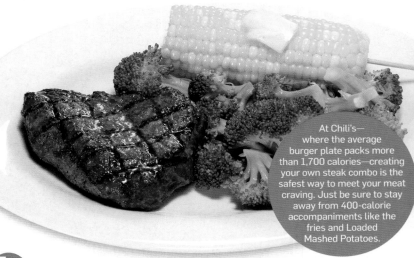

At Chili's—where the average burger plate packs more than 1,700 calories—creating your own steak combo is the safest way to meet your meat craving. Just be sure to stay away from 400-calorie accompaniments like the fries and Loaded Mashed Potatoes.

 Other Picks

Sweet Potato Fries
800 calories
48 g fat
(8 g saturated)
1,080 mg sodium

Margarita Grilled Chicken
610 calories
16 g fat
(4 g saturated)
2,450 mg sodium

Caribbean Salad
with Grilled Chicken
680 calories
27 g fat
(4.5 g saturated)
1,150 mg sodium

1,680 calories
87 g fat
(26 g saturated)
4,590 mg sodium

Not That!
Guacamole Burger
with Homestyle Fries

Veggies and some healthy guac can't save this burger from the Chili's treatment: huge portions, fatty sauces, and a heaping pile of greasy fries. Two days' worth of sodium will have you thirsting for another round of drinks. Hmm, coincidence?

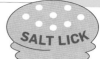

Southern Smokehouse Burger
with Fries

5,500 mg sodium
1,960 calories

A typical Chili's burger plate packs a shameful 4,500 milligrams of sodium, and this disaster is the worst of the lot. Putting even more pressure on your arteries is a calorie load greater than what an adult woman should eat in an entire day.

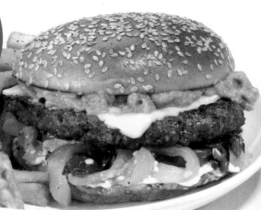

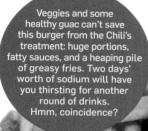

Other Passes

APPETIZER
STACKUP

Classic Nachos
(regular)
820 calories
56 g fat

Loaded Potato Skins
1,110 calories
78 g fat

Texas Cheese Fries
(half order)
1,270 calories
89 g fat

Skillet Queso with Chips
1,590 calories
97 g fat

Boneless Buffalo Chicken Salad

1,030 calories
68 g fat
(14 g saturated)
3,730 mg sodium

Monterey Chicken

940 calories
51 g fat
(19 g saturated)
3,560 mg sodium

Classic Nachos
(large)

1,190 calories
81 g fat
(43 g saturated)
2,990 mg sodium

145

CHIPOTLE MEXICAN GRILL

We've always commended Chipotle for the integrity of its ingredients and the flexibility of its menu. And recent addition of a vegan protein option, Sofritas, in some of its outlets is a big nutritional step forward. But this burrito bar could still do a lot better. After years of telling people to avoid the meal-wrecking chips (570 calories), flour burrito tortillas (300 calories), and vinaigrette (270 calories), we have a challenge for Chipotle: Offer a smaller version of your belly-busting burrito.

SURVIVAL STRATEGY

Chipotle is all about customization. With fresh salsa, beans, lettuce, and grilled vegetables, you can get a nutritionally solid meal. Choose a bowl over a burrito, skip the white rice and sour cream, and you'll do just fine.

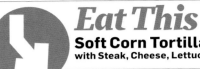

Eat This

Soft Corn Tortilla Tacos
with Steak, Cheese, Lettuce, and Fresh Tomato Salsa

525 calories
14 g fat (7 g saturated)
1,040 mg sodium

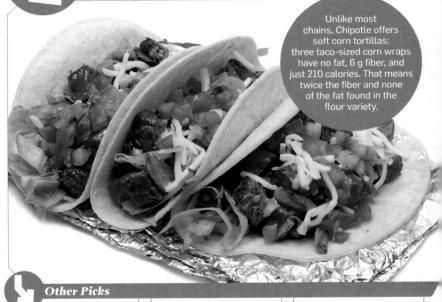

Unlike most chains, Chipotle offers soft corn tortillas; three taco-sized corn wraps have no fat, 6 g fiber, and just 210 calories. That means twice the fiber and none of the fat found in the flour variety.

Other Picks

Burrito Bowl with **Barbacoa Beef, Black Beans, Cheese, Lettuce, and Fresh Tomato Salsa**

410 calories
15.5 g fat
(7.5 g saturated)
1,480 mg sodium

Salad with **Chicken, Black Beans, Cheese, and Fresh Tomato Salsa**

430 calories
15.5 g fat
(8 g saturated)
1,265 mg sodium

Guacamole (side order) and Crispy Corn Taco Shell (3)

410 calories
26.5 g fat
(6 g saturated)
360 mg sodium

146

1,090 calories
40 g fat (15 g saturated)
2,195 mg sodium

Not That!

Burrito with Steak, Black Beans, Cilantro-Lime Rice, Cheese, Sour Cream, and Roasted Chili-Corn Salsa

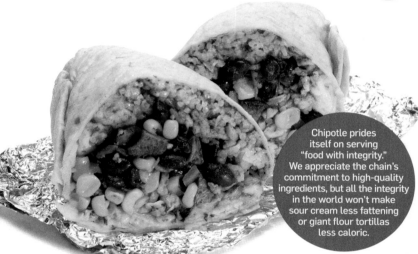

Chipotle prides itself on serving "food with integrity." We appreciate the chain's commitment to high-quality ingredients, but all the integrity in the world won't make sour cream less fattening or giant flour tortillas less caloric.

Salsa SELECTOR

Green Tomatillo (2 oz)
20 calories
250 mg sodium

Fresh Tomato (3.5 oz)
20 calories
500 mg sodium

Red Tomatillo (2 oz)
25 calories
500 mg sodium

Roasted Chili-Corn (3.5 oz)
80 calories
330 mg sodium

TORTILLA STACKUP

Soft Corn Tortilla (3)
210 calories
0 g fat

Crispy Corn Taco Tortilla (3)
210 calories
7.5 g fat

Flour Taco Tortilla (3)
255 calories
7.5 g fat

Flour Burrito Tortilla
300 calories
10 g fat

Other Passes

Chips with Fresh Tomato Salsa
590 calories
27 g fat
(3.5 g saturated)
920 mg sodium

Salad with Chicken, Black Beans, Cheese, and Vinaigrette
680 calories
40.5 g fat
(12.5 g saturated)
1,615 mg sodium

Soft Flour Tacos with Barbacoa Beef, Black Beans, Cheese, Lettuce, and Fresh Tomato Salsa
685 calories
23 g fat
(10.5 g saturated)
1,050 mg sodium

COLD STONE CREAMERY

What makes Cold Stone novel is also what makes it so dangerous. The regular ice cream is fatty enough, but calorie and, perhaps more important, sugar counts escalate quickly when the mix-ins and toppings come into play. Sundaes are a total mess; even small shakes average more than 750 calories; and cakes and plated desserts don't fare much better. Stick to sorbet, frozen yogurt, or Skinny Vanilla ice cream, or save this spot for (very) special occasions.

SURVIVAL STRATEGY

Keep your intake under 400 calories by filling a Like It–size cup with one of the lighter scoops, and then sprinkle fresh fruit on top. Or opt for one of the creamery's real-fruit smoothies, which average just 242 calories apiece.

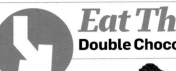

Eat This

Double Chocolate Devotion Cupcake

360 calories
19 g fat (13 g saturated)
40 g sugars

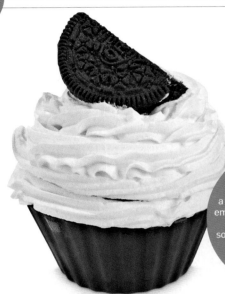

It's a sure sign that a menu is serious trouble when a big, choco-tastic cupcake emerges on the Eat This side of the page. Beyond the sorbets, you won't find many "Love It"–sized items with fewer than 360 calories.

Other Picks

Pumpkin Ice Cream
with Whipped Topping
(Like It size)

335 calories
17.5 g fat
(11 g saturated)
30 g sugars

Cookies & Creamery
Frozen Yogurt
(Like It size)

210 calories
2 g fat
(0.5 g saturated)
33 g sugars

Sweet Cream
Cupcake

390 calories
21 g fat
(15 g saturated)
44 g sugars

810 calories
55 g fat (21 g saturated, 0.5 g trans)
75 g sugars

Not That!
Brownie a La Cold Stone

1,262
The average number of calories in one of Cold Stone Creamery's Love It size milk shakes

We've rarely seen a brownie that can earn our approval, much less a brownie smothered in hot fudge, caramel, and whipped cream that can. The net result delivers nearly as much saturated fat as you'd find in a cup of mayonnaise. Why do the damage when you can satisfy your chocolate craving for so much less?

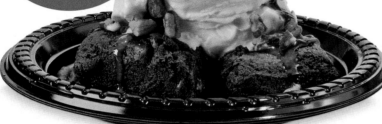

THE TOPPING STACKUP

Blueberries
10 calories, 0 g fat
2 g sugars

Chocolate Sprinkles
25 calories, 0 g fat
6 g sugars

Cherry Pie Filling
50 calories, 0 g fat
0 g sugars

Fudge
90 calories, 2 g fat
16 g sugars

Reese's Peanut Butter Cup (1 piece)
90 calories, 5 g fat
8 g sugars

Kit Kat Candy Bar
110 calories, 5 g fat
10 g sugars

Cookie Dough
180 calories, 8 g fat
26 g sugars

Peanuts
210 calories, 18 g fat
0 g sugars

Other Passes

Hot for Cookie Warm Dessert
730 calories
38 g fat
(23 g saturated, 0.5 g trans)
67 g sugars

Oreo Crème Ice Cream (Like It size)
440 calories
31 g fat
(14 g saturated, 0.5 g trans)
38 g sugars

Oh Fudge! Shake (Like It size)
820 calories
47 g fat
(32 g saturated, 1 g trans)
89 g sugars

COSÌ

Although it's one of the best chains to cozy up to, some of Così's best fare is available only during certain seasons. The year-round items are relatively light, especially in sodium, compared with the industry status quo, but the majority could stand to shed a couple hundred calories. This includes a handful of sandwiches and salads; all of the melts, omelet sandwiches, muffins, and scones; and especially the flatbread pizzas, which average 737 calories per serving.

SURVIVAL STRATEGY

Everything on Così's Lighter Side menu is below the 550-calorie mark, making it your best bet for a low-calorie lunch or dinner. As for breakfast, oatmeal, parfaits, and wraps are all sound starts to your day.

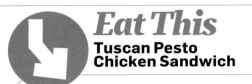

Eat This
Tuscan Pesto Chicken Sandwich

503 calories
13.5 g fat (4.5 g saturated)
967 mg sodium

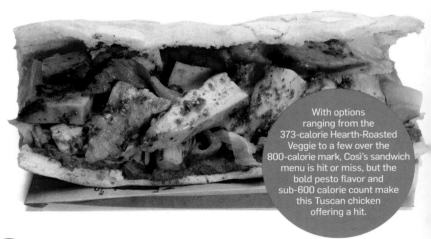

With options ranging from the 373-calorie Hearth-Roasted Veggie to a few over the 800-calorie mark, Cosi's sandwich menu is hit or miss, but the bold pesto flavor and sub-600 calorie count make this Tuscan chicken offering a hit.

Other Picks

Turkey Avocado Sandwich

447 calories
14 g fat
(1 g saturated)
422 mg sodium

Santa Fe Breakfast Wrap

471 calories
28 g fat
(12 g saturated)
1,053 mg sodium

Chai Tea Latte

220 calories
5 g fat
(3 g saturated)
34 g sugars

882 calories
32 g fat (16 g saturated)
1,086 mg sodium

Not That!
Chicken Margherita
Flatbread Pizza (individual)

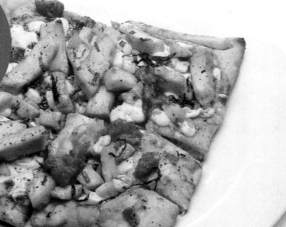

An average pizza at Così contains 737 calories, a good chunk of which is owed to the heavy load of refined carbohydrates in the flatbread crust. All those empty calories leave your stomach feeling empty and your gut looking full. Satisfy your pizza cravings elsewhere.

ALL THIS
- **Regular Oatmeal**
- **Fruit Cup**

and

- **Cranberry Scone**

OR THAT!
- **Asiago Cheese Squagel with Cream Cheese**

582 calories

CHICKEN SALAD
STACKUP

Shanghai Chicken Salad
295 calories
11 g fat

Smart Fit Salad
381 calories
15 g fat

Adobo Lime Chicken Salad
450 calories
19 g fat

Grilled Chicken Caesar Salad
564 calories
36 g fat

Così Cobb Salad
703 calories
53 g fat

Other Passes

Hot Chocolate
422 calories
13 g fat
(8 g saturated)
57 g sugars

T.B.M. Squagel Sandwich
627 calories
26 g fat
(13 g saturated)
751 mg sodium

Grilled Chicken Caesar Salad
564 calories
37 g fat
(7.5 g saturated)
1,575 mg sodium

DAIRY QUEEN

By offering a few decent sandwiches, a Mini Blizzard, and reasonable-size 300-calorie sundaes, DQ has inched their way into C territory. Still, a wide array of bad burgers, bulging chicken baskets, and blindingly sweet concoctions leave plenty of room for error. Here's a look at one hypothetical meal: a Mushroom Swiss Burger with regular onion rings and a small Snickers Blizzard—a hefty 1,530 calories.

SURVIVAL STRATEGY

Your best offense is a solid defense: Skip elaborate burgers, fried sides, and specialty ice cream concoctions. Order a Grilled Chicken Sandwich or an Original Cheeseburger, and if you must have a treat, stick to a soft-serve cone or a small sundae.

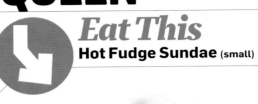

Eat This

Hot Fudge Sundae (small)

300 calories
10 g fat (8 g saturated)
36 g sugars

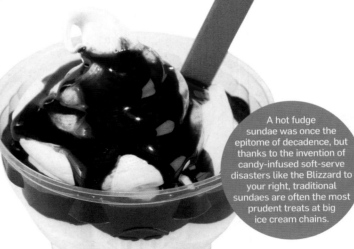

A hot fudge sundae was once the epitome of decadence, but thanks to the invention of candy-infused soft-serve disasters like the Blizzard to your right, traditional sundaes are often the most prudent treats at big ice cream chains.

Other Picks

Original Cheeseburger

380 calories
19 g fat
(8 g saturated)
930 mg sodium

Grilled Chicken Sandwich

360 calories
16 g fat
(2.5 g saturated)
1,040 mg sodium

DQ Sandwich

190 calories
5 g fat
(3 g saturated)
18 g sugars

660 calories
34 g fat (13 g saturated, 0.5 g trans)
61 g sugars

Not That!
Georgia Mud Fudge Blizzard (small)

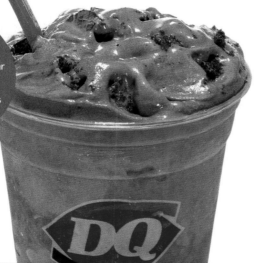

Same fudgy flavor with more than triple the fat and roughly double the sugar and calories. Blizzard, McFlurry, 31° Below—whatever you call it, it's not worth the caloric investment.

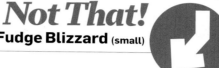

1,250
CALORIE BOMB
Chicken Strip Basket
(6 strips) with Country Gravy

65 g fat
(10 g saturated,
0.5 g trans)
3,210 mg sodium

This bird basket houses more calories than a Bacon Cheese Grill Burger with a large order of fries. Here's some quick math: Fried chicken + a pile of greasy fries + a cup of creamy gravy + 2 slices of butter-drenched toast = one of the worst chicken meals in America.

Guilty Pleasure

Corn Dog with Fries
(regular)

620 calories
30 g fat (5.5 g saturated)
1,180 mg sodium

A battered and deep-fried hot dog doesn't exactly scream "healthy," but compared with DQ's 1,200-calorie basket meals, this corn-dog-and-fry combo is surprisingly sensible.

Other Passes

Buster Bar
460 calories
28 g fat
(16 g saturated)
36 g sugars

Iron Grilled Turkey Sandwich
550 calories
23 g fat
(7 g saturated)
1,510 mg sodium

¼ Pound GrillBurger
with Cheese
520 calories
28 g fat
(11 g saturated, 1 g trans)
1,100 mg sodium

DENNY'S

At least Denny's deserves kudos for giving its calorically overleveraged breakfasts descriptive names that alert us to their dangers. The Lumberjack Slam will hit you with the force of 1,000 calories, and while the Peanut Butter Cup Pancake Breakfast may boast 1,500 calories, at least no one can claim they didn't see that one coming. Fortunately, Denny's offers a small Fit Fare menu with calorie counts under 600.

SURVIVAL STRATEGY

There are two ways to hack the Denny's calorie system. One is to build your own, and choose lean proteins, fruits, and vegetables, like the Grand Slam at the right. The other is to fake your ID and order off the 55+ Menu, as Senior versions tend to have about 15 percent fewer calories.

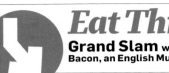

Eat This

Grand Slam with 2 Eggs, 2 Strips of Turkey Bacon, an English Muffin, and Seasonal Fruit

510 calories
26 g fat
(6 g saturated)
822 mg sodium

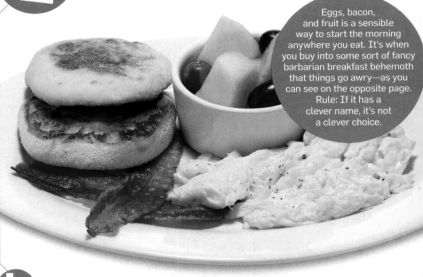

Eggs, bacon, and fruit is a sensible way to start the morning anywhere you eat. It's when you buy into some sort of fancy barbarian breakfast behemoth that things go awry—as you can see on the opposite page. Rule: If it has a clever name, it's not a clever choice.

Other Picks

Fit Fare Sirloin Steak
590 calories
12 g fat
(5 g saturated, 0.5 trans)
1,370 mg sodium

Pancake Puppies
(6 pieces)
490 calories
8 g fat
(2 g saturated)
1,020 mg sodium

Veggie Skillet
340 calories
11 g fat
(2 g saturated)
1,360 mg sodium

154

Not That!
The Grand Slamwich
with Hash Browns

1,340 calories
89 g fat
(28 g saturated, 1 g trans)
3,390 mg sodium

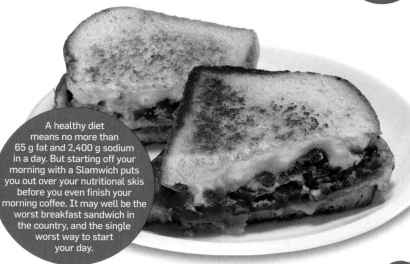

A healthy diet means no more than 65 g fat and 2,400 g sodium in a day. But starting off your morning with a Slamwich puts you out over your nutritional skis before you even finish your morning coffee. It may well be the worst breakfast sandwich in the country, and the single worst way to start your day.

STARCH STACKUP

Hash Browns
210 calories
2 g fiber

Grits with Margarine
220 calories
3 g fiber

Oatmeal
(with milk and brown sugar)
240 calories
3 g fiber

Toast with Margarine (2 slices)
270 calories
1 g fiber

Buttermilk Pancakes (2)
340 calories
2 g fiber

Other Passes

Ultimate Skillet
740 calories
56 g fat
(17 g saturated)
1,470 mg sodium

Zesty Nachos
1,320 calories
65 g fat
(34 g saturatedå)
2,260 mg sodium

Prime Rib Philly Melt (without sides)
670 calories
34 g fat
(13 g saturated)
2,010 mg sodium

DOMINO'S

Domino's has been busy these past few years, first successfully rolling out bolder sauce and better-seasoned dough, then adding the new Artisan line of pizzas, which, along with the Crunchy Thin Crust pizzas, provide some of the lightest slices in America. But there is still plenty of trouble afoot at the pizza juggernaut—namely, a line of high-calorie specialty pies and breadsticks and Domino's appalling line of pasta bread bowls and oven-baked sandwiches.

SURVIVAL STRATEGY

The more loaded a pie is at Domino's, the fewer calories it tends to pack. That's because more vegetables and lean meats mean less space for cheese. It doesn't hold true for greasy meats, so choose wisely.

Eat This

Brooklyn Style Crust Grilled Chicken and Jalapeño Pepper Pizza
(2 slices, large pie)

540 calories
22 g fat (10 g saturated)
1,700 mg sodium

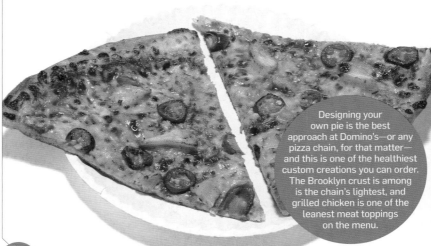

Designing your own pie is the best approach at Domino's—or any pizza chain, for that matter—and this is one of the healthiest custom creations you can order. The Brooklyn crust is among is the chain's lightest, and grilled chicken is one of the leanest meat toppings on the menu.

Other Picks

Hand Tossed Crust Chorizo and Bacon Pizza (2 slices, large pie)

620 calories
24 g fat (10 g saturated)
1,530 mg sodium

Crunchy Thin Crust Sliced Sausage, Onions, and Green Peppers Pizza (2 slices, large pie)

480 calories
26 g fat (9 g saturated)
890 mg sodium

Fire Chicken Wings (4)

200 calories
13 g fat (3.5 g saturated)
1,350 mg sodium

700 calories
34 g fat (17 g saturated)
1,760 mg sodium

Not That!
Hand Tossed Crust Buffalo Chicken American Legends Pizza
(2 slices, large pie)

This is why specialty pizzas fail our nutrition test. You have essentially the same flavor as the pizza on the left, but superfluous additions like multiple cheeses and a whey-infused crust translate to nearly 160 additional calories and 12 extra grams of fat. The novelty's just not worth it.

Grade
B

Chicken Carbonara Breadbowl Pasta
1,480 calories
57 g fat (24 g saturated)
2,220 mg sodium

Domino's already doubled down on carbs with this bready pasta vessel, but by brushing it with an oil blend, the chain adds 44 supernatural ingredients like "disodium inosinate" and "lipolyzed butter oil" to the mix. Consider this a science experiment gone horribly wrong.

ALL THIS
- 9 pieces Boneless Chicken
- 1 slice medium Crunchy Thin Crust Ham Pineapple Pizza

and
- 1 Garden Fresh Salad with Light Italian dressing

OR THAT!
- Italian Sausage and Peppers Sandwich

860 calories

Other Passes

Stuffed Cheesy Bread (4)
555 calories
22 g fat
(12 g saturated, 1 g trans)
960 mg sodium

Italian Sausage Marinara Breadbowl Pasta
1,470 calories
53 g fat
(20 g saturated)
2,770 mg sodium

Hand Tossed Crust MeatZZa Feast Pizza (2 slices, large pie)
760 calories
38 g fat (16 g saturated)
2,060 mg sodium

157

DUNKIN' DONUTS

The doughnut king cast out the trans fats in 2007, and it's been pushing the menu toward healthier options ever since—including the DDSmart Menu, which emphasizes the menu's nutritional champions. With a line of low-fat and protein-packed flatbread sandwiches, there's no excuse to settle for bagels, muffins, doughnuts, and oversweetened coffee drinks, which are as bad as ever.

SURVIVAL STRATEGY

Use the DDSmart Menu as a starting point, or stick to the sandwiches served on flatbread or English muffins. Beware: Beverages like Coolattas and souped-up coffee drinks can do even more damage than the food here, so keep your joe as plain as possible.

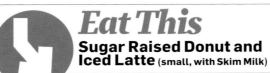

Eat This

Sugar Raised Donut and Iced Latte (small, with Skim Milk)

300 calories
14 g fat
(6 g saturated)
14 g sugars

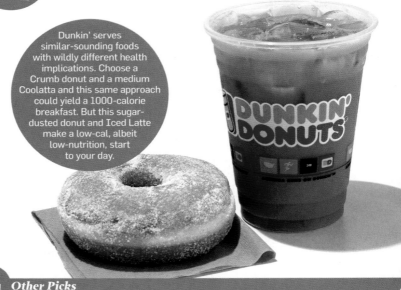

Dunkin' serves similar-sounding foods with wildly different health implications. Choose a Crumb donut and a medium Coolatta and this same approach could yield a 1000-calorie breakfast. But this sugar-dusted donut and Iced Latte make a low-cal, albeit low-nutrition, start to your day.

Other Picks

Apple 'n Spice Donut

270 calories
14 g fat
(6 g saturated)
8 g sugars

Caramel Mocha Iced Coffee
with Cream (medium)

260 calories
9 g fat
(6 g saturated)
36 g sugars

Oatmeal Raisin Cookie

160 calories
5 g fat
(2.5 g saturated)
19 g sugars

500 calories
19.5 g fat
(10 g saturated, 0.5 g trans)
880 mg sodium

Not That!
Sesame Seed Bagel
with Plain Cream Cheese

Another reminder of why bagels are shaped like zeroes: They offer no real nutritional value whatsoever. Even if you went for reduced-fat cream cheese, you'd still be consuming 150 calories more than the donut-latte combo to the left.

Iced Coffee DECODER

Regular Iced Coffees
10 to 250 calories, up to 35 grams of sugars

Regular Iced Latte
70 to 240 calories, up to 20 grams of sugars

Flavored Iced Coffees
110 to 350 calories, up to 48 grams of sugars

Flavored Iced Lattes
170 to 450 calories, up to 68 grams of sugars

MUNCHKIN MOSHPIT

Cinnamon Cake
60 calories
3 g sugars

Glazed Chocolate Cake
70 calories
4 g sugars

Glazed Cake
70 calories
4 g sugars

Jelly Filled
80 calories
2 g sugars

Other Passes

Chocolate Chip Muffin
550 calories
21 g fat
(6 g saturated)
50 g sugars

Coffee Coolatta with Cream (medium)
600 calories
35 g fat
(22 g saturated, 1 g trans)
65 g sugars

Apple Crumb Donut
490 calories
18 g fat
(9 g saturated)
49 g sugars

159

FIVE GUYS

Without much more than burgers, hot dogs, and french fries on the menu, it's difficult to find anything nutritionally redeeming about Five Guys. The only option geared toward health-conscious consumers is the Veggie Sandwich. The burgers range from 480 to 920 calories, so how you order can make a big difference to your waistline. Keep your burgers small, choose your topping wisely, and skip the fries.

SURVIVAL STRATEGY

The regular hamburger is actually a double, so order a Little Hamburger and load up on the vegetation. Or skip the patty entirely and play around with the huge variety of toppings—it's not hard to create a solid sandwich.

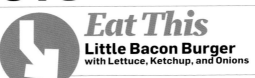

Eat This

Little Bacon Burger
with Lettuce, Ketchup, and Onions

594 calories
33 g fat
(14.5 g saturated)
805 mg sodium

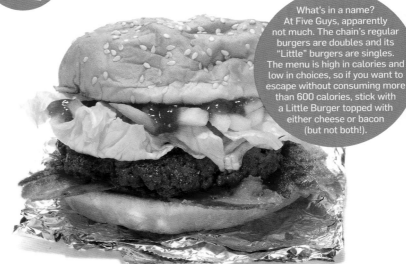

What's in a name? At Five Guys, apparently not much. The chain's regular burgers are doubles and its "Little" burgers are singles. The menu is high in calories and low in choices, so if you want to escape without consuming more than 600 calories, stick with a Little Burger topped with either cheese or bacon (but not both!).

 Other Picks

Hot Dog
545 calories
35 g fat
(15.5 g saturated)
1,130 mg sodium

Little Cheeseburger
550 calories
32 g fat
(15 g saturated)
690 mg sodium

Veggie Sandwich
440 calories
15 g fat
(6 g saturated)
1,040 mg sodium

160

953 calories
41 g fat
(7 g saturated)
962 mg sodium

Not That!
Five Guys Style Fries (regular)

MEET YOUR MATCH

Five Guys Style Fries (large) | 29 Wendy's Chicken Nuggets

1,474 calories

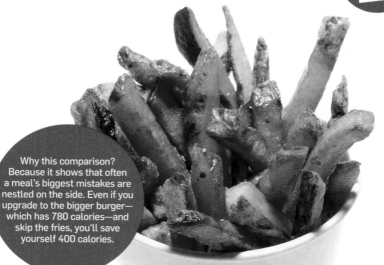

Why this comparison? Because it shows that often a meal's biggest mistakes are nestled on the side. Even if you upgrade to the bigger burger—which has 780 calories—and skip the fries, you'll save yourself 400 calories.

ALL THIS
• Cheese
• Onions
• Grilled Mushrooms
and
• A.1. Steak Sauce

OR THAT!
• Mayonnaise
100 calories

Other Passes

Grilled Cheese
470 calories
26 g fat
(9 g saturated)
715 mg sodium

Cheese Dog
615 calories
41 g fat
(19 g saturated)
1,440 mg sodium

Hamburger
700 calories
43 g fat
(19.5 g saturated)
430 mg sodium

250K
Number of possible burger combinations you could order at Five Guys

161

FRIENDLY'S

For the health-conscious eater, there's nothing particularly friendly about this joint. Breakfast is a sordid affair of fat and refined carbs with few options under 1,000 calories, while lunch and dinner are headlined by a roster of hypercaloric sandwiches, salads, and chicken dishes. Friendly's does offer an Under 565 Calories menu, but still, the best thing we can say about Friendly's is it has good sides.

SURVIVAL STRATEGY

Take advantage of Friendly's massive menu by honing in on the few relatively safe zones. For breakfast, that means eggs à la carte with a side of bacon or ham. For lunch and dinner, try the Make Your Own burger, or combine a cup of soup with a small salad or a few sides.

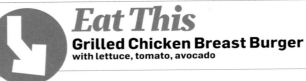

Eat This
Grilled Chicken Breast Burger
with lettuce, tomato, avocado

570 calories
13 g fat
(7 g saturated)
1,450 mg sodium

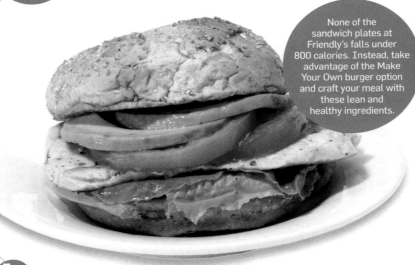

None of the sandwich plates at Friendly's falls under 800 calories. Instead, take advantage of the Make Your Own burger option and craft your meal with these lean and healthy ingredients.

Other Picks

Chicken Soup (crock)

120 calories
3 g fat
(1 g saturated)
270 mg sodium

Grilled Salmon
(with Onion, Potatoes, Peppers)

540 calories
26 g fat
(4 g saturated)
1,190 mg sodium

Strawberry Shortcake Sundae

580 calories
27 g fat
(16 g saturated)
190 mg sodium

1,250 calories
69 g fat
(16 g saturated)
2,250 mg sodium

Not That!
Citrus Grilled
Chicken Sandwich

1,550
CALORIE BOMB
**Honey BBQ
Chicken
SuperMelt
Sandwich**

81 g fat
(24 g saturated)
2,840 mg sodium
37 g sugars

This sandwich attacks
your body from all
angles: three-quarters
of a day's calories, more
than a day's worth of
saturated fat and sodium,
and as much sugar as
you'd find in 123 Honey
Teddy Grahams. If you
want any chance of melt-
ing fat, stay away from
the SuperMelt menu.

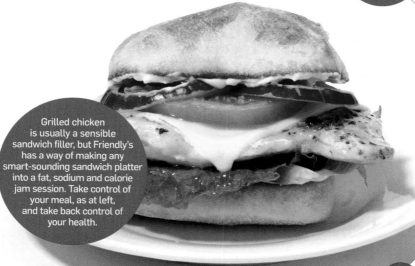

Grilled chicken
is usually a sensible
sandwich filler, but Friendly's
has a way of making any
smart-sounding sandwich platter
into a fat, sodium and calorie
jam session. Take control of
your meal, as at left,
and take back control of
your health.

Other Passes

Chocolate
Fribble Shake

810 calories
34 g fat
(20 g saturated)
330 mg sodium

Grilled Chicken
Salad (with Honey
Mustard Dressing)

830 calories
54 g fat
(13 g saturated)
1,650 mg sodium

Homestyle Clam
Chowder (crock)

470 calories
31 g fat
(17 g saturated)
1,790 mg sodium

PROTEIN
STACKUP

**Grilled Chicken
Breast**
160 calories
5 g fat (1 g saturated)

**Boca Burger
Patty**
180 calories
7 g fat (2 g saturated)

**Fresh Choice
Burger**
250 calories
17 g fat (7 g saturated)

HARDEE'S

Hardee's earns its reputation as one of the most perilous fast-food chains by continuing to sire one crazily caloric burger after the next (and by failing to offer many impressive breakfast options). A recent line of lean turkey burgers has, sadly, been rolled back to just one, leaving diners with fewer options to squash their hunger without breaking the caloric bank.

SURVIVAL STRATEGY

The Sunrise Croissant and the Frisco Breakfast Sandwich are two of your best options in the early hours. For lunch, look to the roast beef, the Big Hot Ham 'N' Cheese, or the Charbroiled BBQ Chicken Sandwich. The Original Turkey Burger is a safe, 390-calorie go-to, or else take the bull by the horns and customize your own burger, as we've done on these pages.

164

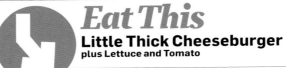

Eat This

Little Thick Cheeseburger
plus Lettuce and Tomato

440 calories
23 g fat
(9 g saturated)
1,150 mg sodium

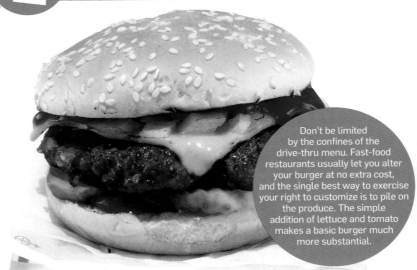

Don't be limited by the confines of the drive-thru menu. Fast-food restaurants usually let you alter your burger at no extra cost, and the single best way to exercise your right to customize is to pile on the produce. The simple addition of lettuce and tomato makes a basic burger much more substantial.

Other Picks

Charbroiled BBQ Chicken Sandwich

330 calories
6 g fat
(0 g saturated)
1,160 mg sodium

Hand Breaded Chicken Tenders
(3 pieces)

260 calories
13 g fat
(2.5 g saturated)
770 mg sodium

Ham, Egg & Cheese Biscuit

450 calories
24 g fat
(8 g saturated)
1,440 mg sodium

580 calories
39 g fat
(12 g saturated)
1,190 mg sodium

Not That!
¼ lb. Little Thickburger

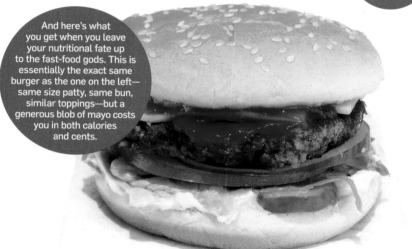

And here's what you get when you leave your nutritional fate up to the fast-food gods. This is essentially the exact same burger as the one on the left—same size patty, same bun, similar toppings—but a generous blob of mayo costs you in both calories and cents.

HEALTH-FOOD FRAUD

Low Carb Breakfast Bowl

660 calories
52 g fat
(20 g saturated)
1,550 mg sodium

Sure, it's low-carb, but it's nearly a day's worth of fat. This meal is like putting the entire barn-yard—chickens, cows and pigs—onto one heart-stopping combination of eggs, ham, two types of sausage, bacon, and a triple dose of cheese.

Guilty Pleasure

Jumbo Chili Dog

370 calories
25 g fat
(8 g saturated)
1,210 mg sodium

Ironically, the Jumbo Chili Dog is one of the smallest threats at Hardee's. With 15 grams of protein and fewer calories than all but the smallest burger, you could do a lot worse than this spicy dog.

Other Passes

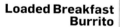

Loaded Breakfast Burrito

580 calories
30 g fat
(12 g saturated)
1,320 mg sodium

Natural-Cut French Fries
(medium)

490 calories
24 g fat
(4.5 g saturated)
970 mg sodium

Charbroiled Chicken Club Sandwich

540 calories
31 g fat
(8 g saturated)
1,510 mg sodium

IHOP

IHOP was one of the last chains to release its nutritional numbers, and given the national-debt-level calorie counts on much of its menu, we see why. Factor in the new line of bacon burgers and the absolute worst breakfast menu in America and it's hard to find much to like about IHOP. The best thing we can say is that lunch and dinner aren't nearly as calamitous as breakfast.

SURVIVAL STRATEGY

IHOP's full name includes the word "cake," and it seems to take that seriously, piling on the carbs at every turn. You'll have a hard time finding a regular breakfast with fewer than 700 calories and a lunch or dinner with fewer than 1,000 calories. Your only safe bet is to stick to the Simple & Fit menu, where you'll find a small selection of healthier items.

166

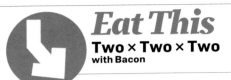

Eat This
Two × Two × Two
with Bacon

680 calories
39 g fat
(13 g saturated, 0.5 g trans)
1,790 mg sodium

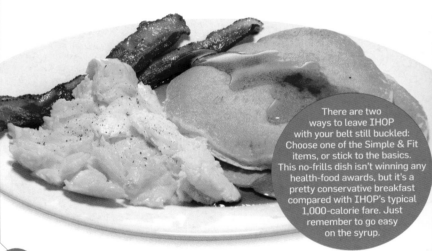

There are two ways to leave IHOP with your belt still buckled: Choose one of the Simple & Fit items, or stick to the basics. This no-frills dish isn't winning any health-food awards, but it's a pretty conservative breakfast compared with IHOP's typical 1,000-calorie fare. Just remember to go easy on the syrup.

Other Picks

Honey-Lime Chicken Salad

410 calories
21 g fat (4 g saturated)
1,160 mg sodium

Simple & Fit Blueberry Harvest Grain 'N Nut Combo

500 calories
24 g fat (4 g saturated)
1,250 mg sodium

Double BLT

690 calories
48 g fat (12 g saturated)
2,139 mg sodium

910 calories
58 g fat
(19 g saturated, 0.5 g trans)
1,420 mg sodium

Not That!
Quick Two-Egg Breakfast
with Bacon

53

The number of
breakfast entrées
with more than
1,000 calories

Sounds innocuous
enough, yet it packs nearly
a third more calories and fat
of the Two × Two × Two.
The principal difference between
this plate and the breakfast on the
opposite page is the double dose
of starch. It's never a good idea to
double up on empty carbs,
especially when one of them
comes in the form of oil-
drenched potatoes.

4 FLAPJACKS STACKUP

Original Buttermilk
624 calories
17 g sugars

Double Blueberry
690 calories
37 g sugars

Chocolate Chip
730 calorie
32 g sugars

Strawberry Banana
760 calories
41 g sugars

Harvest Grain 'N Nut
740 calories
34 g sugars

CINN-A-STACK
900 calories
61 g sugars

New York Cheesecake
1,100 calories
53 g sugars

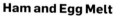

Other Passes

Ham and Egg Melt
1,190 calories
75 g fat
(37 g saturated, 1.5 g trans)
2,800 mg sodium

Whole Wheat Pancake w/Bananas and Sausage
990 calories
60 g fat
(17 g saturated, 0.5 g trans)
1,780 mg sodium

Crispy Chicken Cobb Salad w/ Grilled Chicken
1,130 calories
89 g fat
(27 g saturated, 1.5 g trans)
2,880 mg sodium

IN-N-OUT BURGER

In-N-Out has the most pared-down menu in America. Wander in to the West Coast powerhouse and you'll find nothing more than burgers, fries, shakes, and sodas. While that's certainly nothing to build a healthy diet on, In-N-Out earns points for offering plenty of calorie-saving menu tweaks, like the Protein-Style Burger, which replaces the bun with lettuce and saves you 150 calories.

SURVIVAL STRATEGY

A single cheeseburger and a glass of iced tea or H20 make for a reasonable lunch, while the formidable Double-Double is an option for an occasional splurge (especially if you use a few of the calorie-lowering secret menu options). Or ask them to customize a grilled cheese off the "secret" menu.

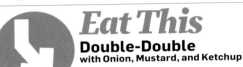

Eat This

Double-Double
with Onion, Mustard, and Ketchup

590 calories
32 g fat
(17 g saturated, 0.5 g trans)
1,520 mg sodium

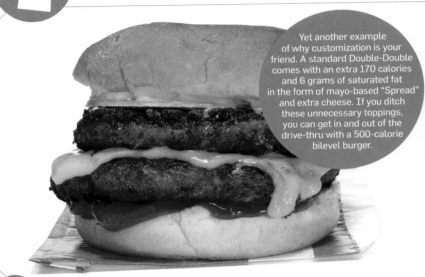

Yet another example of why customization is your friend. A standard Double-Double comes with an extra 170 calories and 6 grams of saturated fat in the form of mayo-based "Spread" and extra cheese. If you ditch these unnecessary toppings, you can get in and out of the drive-thru with a 500-calorie bilevel burger.

Other Picks

Cheeseburger Protein Style

330 calories
25 g fat
(9 g saturated)
720 mg sodium

Grilled Cheese

470 calories
28 g fat
(12 g saturated)
1,260 mg sodium

Minute Maid Light Lemonade (16 fl oz)

8 calories
0 g fat
0 g sugars

875 calories
45 g fat
(15 g saturated, 0.5 g trans)
1,245 mg sodium

Not That!
Cheeseburger
with Onions and French Fries

Menu Magic

Customizing is key in the fast-food world. If you swap Spread for mustard and ketchup, you'll save 80 calories and an impressive 9 grams of fat. Your calorie savings if you opt for a sans-bun Protein Style burger? 150.

We're not sure why fries became the gold standard of fast-food sides. The deep-fried potato sticks account for nearly half of this meal's calories, and what do they bring to the plate? Nothing but empty carbs and fat. For 375 fewer calories, you'll be fuller for longer if you opt for the bigger burger on the left.

Guilty Pleasure

Grilled Cheese

470 calories
28 g fat (12 g saturated)
1,260 mg sodium

You won't find Grilled Cheese on the menu, but it's a custom order worth knowing about, as it's one of the lightest things you can order. If you order it without Spread, you can bring it down to 390 calories. Not bad for a cheesy comfort food.

Other Passes

7Up (16 fl oz)
200 calories
0 g fat
54 g sugars

Chocolate Shake
590 calories
29 g fat
(19 g saturated, 1 g trans)
320 mg sodium

Cheeseburger
480 calories
27 g fat
(10 g saturated)
1,000 mg sodium

Grade B–

19,490
Number of calories in record-setting 100 × 100 burger ordered in 2004

JACK IN THE BOX

Jack in the Box's menu has come a long way in the past few years, but a few major changes still need to be made: banishing anything in a bowl or burrito, offering six burgers with fewer than than 500 calories, and eliminating all partially hydrogenated oils once and for all. Jack might have taken the harmful oils out of the fryer, but partially hydrogenated oils still can be found all over the ingredients lists, including in the sirloin beef patty seasoning.

SURVIVAL STRATEGY

Keep your burger small, or order a Whole Grain Chicken Fajita Pita with an order of Apple Bites with Caramel on the side. For breakfast, order any Breakfast Jack without sausage. Your safest bet is to not touch the fried foods.

Eat This
Jack's Spicy Chicken

530 calories
20 g fat (3 g saturated)
820 mg sodium

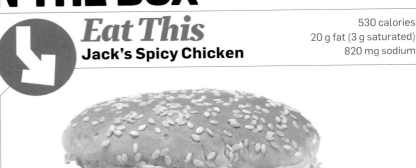

Seems that nearly every major fast-food player needs a spicy chicken sandwich on its menu. Jack's version is surprisingly gentle on the waistline, especially for a place known for producing some of the greasiest grub in the business. Plus, we love that it has fewer than 1,000 milligrams of sodium—a rarity in the realm of fast-food chicken.

Other Picks

Cheeseburger

320 calories
14 g fat
(6 g saturated, 1 g trans)
820 mg sodium

Chicken Fajita Pita

360 calories
13 g fat
(6 g saturated)
1,000 mg sodium

Breakfast Jack
with Bacon

310 calories
14 g fat
(5 g saturated)
790 mg sodium

710 calories
36 g fat (9 g saturated)
1,910 mg sodium

Not That!
Homestyle Ranch Chicken Club

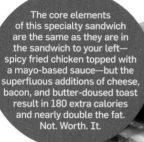

The core elements of this specialty sandwich are the same as they are in the sandwich to your left—spicy fried chicken topped with a mayo-based sauce—but the superfluous additions of cheese, bacon, and butter-doused toast result in 180 extra calories and nearly double the fat. Not. Worth. It.

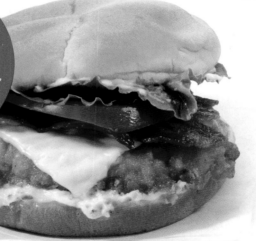

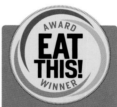

AWARD
EAT THIS!
WINNER

Chicken Fajita Pita
(with salsa)

370 calories
13 g fat
(6 g saturated)
1,120 mg sodium

One of the best entrées in the entire fast-food universe. Low in calories, packed with protein and fiber, this one would be hard to top in your own kitchen.

Other Passes

Meaty Breakfast Burrito
600 calories
36 g fat
(14 g saturated, 0.5 g trans)
1,700 mg sodium

Sourdough Grilled Chicken Club
540 calories
26 g fat
(7 g saturated)
1,490 mg sodium

Sirloin Cheeseburger
930 calories
65 g fat
(21 g saturated, 2.5 g trans)
1,890 mg sodium

JAMBA JUICE

Jamba Juice makes more than a few faux-fruit blends—beverages unnecessarily weighed down with sherbet, sorbet, and other added sugars—but its menu has a ton of real-deal smoothies, as well. Jamba's incredible line of Fruit & Veggie smoothies and its low-calorie food menu are unrivaled by other American chains. But order what's on the opposite page and you could be drinking down the equivalent of more than 24 packets of sugar.

SURVIVAL STRATEGY

For a perfectly guilt-free treat, opt for a Jamba Light or an All Fruit Smoothie in a 16-ounce cup. And unless you're looking to put on weight for your latest movie role, don't touch the Peanut Butter Moo'd or any of the other Creamy Treats.

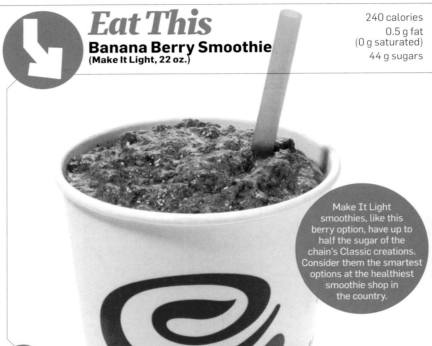

Eat This
Banana Berry Smoothie
(Make It Light, 22 oz.)

240 calories
0.5 g fat
(0 g saturated)
44 g sugars

Make It Light smoothies, like this berry option, have up to half the sugar of the chain's Classic creations. Consider them the smartest options at the healthiest smoothie shop in the country.

Other Picks

Mega Mango Smoothie (16 oz)

230 calories
0 g fat (0 g saturated)
52 g sugars

Blueberry & Blackberry Oatmeal

290 calories
3.5 g fat
(1 g saturated)
25 g sugars

Spinach 'N Cheese Breakfast Wrap

240 calories
8 g fat
(6 g saturated)
1 g sugars

450 calories
1.5 g fat
(0.5 g saturated)
98 g sugars

Not That!
Strawberry Surf Rider
(regular, 22 oz.)

Smoothies have a reputation as a health food, but sugary add-ins turn many frozen-fruit blends into glorified desserts. The fruit in this cup is mixed with sherbet—no wonder it has more sugar than two McDonald's Hot Fudge Sundaes.

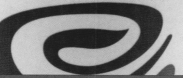

Other Passes

TWISTED DOUGH
TORNADO

Cheddar Tomato Twist
240 calories
3 g sugars

Pesto Twist
290 calories
3 g sugars

Cheesy Pretzel
310 calories
6 g sugars

Apple Cinnamon Pretzel
380 calories
14 g sugars

Sourdough Parmesan Pretzel
410 calories
4 g sugars

STEALTH
HEALTH

Berry UpBEET
(Original size, 22 fl oz)

340 calories
56 g sugars
13 g fiber

True to their name, Jamba's Fruit & Veggie smoothies contain nothing but fruit, fruit juice, and vegetable juice. This berry option packs the most belly-filling fiber, but all four of the flavors are decent—not to mention tasty—ways to meet your veggie quota.

Sweet Belgian Waffle
310 calories
15 g fat
(8 g saturated)
21 g sugars

Coconut Water Pina Colada (medium)
380 calories
8 g fat
(7 g saturated)
68 g sugars

Mango-a-Go-Go Smoothie (16 oz)
300 calories
1.5 g fat
(0 g saturated)
66 g sugars

KFC

Hold on a second! KFC gets a B+? Surprisingly enough, KFC has more than a few things going for it. The menu's crispy bird bits are offset by skinless chicken pieces, low-calorie sandwich options, and a host of sides that come from beyond the fryer. Plus, the fact that KFC has stuck with its grilled chicken line shows that its determined to cast aside the Kentucky fried nutritional demons of their past.

SURVIVAL STRATEGY

Avoid the bowls and pot pies, and choose your chicken wisely: The difference between an Original Recipe breast and an Extra Crispy is 170 calories; order Kentucky Grilled and you'll save another 100 calories. Then adorn your plate with one of the Colonel's healthy sides.

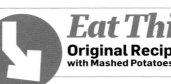

Eat This
Original Recipe Chicken Breast
with Mashed Potatoes and Gravy and Sweet Kernel Corn

540 calories
18.5 g fat (4 g saturated)
1,660 mg sodium

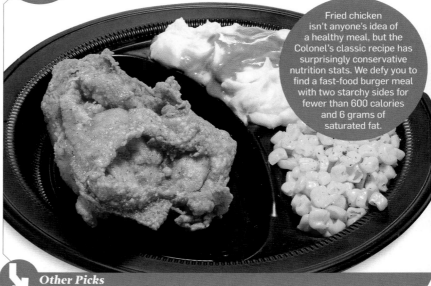

Fried chicken isn't anyone's idea of a healthy meal, but the Colonel's classic recipe has surprisingly conservative nutrition stats. We defy you to find a fast-food burger meal with two starchy sides for fewer than 600 calories and 6 grams of saturated fat.

Other Picks

Doublicious
with Original Recipe Fillet
530 calories
27 g fat
(7 g saturated)
1,390 mg sodium

Hot Wings
Value Box
490 calories
27 g fat
(4.5 g saturated)
1,290 mg sodium

Sweet Life
Chocolate Chip
Cookie
160 calories
8 g fat (3.5 g saturated)
22 g sugars

790 calories
45 g fat (37 g saturated)
1,970 mg sodium

Not That!
Chunky Chicken Pot Pie

Green Beans
25 calories
0 g fat (0 g saturated)

Corn on the Cob (3")
70 calories
0.5 g fat (0 g saturated)

Sweet Kernal Corn
100 calories
5 g fat (0.5 g saturated)

Cole Slaw
170 calories
10 g fat (1.5 g saturated)

This is the single worst option on KFC's menu. Chunky Chicken Pot Pie is stuffed with veggies and never touches the deep fryer, but it remains one of the worst chicken dishes of all time. The main calorie culprit is its buttery shell, but the creamy sauce that binds the filling together certainly doesn't help matters.

CHICKEN STACKUP

Kentucky Grilled Chicken
80 to 220 calories
4 to 10 g fat

Original Recipe
120 to 320 calories
2 to 21 g fat

Extra Crispy
160 to 490 calories
10 to 29 g fat

Spicy Crispy
150 to 520 calories
10 to 34 g fat

Other Passes

Cafe Valley Bakery Mini Chocolate Chip Cake
300 calories
12 g fat
(2.5 g saturated)
35 g sugars

EC Thigh Value Box
660 calories
41 g fat
(7 g saturated)
1,560 mg sodium

Crispy Twister
620 calories
32 g fat
(6 g saturated)
1,260 mg sodium

KRISPY KREME

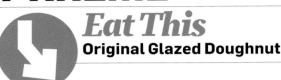

In some parts of the U.S., Krispy Kreme has expanded its food menu beyond doughnuts. The bad news is that most of the new additions are primarily sugar calories—mostly bagels—the same type of nutrient-devoid, carb-heavy fare the bakery has always specialized in. The rule of thumb at Krispy Kreme is to avoid anything that's filled with custard, cream or whatever the berry flavoring is made from. A simple round doughnut is the closest you'll get to a square meal.

SURVIVAL STRATEGY

To stay under 500 calories, keep your doughnuts simple and your coffee drinks even more so. The Kreme's specialty drinks are sweeter than a YouTube puppy video.

Eat This
Original Glazed Doughnut

190 calories
11 g fat (5 g saturated)
10 g sugars

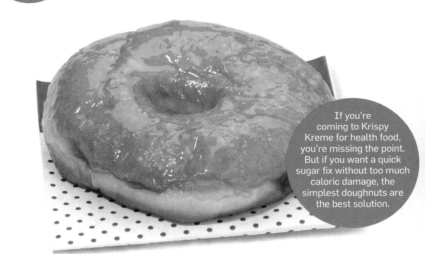

If you're coming to Krispy Kreme for health food, you're missing the point. But if you want a quick sugar fix without too much caloric damage, the simplest doughnuts are the best solution.

Other Picks

Cinnamon Bun Doughnut

222 calories
12 g fat (5 g saturated)
13 g sugars

Deep Chocolate Cone

310 calories
9 g fat (6 g saturated)
33 g sugars

Iced Latte with 2% Milk **(20 fl oz)**

180 calories
7 g fat (4.5 g saturated)
18 g sugars

400 calories
20 g fat (9 g saturated)
28 g sugars

Not That!
Apple Fritter

You came for a doughnut. Have a doughnut. Don't fritter your time away on this meteorite-shaped lump of sugar and fat.

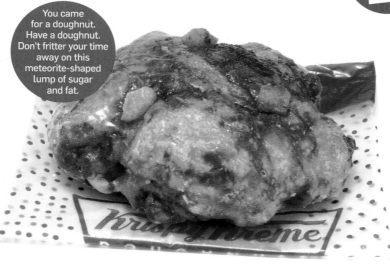

Krispy Kreme

MEET YOUR MATCH

Hazelnut Iced Coffee (20 fl oz)	14 Sugar Dough-nuts
126 g sugars	

Donut DECODER

Doughnut Holes (4 holes)
190 to 210 calories
as much as 11 g fat

Original or Sugar
200 calories
12 g fat

Cinnamon
210 to 290 calories
as much as 16 g fat

Cake
230 to 290 calories
as much as 14 g fat

Iced (but not filled)
240 to 280 calories
as much as 14 g fat

Filled
290 to 350 calories
as much as 20 g fat

Other Passes

Vanilla Iced Coffee (20 fl oz)
540 calories
2.5 g fat (1.5 g saturated)
125 g sugars

Chocolate Kool Kreme Shake
750 calories
24 g fat
(16 g saturated, 0.5 g trans)
90 g sugars

Classic Cinnamon Roll
670 calories
38 g fat
(18 g saturated, 1 g trans)
41 g sugars

LONG JOHN SILVER'S

For years, we've been battling LJS to remove all of the trans fats from its deep fryers. And then, quietly, it did—and we're happy to say it's safe to go back there again. While fried foods—even fish —are high in omega-6 fatty acids, instead of the omega-3s you really want, there are more than enough grilled or baked options to choose from. But Long John still seems to be hiding something: Go to their website and, incredibly enough, the "nutrition information" link has been crossed out. WTF, LJS?

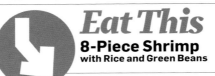

Eat This
8-Piece Shrimp
with Rice and Green Beans

267 calories
1 g fat (1 g saturated)
1,075 mg sodium

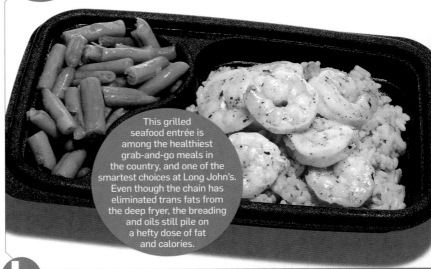

This grilled seafood entrée is among the healthiest grab-and-go meals in the country, and one of the smartest choices at Long John's. Even though the chain has eliminated trans fats from the deep fryer, the breading and oils still pile on a hefty dose of fat and calories.

SURVIVAL STRATEGY

Avoid tortillas at all costs. Avoid breading if possible. Then pair your selection with a cocktail or sweet and sour sauce and some of Long John's healthy side dishes.

Other Picks

Baked Cod
(2 pieces, with Corn on the Cob, No Butter, and Rice)
590 calories
5 g fat
(2 g saturated)
1,250 mg sodium

Seafood Salad
310 calories
23 g fat
(5 g saturated)
760 mg sodium

Crab Cakes (1)
with Green Beans and Rice
489 calories
16 g fat
(7 g saturated)
1,712 mg sodium

980 calories
70 g fat (24 g saturated)
2,020 mg sodium

Not That!
Fish Tacos (2)

Fat in the breading, fat in the tortillas, fat in the sauce—and none of it the healthy kind. It all adds up to a full day's worth of the stuff, plus nearly a full day's allotment of salt. While Long John has come a long way in recent years, there are still plenty of fried entrées that could sink your battleship.

DIPPIN SAUCE STACKUP

Cocktail Sauce
(1 oz)
25 calories
0 g fat

Tartar Sauce
(1 oz)
40 calories
4 g fat (1 g saturated)

Sweet & Sour Sauce
(1 dipping cup)
45 calories
0 g fat

Honey Mustard Sauce (1 dipping cup)
100 calories
6 g fat (2 g saturated)

Ranch Sauce
(1 dipping cup)
160 calories
17 g fat
(3 g saturated)

SIDESWIPED

Crumblies

150 calories
13 g fat
(5 g saturated)
360 mg sodium

Crumblies are simply deep-fried bits of batter, and while they may not have the most overwhelming calorie counts, they are 100 percent nutrition free.

Other Passes

Chicken Tacos (2)
1,060 calories
66 g fat
(22 g saturated)
2,400 mg sodium

Fish Sandwich
550 calories
30 g fat
(10 g saturated)
1,300 mg sodium

Breaded Clam Strips Snack Box
320 calories
19 g fat
(4.5 g saturated, 7 g trans)
1,190 mg sodium

McDONALD'S

The world-famous burger baron has come a long way since the publication of *Fast Food Nation*—at least nutritionally speaking. The trans fats are gone from its oils, the number of calorie bombs has been reduced, and there are more healthy options, such as salads and yogurt parfaits, than ever. Still, too many of the breakfast and lunch items still top the 500-calorie mark, and the dessert menu is a total mess.

SURVIVAL STRATEGY

At breakfast, look no further than the Egg McMuffin—it remains one of the best ways to start your day in the fast-food world. Grilled chicken and Snack Wraps make for a sound lunch. Splurge on a Big Mac or Quarter Pounder, but only if you skip the fries and soda.

Eat This
Premium Grilled Chicken Ranch BLT Sandwich

450 calories
15 g fat
(4.5 g saturated)
1,230 mg sodium

The beauty of a grilled chicken breast: Its super-low calorie count leaves room for splurge-worthy toppings like bacon and ranch dressing. Just be sure to stay away from the Crispy version of this sandwich. The price you pay for going fried over grilled at Mickey D's is an extra 160 calories and 13 grams of fat.

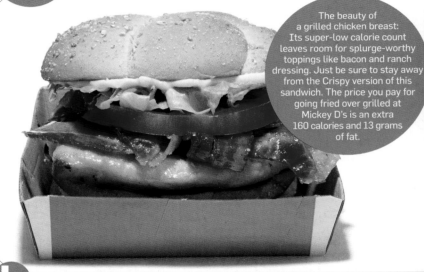

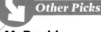
Other Picks

McDouble

380 calories
17 g fat
(8 g saturated, 1 g trans)
840 mg sodium

Chicken McNuggets
(6) with Tangy Barbecue Sauce

330 calories
18 g fat (3 g saturated)
800 mg sodium

Bacon, Egg & Cheese McGriddles

460 calories
21 g fat (9 g saturated)
1,250 mg sodium

610 calories
28 g fat
(6 g saturated)
1,400 mg sodium

Not That!
Premium Crispy Chicken Ranch BLT Sandwich

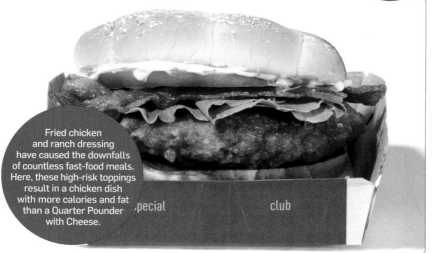

Fried chicken and ranch dressing have caused the downfalls of countless fast-food meals. Here, these high-risk toppings result in a chicken dish with more calories and fat than a Quarter Pounder with Cheese.

special   *club*

Other Passes

Bacon, Egg & Cheese Bagel
620 calories
31 g fat
(11 g saturated, 0.5 g trans)
1,480 mg sodium

Southwest Crispy McWrap
670 calories
33 g fat
(8 g saturated, 0.5 g trans)
1,480 mg sodium

Cheeseburger (2)
580 calories
22 g fat
(10 g saturated, 1 g trans)
1,360 mg sodium

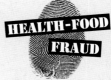

HEALTH-FOOD FRAUD

Mango Pineapple Smoothie (small)

210 calories
0.5 g fat
40 mg sodium
46 g sugar

Even a small version of Ronald's smoothie has more sugar than a Hot Caramel Sundae. Smoothies tend to be health food imposters at most major chains, and at Mickey D's it's no different.

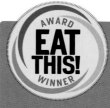

AWARD EAT THIS! WINNER

Egg McMuffin

300 calories
13 g fat (5 g saturated)
750 mg sodium

Few on-the-go breakfasts offer a better balance of protein, carbs and fat than McDonald's legendary breakfast sandwich.

OLIVE GARDEN

Olive Garden is in desperate need of a menu makeover. The chicken and beef entrées are saddled with huge calorie and fat counts, the seafood is swimming in sodium, and the average dinner-size plate of pasta packs a staggering 976 calories. All of this is before you tack on the breadsticks and salad. Olive Garden cooks need to learn to lay off the oil and the salt, then maybe we'll bump them up to a C.

SURVIVAL STRATEGY

Most pasta dishes are burdened with at least a day's worth of sodium and more than 1,000 calories, but the Lighter Italian Fare menu goes easier on your waistline. As for chicken and seafood, stick with the Herb-Grilled Salmon or Parmesan-Crusted Tilapia. And lay off the breadsticks!

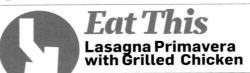

Eat This
Lasagna Primavera with Grilled Chicken

560 calories
29 g fat (7 g saturated)
1,700 mg sodium

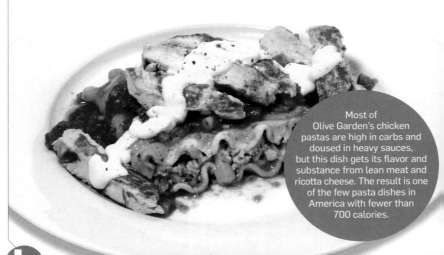

Most of Olive Garden's chicken pastas are high in carbs and doused in heavy sauces, but this dish gets its flavor and substance from lean meat and ricotta cheese. The result is one of the few pasta dishes in America with fewer than 700 calories.

Other Picks

Caprese Flatbread
600 calories
34 g fat
(10 g saturated)
1,430 mg sodium

Baked Tilapia
with Shrimp
360 calories
12 g fat
(6 g saturated)
980 mg sodium

Chicken Meatballs
260 calories
9 g fat
(3 g saturated)
910 mg sodium

1,310 calories
76 g fat (20 g saturated)
1,850 mg sodium

Not That!
Chicken Scampi

Other than the choice of noodles, what's the difference between this plate and the lasagna? The simple addition of garlic cream sauce gives it almost double the calories and nearly three times the saturated fat.

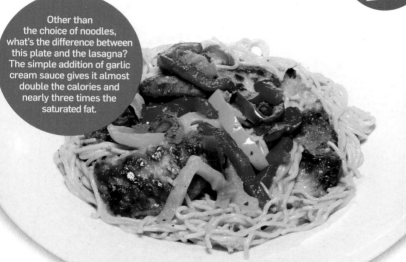

TEST TUBE FOODS

Lasagna Fritta
1,070 calories
71 g fat
(29 g saturated, 1.5 g trans)
1,650 mg sodium

Olive Garden's battered, deep-fried lasagna invention will set you back a day's worth of saturated fat. Just because you can deep-fry something doesn't mean you should.

SOUP STACKUP

Minestrone
110 calories
1.5 g fat (0 g saturated)
840 mg sodium

Pasta e Fagioli
180 calories
6 g fat (0 g saturated)
840 mg sodium

Zuppa Toscana
220 calories
15 g fat (0 g saturated)
840 mg sodium

Chicken & Gnocchi
250 calories
14 g fat (5 g saturated)
1,400 mg sodium

Other Passes

Artichoke Fritti
650 calories
31 g fat
(15 g saturated)
1,430 mg sodium

Seafood Alfredo
1,210 calories
71 g fat
(42 g saturated, 1.5 g trans)
3,200 mg sodium

Grilled Chicken Flatbread
760 calories
44 g fat
(15 g saturated)
1,500 mg sodium

ON THE BORDER

On the Border continues to make tweaks to its menu, but those tweaks only reinforce what we already know about this place: that its Tex-Mex fare is some of the fattiest, saltiest food in the chain restaurant world. The massive menu suffers from appetizers with 134 grams of fat, salads with a full day's worth of sodium, and fish taco entrées with up to 1,950 calories. À la carte items offer the only real hope here.

SURVIVAL STRATEGY

The Border Smart Menu highlights just three items with fewer than 600 calories and 25 grams of fat each (and an average of 1,490 milligrams of sodium). Create your own combo plate with two individual items, but be sure to pass on the sides.

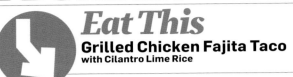

Eat This
Grilled Chicken Fajita Taco
with Cilantro Lime Rice

500 calories
10.5 g fat
(5 g saturated)
1,560 mg sodium

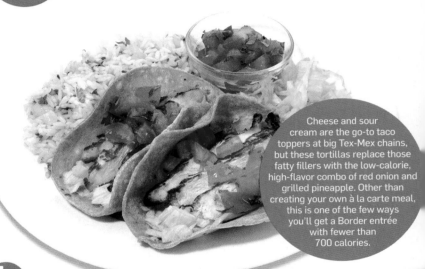

Cheese and sour cream are the go-to taco toppers at big Tex-Mex chains, but these tortillas replace those fatty fillers with the low-calorie, high-flavor combo of red onion and grilled pineapple. Other than creating your own à la carte meal, this is one of the few ways you'll get a Border entrée with fewer than 700 calories.

Other Picks

Chicken Salsa Fresca

450 calories
6 g fat
(5 g saturated)
1,830 mg sodium

Seasoned Ground Beef Enchiladas (2)
with Chile con Carne

500 calories
28 g fat
(12 g saturated)
1,220 mg sodium

Flan

420 calories
17 g fat
(15 g saturated)
210 mg sodium

1,160 calories
44.5 g fat
(14 g saturated)
2,340 mg sodium

Not That!
Street-Style Mini Chicken Tacos
with Rice

There are far worse taco options at On the Border—like the 1,950-calorie Dos XX Fish Tacos—but for a few basic chicken tacos accompanied by avocado slices and pico de gallo, this plate's calorie count is unacceptable and far from "mini."

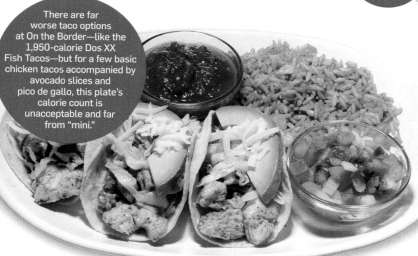

SMART SIDES

Pico de Gallo
10 calories
1 g fat (0 g saturated)
130 mg sodium

Guacamole
45 calories
4 g fat (0 g saturated)
90 mg sodium

Grilled Vegetables
50 calories
0 g fat (0 g saturated)
25 mg sodium

Black Beans
170 calories
1.5 g fat (0 g saturated)
500 mg sodium

ALL THIS
- 1 Chicken Soft Taco
- 2 Ground Beef Tostadas
- 1 order of Chicken Flautas with Chile con Queso
- 1 cup of Chicken Tortilla Soup
- 2 Flan

and

- a side of Guacamole

OR **THAT!**
- Border Sampler

2,060 calories

Other Passes

Kahlua Ice Cream Pie
820 calories
39 g fat
(19 g saturated)
490 mg sodium

Ground Beef Empanadas (2)
with Original Queso
1,240 calories
92 g fat
(32 g saturated)
1,740 mg sodium

Dos XX Fish Tacos
1,670 calories
114 g fat
(23 g saturated)
2,990 mg sodium

OUTBACK STEAKHOUSE

Outback has made some respectable strides in recent years, lightening up existing fare (the Alice Springs Chicken Quesadilla shrank from 2,140 calories down to 1,554) and offering a range of items under 500 calories. Many of the steaks now fall below 800 calories, and more than half of the side dishes come in under 350 calories.

SURVIVAL STRATEGY

Curb your desire to order the Porterhouse (1,009 calories). Start with a small Seared Ahi Tuna (331 calories), then have the decadent-sounding Sirloin and Grilled Shrimp (494 calories). If you skip the bread and house salad (590 calories) and choose steamed veggies as your side, you can escape for less than 1,000 calories.

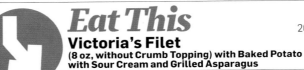

Eat This

Victoria's Filet
(8 oz, without Crumb Topping) with Baked Potato with Sour Cream and Grilled Asparagus

620 calories
20 g fat (8 g saturated)
1,200 mg sodium

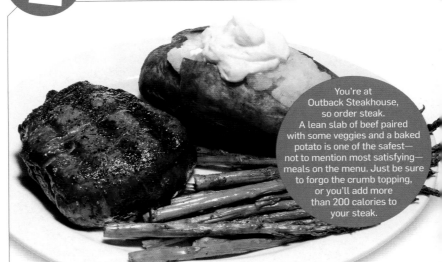

You're at Outback Steakhouse, so order steak. A lean slab of beef paired with some veggies and a baked potato is one of the safest—not to mention most satisfying—meals on the menu. Just be sure to forgo the crumb topping, or you'll add more than 200 calories to your steak.

Other Picks

Sweet Glazed Pork Tenderloin with Baked Potato with Sour Cream and Fresh Steamed French Green Beans

625 calories
15 g fat (7 g saturated)
1,672 mg sodium

Simply Grilled Mahi (8 oz) with Rice Garnish and Steamed Veggies

475 calories
7 g fat (3 g saturated)
1,178 mg sodium

Asian Sesame Salad with Seared Ahi and Sesame Vinaigrette

490 calories
37.8 g fat (4.3 g saturated)
1,243 mg sodium

1,235 calories
72 g fat (33 g saturated)
2,007 mg sodium

Not That!
The Outback Burger
with American Cheese and Sweet Potato Fries

Burgers can be a sensible, protein-packed meal, but sit-down chains squash their nutritional potential by serving them up in jumbo portions alongside heaping piles of fried potatoes. All of the burger-and-fry combos at Outback pack more than 1,000 calories.

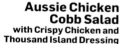

MEET YOUR MATCH

Wings with Mild Sauce	16 KFC Original Recipe Chicken Drumsticks
1,919 calories	

Other Passes

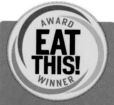

AWARD
EAT THIS!
WINNER

Grilled Shrimp on the Barbie

312 calories
19.7 g fat (4.6 g saturated)
587 mg sodium

On too many chain menus, the word "appetizer" is nothing but a formality—1,000-calorie nachos and plates of french fries smothered in cheese and bacon are hardly a way to warm up the appetite. A true appetizer should be light on fat and low in calories so you're not stuffed when your entrée arrives. This shrimp plate delivers.

Aussie Chicken Cobb Salad
with Crispy Chicken and Thousand Island Dressing

1,296 calories
100 g fat (31 g saturated)
2,023 mg sodium

Hearts of Gold Mahi
with Fresh Seasonal Mixed Veggies

694 calories
29 g fat (17 g saturated)
1,624 mg sodium

Baby Back Ribs
(½ order) with Garlic Mashed Potatoes

986 calories
60 g fat (24 g saturated)
1,953 mg sodium

PANDA EXPRESS

Oddly enough, it's not the wok-fried meat or the viscous sauces that do the most harm on this menu—it's the more than 400 calories of rice and noodles that form the foundation of each meal. Scrape these starches from the plate, and Panda Express starts to look a lot healthier. Only one entrée item has more than 500 calories, and there's hardly a trans fat on the menu. Problems arise when multiple entrées and sides start piling up on one plate, though, so bring some self-restraint to the table.

SURVIVAL STRATEGY

Avoid these entrées: Orange Chicken, Sweet & Sour Chicken, Beijing Beef, and anything with pork. Then swap in Mixed Veggies for the scoop of rice.

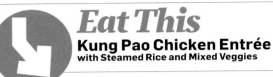

Eat This
Kung Pao Chicken Entrée
with Steamed Rice and Mixed Veggies

690 calories
18.5 g fat
(3 g saturated)
1,450 mg sodium

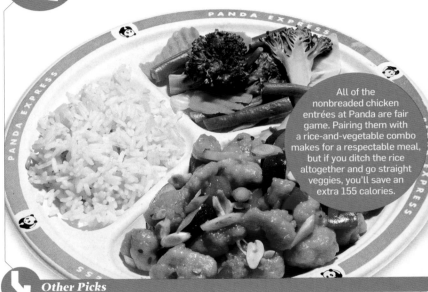

All of the nonbreaded chicken entrées at Panda are fair game. Pairing them with a rice-and-vegetable combo makes for a respectable meal, but if you ditch the rice altogether and go straight veggies, you'll save an extra 155 calories.

Other Picks

Golden Treasure Shrimp

230 calories
10 g fat
(1.5 g saturated)
250 mg sodium

Chicken Pot Stickers (3)

220 calories
6 g fat
(1.5 g saturated)
250 mg sodium

Fortune Cookies (3)

96 calories
0 g fat
9 g sugars

910 calories
40 g fat
(7.5 g saturated)
1,600 mg sodium

Not That!
Orange Chicken Entrée
with Chow Mein

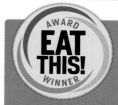

Grade

C+

Broccoli Beef

120 calories
9 g fat (1.5 g saturated)
660 mg sodium

The lowest-calorie entrée on Panda's menu, Broccoli Beef is a standout. Pair an order with an appetizer and you'll have a satisfying meal for a scant amount of calories. PF Chang's version, by comparison, packs 870 calories and more than 4,500 milligrams of sodium.

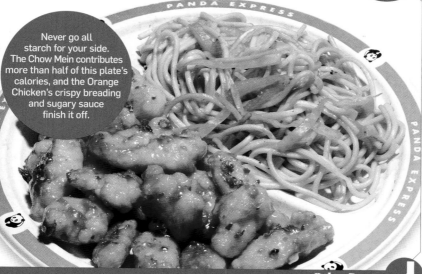

Never go all starch for your side. The Chow Mein contributes more than half of this plate's calories, and the Orange Chicken's crispy breading and sugary sauce finish it off.

Other Passes

Chocolate Chunk Cookie

160 calories
7 g fat
(3 g saturated)
14 g sugars

Chicken Egg Rolls (2)

400 calories
24 g fat
(8 g saturated)
780 mg sodium

Honey Walnut Shrimp

370 calories
23 g fat
(4 g saturated)
470 mg sodium

SIDE STACKUP

Mixed Veggies
70 calories
0.5 g fat

Steamed Rice
380 calories
0 g fat

Fried Rice
470 calories
19 g fat

Chow Mein
490 calories
22 g fat

189

PANERA BREAD

Panera's menu still features a roster of mostly great salads and soups, and between the 340-calorie Power Sandwich and the steel-cut oatmeal, a first-rate breakfast is there for the taking. But only 6 out of 18 sandwiches have 600 calories or fewer, and the bakery puts out little not tainted by refined carbs. Even its "whole-wheat" bread is more than 50 percent white flour. Until we see real progress, this B- is as good as Panera can hope for.

SURVIVAL STRATEGY

For breakfast, choose between the Egg & Cheese breakfast sandwich and 310-calorie granola parfait. Skip the stand-alone sandwich lunch. Instead, pair soup and a salad, or order the soup and half-sandwich combo.

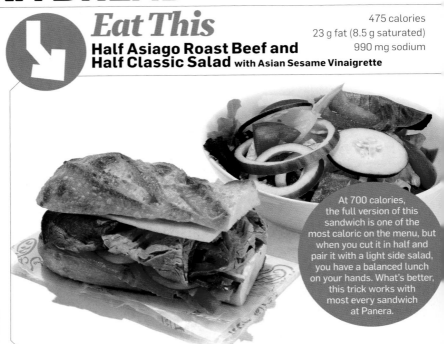

Eat This

Half Asiago Roast Beef and Half Classic Salad with Asian Sesame Vinaigrette

475 calories
23 g fat (8.5 g saturated)
990 mg sodium

At 700 calories, the full version of this sandwich is one of the most caloric on the menu, but when you cut it in half and pair it with a light side salad, you have a balanced lunch on your hands. What's better, this trick works with most every sandwich at Panera.

 Other Picks

Smoked Turkey Breast on Country

430 calories
3.5 g fat (1 g saturated)
1,790 mg sodium

Full Strawberry Poppyseed & Chicken Signature Salad

350 calories
13 g fat (1.5 g saturated)
290 mg sodium

Breakfast Power Sandwich

340 calories
15 g fat (7 g saturated)
710 mg sodium

710 calories
53 g fat (16 g saturated)
1,280 mg sodium

Not That!
Chicken Cobb
with Avocado and Buttermilk Ranch

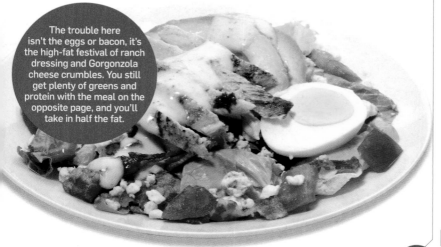

The trouble here isn't the eggs or bacon, it's the high-fat festival of ranch dressing and Gorgonzola cheese crumbles. You still get plenty of greens and protein with the meal on the opposite page, and you'll take in half the fat.

T U B E
T E S T   F O O D S

Sourdough Bread Bowl

590 calories
2.5 g fat (0 g saturated)
1,210 mg sodium

Sure, you could eat your lunch out of a bowl made entirely of bread. You could also eat your breakfast off of a pancake plate, but why would you? Bread bowls are just another wacky invention designed to get your novelty neurons firing, and they offer nothing but empty carbs.

Guilty Pleasure

Pumpkin Muffie

290 calories
11 g fat (2 g saturated)
26 g sugars

Lop off the bottom of a muffin and you get a pretty good treat. A regular pumpkin muffin, for example, has double the calories and sugars as this mini muffin. Plus, the top is the tastiest part.

Other Passes

Asiago Cheese Bagel with Bacon

610 calories
28 g fat
(13 g saturated, 0.5 g trans)
1,350 mg sodium

Full Roasted Turkey Fuji Apple Signature Salad

550 calories
34 g fat (7 g saturated)
620 mg sodium

Sierra Turkey
on Asiago Cheese Focaccia

810 calories
37 g fat
(9 g saturated)
1,950 mg sodium

PAPA JOHN'S

We're glad that Papa John's struck its disastrous pan crust pizza from the menu. But with it also went its whole-wheat crust option. Now, very little separates Papa from the rest of the pizza competition. It still has some high-quality toppings, but they're nothing you can't get elsewhere. What hasn't changed? The breadsticks still deliver far too many calories and the Special Garlic sauce can wreck even the healthiest slice.

SURVIVAL STRATEGY

As with any other pizza place, it's best to start with a thin base, ask for light cheese, and cover it with anything other than sausage, pepperoni, or bacon. The Spinach Alfredo remains the pie to pick at Papa John's.

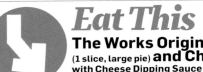

Eat This

400 calories
26 g fat (8.5 g saturated)
1,060 mg sodium

The Works Original Crust Pizza
(1 slice, large pie) **and Chickenstrips** (3)
with Cheese Dipping Sauce

The best defense is a good offense, so start the meal off with a few pieces of belly-filling protein in the form of wings or chicken strips. Consider it insurance against scarfing too many slices later on in the meal.

Other Picks

Spinach Alfredo Original Crust Pizza
(2 slices, medium pie)

400 calories
16 g fat
(7 g saturated)
1,000 mg sodium

Sausage Original Crust Pizza
(2 slices, medium pie)

480 calories
22 g fat
(9 g saturated)
1,200 mg sodium

Honey Chipotle Wings (2)

190 calories
12 g fat
(3 g saturated)
730 mg sodium

715 calories
43 g fat (13.5 g saturated)
1,720 mg sodium

Not That!

Spicy Italian Original Crust Pizza
(1 slice, large pie) and Cheesesticks (2)
with Special Garlic Dipping Sauce

560 CALORIE BOMB
Cinnapie
(4 sticks)

19 g fat (6 g saturated)
39 g sugars

After a dinner of refined carbs, do you really need more of the same? Just four of these cinnamon sticks pretty much guarantee that your delivered dinner will cross the 1,000-calorie mark.

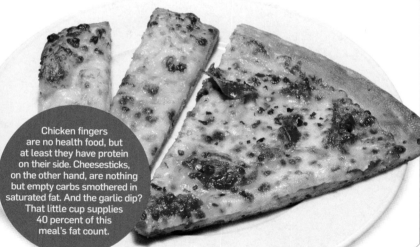

Chicken fingers are no health food, but at least they have protein on their side. Cheesesticks, on the other hand, are nothing but empty carbs smothered in saturated fat. And the garlic dip? That little cup supplies 40 percent of this meal's fat count.

DIPPING SAUCE
(1 cup)
STACKUP

Buffalo Sauce
15 calories
0.5 g fat

Pizza Sauce
20 calories
1 g fat

Cheese Sauce
40 calories
3.5 g fat

Honey Mustard
150 calories
15 g fat

Special Garlic
150 calories
17 g fat

Blue Cheese
160 calories
16 g fat

Other Passes

Parmesan Breadsticks (2)

340 calories

10 g fat
(1.5 g saturated)

720 mg sodium

The Meats Thin Crust Pizza
(2 slices, large pie)

620 calories

38 g fat
(14 g saturated)

1,420 mg sodium

Tuscan Six Cheese Thin Crust Pizza
(2 slices, large pie)

640 calories

26 g fat
(12 g saturated)

1600 mg sodium

193

PERKINS

Of the more than 90 dishes at Perkins, only five qualify for the Calorie Counter menu. Outside of that you'll find entrées with more than 4,000 milligrams of sodium, pasta plates with more than 100 grams of fat, and an all-day omelet menu that averages more than 1,500 calories per order. Currently the chain has stores in 34 states. Hopefully it cleans up its nutritional act before it hits the other 16.

SURVIVAL STRATEGY

Stick with the steak pictured here or choose something off the Calorie Counter menu. Elsewhere on the menu, unexpected calories lurk at every turn. Even the Grilled Salmon with broccoli, a dish that seems impossible to screw up, packs 750 calories.

Eat This

Steak Medallions and Portabella Mushrooms Dinner with broccoli and garlic butter

520 calories
29 g fat (8 g saturated)
1,050 mg sodium

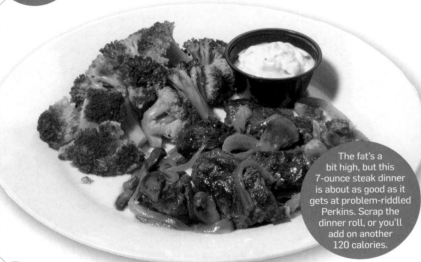

The fat's a bit high, but this 7-ounce steak dinner is about as good as it gets at problem-riddled Perkins. Scrap the dinner roll, or you'll add on another 120 calories.

Other Picks

French Dip Sandwich

610 calories
31 g fat
(9 g saturated)
2,150 mg sodium

Classic Eggs and Bacon with Breakfast Potatoes and Seasonal Fresh Fruit

610 calories
37 g fat
(11.5 g saturated)
1,220 mg sodium

White Chocolate Macadamia Nut Cookie

340 calories
19 g fat
(8 g saturated)
14 g sugars

810 calories
37 g fat (12 g saturated)
2,440 mg sodium

Not That!
Butterball Turkey & Dressing
with Mashed Potatoes with Gravy and Broccoli and Cranberry Sauce

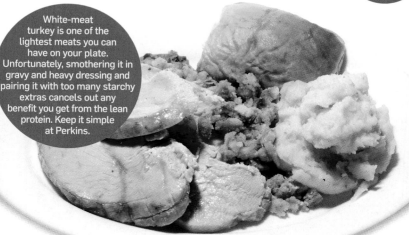

White-meat turkey is one of the lightest meats you can have on your plate. Unfortunately, smothering it in gravy and heavy dressing and pairing it with too many starchy extras cancels out any benefit you get from the lean protein. Keep it simple at Perkins.

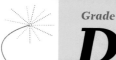

1,390 CALORIE BOMB
Country Sausage Biscuit Platter

90 g fat (46 g saturated)
3,680 mg sodium

Two sausage and cheese biscuits, two eggs, a pile of fried potatoes, a stack of bacon, and a smothering of cream gravy combine to give you a plate with nearly two days' worth of saturated fat and sodium. The scariest part? This isn't the worst breakfast plate on the menu! (That honor goes to their 1,860-calorie Southern Fried Chicken Biscuit Platter.)

Other Passes

Banana Nut Mammoth Muffin
with Whipped Butter Blend

700 calories
40 g fat (9 g saturated)
42 g sugars

Smoked Bacon & Ham Omelette
with Hash Browns and Seasonal Fresh Fruit

1,410 calories
73 g fat (23.5 g saturated)
3,380 mg sodium

Triple Decker Club Sandwich

890 calories
55 g fat (11 g saturated)
2,070 mg sodium

SIDE STACKUP

Sautéed Spinach
70 calories
3.5 g fat

Buttered Corn
150 calories
8 g fat

Mashed Potatoes
150 calories
7 g fat

Baked Potato
with Lite Sour Cream
210 calories
2.5 g fat

195

P.F. CHANG'S

It's now considerably easier to put together a nutritionally respectable meal at P.F. Chang's than it was a few years ago, thanks in part to a solid line of low-calorie salads. But noodle dishes and nearly anything from the grill still come with dangerously high fat and calorie counts, while the entire menu is saltier than a Chris Rock monologue.

SURVIVAL STRATEGY

Order a lean appetizer like an order of dumplings or the Seared Ahi Tuna for the table, and resolve to avoid anything that's prepared breaded. Servings are generous enough that you can even split one of the more reasonable entrées between two people. Earn bonus points by tailoring your dish to be light on the oil and sauce.

Eat This
Shrimp with Lobster Sauce

360 calories
18 g fat (3.5 g saturated)
2,700 mg sodium

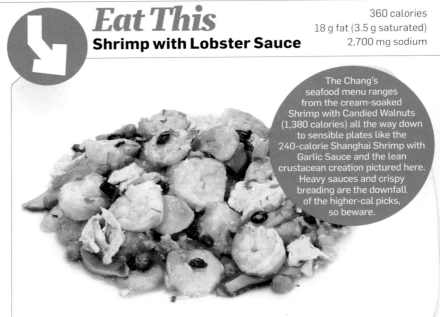

The Chang's seafood menu ranges from the cream-soaked Shrimp with Candied Walnuts (1,380 calories) all the way down to sensible plates like the 240-calorie Shanghai Shrimp with Garlic Sauce and the lean crustacean creation pictured here. Heavy sauces and crispy breading are the downfall of the higher-cal picks, so beware.

Other Picks

Ginger Chicken
with Broccoli

460 calories
10 g fat
(2 g saturated)
2,320 mg sodium

Ahi Tuna with Avocado

320 calories
14 g fat
(2 g saturated)
530 mg sodium

Sweet and Sour Pork

710 calories
25 g fat
(6 g saturated)
1,460 mg sodium

1,000 calories
43 g fat (7 g saturated)
3,460 mg sodium

Not That!
Hunan-Style Hot Fish

Menu Magic

A simple way to shave calories off your Chang's plate: Scratch the rice and get a small order of nutrient-packed vegetables instead. Most any vegetable side will save you more than 100 calories over a side of brown rice. One exception: Don't touch the Spicy Eggplant Side (see below)!

Compared with most fish, the tilapia used in this dish contains very little heart-healthy omega-3 fats. Rolled in deep-fried breading, this not-great protein becomes the star of When Bad Fats Happen to Good People.

SALT LICK

Hot & Sour Soup (bowl)

7,980 mg sodium
380 calories
11 g fat (3 g saturated)

Would you like some soup with your salt? There's more than 5 days' worth of sodium in this simple bowl of broth, making it the single saltiest restaurant food we've ever come across— and it's only a side dish!

Other Passes

Chang's Pork Fried Rice

1,370 calories
41 g fat
(8 g saturated)
2,130 mg sodium

Spicy Eggplant Side

1,010 calories
88 g fat
(13 g saturated)
3,790 mg sodium

Kung Pao Chicken

1,070 calories
64 g fat
(10 g saturated)
2,410 mg sodium

PIZZA HUT

In an attempt to push the menu beyond slices, Pizza Hut expanded into pastas, salads, and something called a P'Zone. Sound like an improvement? Think again. Calzone-like P'Zones all pack more than 1,000 calories each. The salads aren't much better, and the pastas are actually worse. The thin crust and Fit 'N Delicious pizzas offer sub 200-calorie slices and the bone-in wings are a solid start to any meal. Combine those elements and you'll do just fine.

SURVIVAL STRATEGY

This is not the place for pasta. A pan of Chicken Alfredo packs more than 1,000 calories. The key to the Hut lies in the crust: Pan Pizzas cost you 80 more calories per slice over Thin 'N Crispy, and 40 more per slice than the Stuffed Crust.

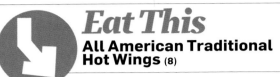

Eat This
All American Traditional Hot Wings (8)

320 calories
20 g fat
(6 g saturated)
1,160 mg sodium

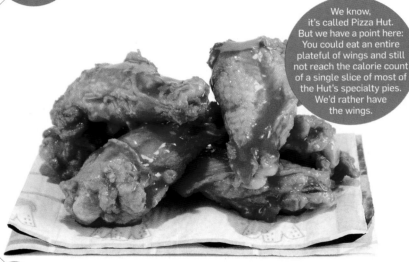

We know, it's called Pizza Hut. But we have a point here: You could eat an entire plateful of wings and still not reach the calorie count of a single slice of most of the Hut's specialty pies. We'd rather have the wings.

Other Picks

Pepperoni Thin 'N Crispy Pizza
(2 slices, medium pie)
420 calories
20 g fat (9 g saturated)
1,400 mg sodium

Chicken Supreme Personal Pan Pizza
590 calories
21 g fat (8 g saturated)
1,370 mg sodium

Lemon Pepper Traditional Wings (2)
150 calories
10 g fat (2 g saturated)
430 mg sodium

470 calories
28 g fat
(10 g saturated)
1,150 mg sodium

Not That!
Meat Lover's Pizza
(1 slice, 14" large pan pizza)

You can love meat without taking in half a day's saturated fat with one slice of pizza. Specialty pizzas are an excuse to go crazy with a ton of high-fat toppings that do virtually nothing for flavor and increase your calorie load considerably. At Pizza Hut, don't be a Lover, be a fighter.

Garlic Parmesan Bone-Out Wings (6)
780 calories
57 g fat (10.5 g saturated)
2,130 mg sodium

Ever seen a chicken without bones? Of course not. Mother Nature put them there for a reason, and it wasn't so multinational food corporations could go removing them for their own twisted purposes. These freakish "bone-out" wings have twice as many calories as Pizza Hut's traditional wings.

Other Passes

Garlic Parmesan Bone-Out Wings (2)
260 calories
19 g fat (3.5 g saturated)
710 mg sodium

Ultimate Cheese Lover's Stuffed Crust Pizza
(2 slices, 14" large pie)
680 calories
30 g fat (16 g saturated)
2,070 mg sodium

Pepperoni P'Zone Pizza with
Marinara Dipping Sauce
980 calories
32 g fat (14 g saturated)
2,340 mg sodium

BREAD STACKUP

Breadstick
140 calories
5 g fat (1 g saturated)
260 mg sodium

Cheese Breadstick
170 calories
6 g fat (2.5 g saturated)
390 mg sodium

Stuffed Pizza Roller
230 calories
10 g fat (4.5 g saturated)
630 mg sodium

POPEYES

For a fried-chicken fix, Popeyes isn't at the front of the line. Its menu features some of the most trans-fat-soaked items in the whole fast-food universe, especially their fish and side dishes. With no grilled chicken options, plus 830-calorie onion rings and 660-calorie cole slaw, we'd like to tell Popeyes patrons to eat their spinach— but there is none!

SURVIVAL STRATEGY

Skip the chicken-and-biscuit combo meals. Popeyes' chicken harbors more fat than the Original Recipe pieces at KFC, and the biscuit adds an extra 260 calories to your plate. Tenders and nuggets are relatively safe, but when it comes time for sides, settle for nothing less than non-fried foods. A large order of fries, for instance, delivers 3.5 grams of trans fatty acids.

Eat This
Loaded Chicken Wrap

310 calories
13 g fat (6 g saturated)
890 mg sodium

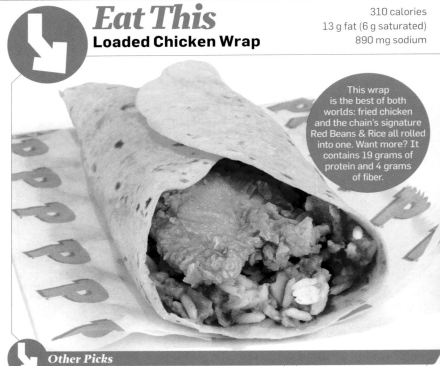

This wrap is the best of both worlds: fried chicken and the chain's signature Red Beans & Rice all rolled into one. Want more? It contains 19 grams of protein and 4 grams of fiber.

Other Picks

Spicy Chicken Leg and Wing

380 calories
24 g fat
(10 g saturated)
770 mg sodium

Louisiana Nuggets (6)

230 calories
14 g fat
(6 g saturated, 1 g trans)
350 mg sodium

Bacon Biscuit

400 calories
25 g fat
(12 g saturated)
780 mg sodium

690 calories
42 g fat (13 g saturated, 1 g trans)
2,165 mg sodium

Not That!
Shrimp Po Boy

Menu Magic

How to put your cardiologist's kids through school: Order the chicken liver sandwich and large fries, and get four days' worth of artery-plugging trans fats! Cha-chinggg!

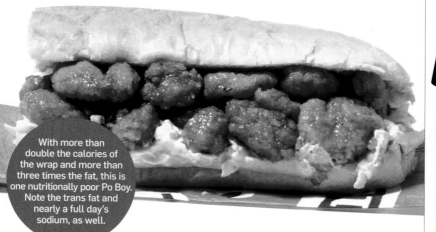

With more than double the calories of the wrap and more than three times the fat, this is one nutritionally poor Po Boy. Note the trans fat and nearly a full day's sodium, as well.

CHICKEN STACKUP

Nuggets (4)
150 calories
9 g fat

Mild Leg
160 calories
9 g fat

Blackened Tenders (3)
170 calories
2 g fat

Mild Wing
210 calories
14 g fat

Mild Thigh
280 calories
21 g fat

Mild Breast
440 calories
27 g fat

Other Passes

Sausage Biscuit
540 calories
36 g fat
(18 g saturated)
1,100 mg sodium

Louisiana Tenders
(mild, 3)
340 calories
14 g fat
(6 g saturated, 1 g trans)
350 mg sodium

Spicy Chicken Breast
420 calories
27 g fat
(9 g saturated, 1 g trans)
830 mg sodium

201

QUIZNOS

Submarine sandwiches can only be so bad, right? We thought so, too, until we saw some of the outrageous offerings on the Quiznos menu. The bigger subs and wraps can easily pack 1,000 calories and a full day's worth of saturated fat, and the oversize salads aren't much better. Sammies used to be the easy way out of trouble at Quiznos, but as their calorie counts continue to climb, options for healthy dining grow ever slimmer.

SURVIVAL STRATEGY

Avoid the salads, large subs, and soups that come in bread bowls. Stick with a small sub (at 360 calories, the Honey Bourbon Chicken is easily the best), or pair a Sammie with a cup of soup.

Eat This
Chicken Bacon Ranch Flatbread (small)

480 calories
24 g fat
(9 g saturated)
1,140 mg sodium

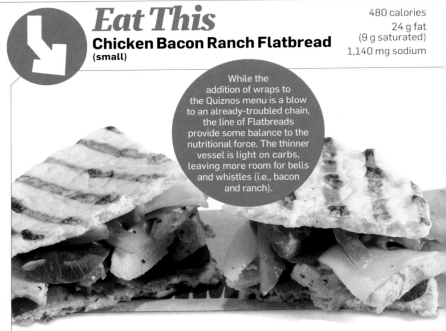

While the addition of wraps to the Quiznos menu is a blow to an already-troubled chain, the line of Flatbreads provide some balance to the nutritional force. The thinner vessel is light on carbs, leaving more room for bells and whistles (i.e., bacon and ranch).

Other Picks

Turkey Ranch & Swiss Sub
on Wheat Bread (small)

470 calories
22 g fat
(7 g saturated)
1,410 mg sodium

Honey Bourbon Chicken Sub (small)

360 calories
6 g fat
(6 g saturated)
1,000 mg sodium

Spicy Monterey Sub (small)

400 calories
13 g fat
(5 g saturated)
1,480 mg sodium

780 calories
35 g fat
(13 g saturated)
1,410 mg sodium

Not That!
Apple Harvest Chicken Wrap
(with Acai Dressing)

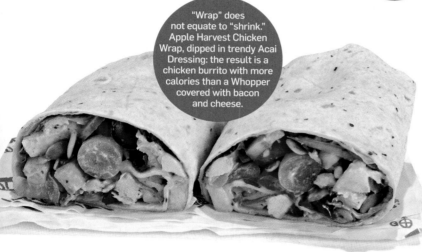

"Wrap" does not equate to "shrink." Apple Harvest Chicken Wrap, dipped in trendy Acai Dressing: the result is a chicken burrito with more calories than a Whopper covered with bacon and cheese.

HEALTH-FOOD FRAUD

Pesto Caesar Sub
(large)

1,070 calories
46 g fat (25 g saturated)
2,690 mg sodium

At first glance this looks like a salad on a roll, and seems healthier than a meat-packed sandwich. But you're saving only 80 calories over the Double Swiss Prime Rib. Creamy dressing and cheese will get you every time.

LOAVES LESSONS

Artisan Wheat
410 calories
4 g fiber

Rosemary Parmesan
410 calories
3 g fiber

Italian White
430 calories
3 g fiber

Garlic Focaccia
480 calories
3 g fiber

Jalapeño Cheddar
500 calories
3 g fat

Other Passes

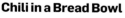

Chili in a Bread Bowl
820 calories
28 g fat
(7 g saturated)
1,910 mg sodium

Mesquite Chicken Sub (small)
550 calories
27 g fat
(13 g saturated)
1,350 mg sodium

Italian Meatball Sub (small)
630 calories
33 g fat
(11 g saturated)
1,450 mg sodium

RED LOBSTER

Compared with the other major sit-down chains, Red Lobster looks like a paradigm of sound nutrition. The new Lighthouse menu features grilled options like the meal pictured here, and the menu is long on low-calorie, high-protein entrées and reasonable vegetable-based sides. That's why Red Lobster is one of America's healthiest chain restaurants. The only flaw you'll find is an overreliance on the deep fryer and the salt shaker.

SURVIVAL STRATEGY

Avoid calorie-heavy Cajun sauces, combo dishes, and anything labeled "crispy." And tell the waiter to keep those biscuits for himself. You'll never go wrong with simple broiled or grilled fish and a vegetable side.

Eat This

Wood-Grilled Fresh Tilapia
with a side of green beans and chilled jumbo shrimp appetizer

515 calories
12.5 g fat (N/A g saturated)
1,750 mg sodium

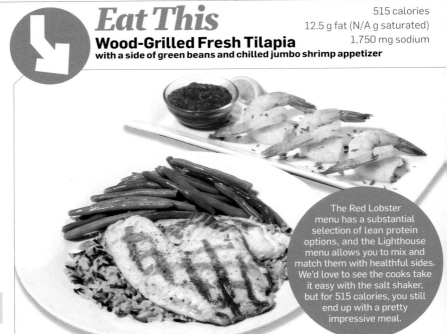

The Red Lobster menu has a substantial selection of lean protein options, and the Lighthouse menu allows you to mix and match them with healthful sides. We'd love to see the cooks take it easy with the salt shaker, but for 515 calories, you still end up with a pretty impressive meal.

Other Picks

Crunchy Popcorn Shrimp

380 calories
18 g fat
(1.5 g saturated)
1,410 mg sodium

Clam Strips

390 calories
24 g fat
(7 g saturated)
2,110 mg sodium

Garden Salad
with Red Wine Vinaigrette (side order)

150 calories
6.5 g fat
(0 g saturated)
580 mg sodium

1,600 calories
90 g fat (37 g saturated)
3,840 mg sodium

Not That!
Crab Linguine Alfredo
(full)

We don't know who Alfredo is, but he must love butter. And salt. With nearly two days' worth of sodium and almost as many calories as an adult woman should eat in a day, this crab dish isn't worth shelling out for.

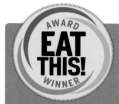

Fresh Fish Menu

Red Lobster may have built its name on crustaceans, but it's the daily rotating selection of fresh fish that represents why this is still the best sit-down chain in America. Try any of the fish (minus the cobia) blackened or grilled with a side of pineapple salsa for an amazing low-cal meal.

ALL THIS

- New England Clam Chowder (bowl)
- Wood-Grilled Tilapia
- Garlic-Grilled Shrimp

and

- Caramel Cheesecake

OR THAT!

- Bar Harbor Lobster Bake

1,530 calories

Other Passes

Caesar Salad
with Caesar Dressing
(side order)

570 calories
57 g fat
(10.5 g saturated)
1,140 mg sodium

Crispy Calamari and Vegetables

1,650 calories
109 g fat
(12 g saturated)
4,170 mg sodium

Parrot Isle Jumbo Coconut Shrimp

880 calories
60 g fat
(15 g saturated)
1,860 mg sodium

ROMANO'S MACARONI GRILL

In 2010, we commended Macaroni Grill's efforts to revamp a pretty miserable menu by cutting calories and adding menu items such as rosemary spiedinis. Shortly thereafter—because no good deed goes unpunished—new ownership swept in to undo most of the progress from before. Lean proteins and prudent pastas have been traded in for the same cheesy, fatty fare it put out so many years ago. It was great while it lasted.

SURVIVAL STRATEGY

The Flatbreads, Pasta, and Classics menus are all serious trouble. Instead, opt for a soup-and-salad combo or a Create Your Own pasta with spaghetti, red sauce, and as many vegetables as you can fit in the bowl. Split a bowl of gelato and call it a day.

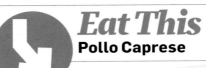

Eat This
Pollo Caprese

560 calories
N/A g fat (11 g saturated)
1,250 mg sodium

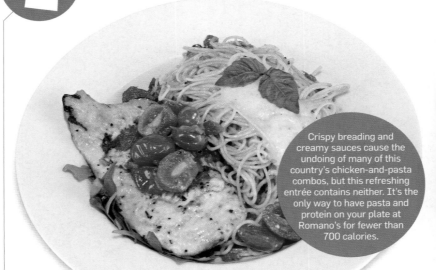

Crispy breading and creamy sauces cause the undoing of many of this country's chicken-and-pasta combos, but this refreshing entrée contains neither. It's the only way to have pasta and protein on your plate at Romano's for fewer than 700 calories.

Other Picks

Lobster Ravioli
600 calories
N/A g fat
(21 g saturated)
1,490 mg sodium

Goat Cheese Peppadew Peppers
350 calories
N/A g fat
(6 g saturated)
710 mg sodium

Tiramisu
600 calories
N/A fat
(24 g saturated)
65 mg sodium

1,590 calories
N/A g fat (31 g saturated)
2,040 mg sodium

Not That!
Chicken Under a Brick

Romano's doesn't make its ingredients public, so we're not sure how roasted chicken and potatoes can bear such a shameful nutritional profile, but knowing it contains more than half a day's calories and nearly a day's worth of sodium is reason enough not to order it.

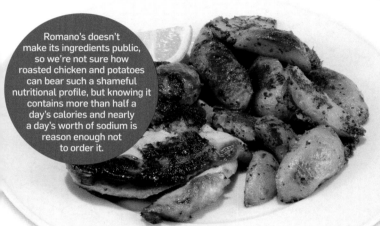

2,040
CALORIE BOMB
Mama's Trio

N/A g fat
(53 g saturated)
4,160 mg sodium

Mama's Trio has the saturated fat content of the Three Tenors. A combination of chicken parmesan, lasagna bolognese, and cannelloni bolognese, it's cheese on meat and meat on cheese, wrapped in a noodle coffin.

SIDESWIPED
Fatbreads!
1,210–1,420 calories

Having embraced its mission of making America's beaches just plain uglier, Romano's recently launched Fatbreads, "the anti-flatbread. Fat on crust. Fat on toppings." Fat on your body. The most industriously caloric of the four is the Farmhouse, which comes with pepperoni, bacon and prosciutto, plus three types of cheese and dipping sauce.

Other Passes

Homemade Chocolate Cake
940 calories
N/A g fat
(29 g saturated)
570 mg sodium

Crispy Fresh Mozzarella
820 calories
N/A g fat
(16 g saturated)
210 mg sodium

Shrimp Portofino
1,120 calories
N/A g fat
(36 g saturated)
1,700 mg sodium

RUBY TUESDAY

The chain built its reputation on a hearty selection of hamburgers. The problem is, the burgers average 75 grams of fat—100 percent of your recommended daily limit. And now that Ruby Tuesday has finally released full sodium counts, it's apparent it's been harboring one of the saltiest menus in America. But with the addition of the Fit & Trim and Petite menus in recent years, Ruby's earns a slight bump up on its report card.

SURVIVAL STRATEGY

Solace lies in the 3 S's: sirloin, salmon, and shrimp all make for relatively innocuous eating, especially when paired with one of Ruby Tuesday's half dozen healthy sides, such as roasted spaghetti squash and fresh green beans.

Eat This

Asiago Peppercorn Sirloin
with garlic cheese biscuit and fresh steamed broccoli

535 calories
23 g fat
1,810 mg sodium

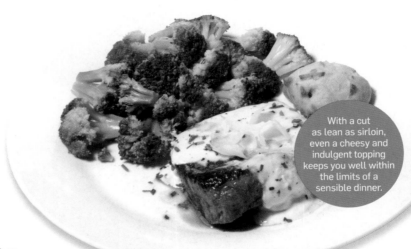

With a cut as lean as sirloin, even a cheesy and indulgent topping keeps you well within the limits of a sensible dinner.

Other Picks

Hickory Bourbon Chicken
250 calories
5 g fat
720 mg sodium

Top Sirloin and Lobster Tail
461 calories
25 g fat
1,337 mg sodium

Fried Mozzarella
(per serving)
135 calories
8 g fat
420 mg sodium

1,254 calories
85 g fat
1,096 mg sodium

Not That!
Ribeye
with baked potato with butter and sour cream

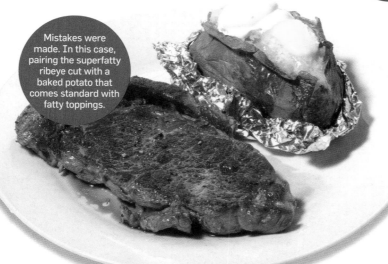

Mistakes were made. In this case, pairing the superfatty ribeye cut with a baked potato that comes standard with fatty toppings.

Avocado Grilled Chicken Sandwich

1,311 calories
64 g fat
2,833 mg sodium

Ruby's makes a habit of corrupting healthy ingredients with fatty toppers and jumbo portions. A sandwich based on lean protein and avocado should be a nutritional no-brainer, but this plate has almost the same calorie count as a Triple Prime Burger.

Other Passes

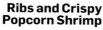

Queso & Chips
(per serving)

288 calories
18 g fat
489 mg sodium

Ribs and Crispy Popcorn Shrimp

1,030 calories
55 g fat
2,335mg sodium

Avocado Turkey Burger

1,381 calories
77 g fat
2,763 mg sodium

SIDE STACKUP

Mashed Potatoes
267 calories
15 g fat

Sweet Potato Fries
330 calories
12 g fat

French Fries
480 calories
24 g fat

Loaded Baked Potato
566 calories
29 g fat

SMOOTHIE KING

Smoothie King, the older and smaller of the two smoothie titans, suffers from portion problems. The smallest adult option is 20 ounces, which makes it that much harder to keep the calories from sugar remotely reasonable. Added sugars and honey don't make things any better. (Isn't fruit sweet enough?) Still, the menu boasts some great all-fruit smoothies, light options, and an excellent portfolio of smoothie enhancers.

SURVIVAL STRATEGY

Stick with the Energy Blends and Slim Blends menus and you'll be okay. And be sure to choose 20-ounce smoothies made from nothing but real fruit. No matter what you do, avoid most anything listed under the Take a Break section —it's pure trouble.

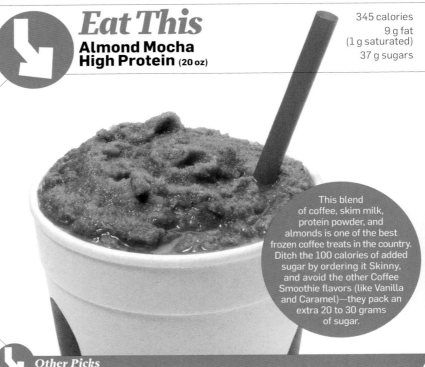

Eat This
Almond Mocha High Protein (20 oz)

345 calories
9 g fat
(1 g saturated)
37 g sugars

This blend of coffee, skim milk, protein powder, and almonds is one of the best frozen coffee treats in the country. Ditch the 100 calories of added sugar by ordering it Skinny, and avoid the other Coffee Smoothie flavors (like Vanilla and Caramel)—they pack an extra 20 to 30 grams of sugar.

Other Picks

Apple Kiwi Kale Smoothie (20 fl oz)

277 calories
0 g fat
62 g sugars

Original High Protein Smoothie, Chocolate (20 fl oz)

366 calories
9 g fat (1 g saturated)
37 g sugars

Blueberry Heaven (20 fl oz)

325 calories
1 g fat (0 g saturated)
64 g sugars

698 calories
26 g fat
(3 g saturated)
63 g sugars

Not That!
Peanut Power Plus, Chocolate (20 oz)

The main difference between these two? The drink on the left lists protein as its first ingredient. The contestant on the right lists sugar before protein.

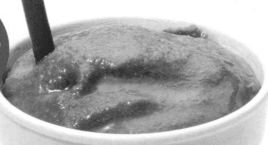

964
Number of calories in a large Hulk Strawberry smoothie

Guilty Pleasure

Yogurt D-Lite Smoothie (20 fl oz)

275 calories
4 g fat (2 g saturated)
34 g sugars

This is the only treat on the Take a Break menu that's worth, well, taking to. It's made with frozen yogurt instead of ice cream, which will save you up to 455 calories and 73 grams of sugar.

Other Passes

Super Punch Plus (20 fl oz)

395 calories
0 g fat
90 g sugars

Chocolate The Hulk Smoothie (20 fl oz)

801 calories
31 g fat (12 g saturated)
90 g sugars

Orange Ka-Bam Smoothie (20 fl oz)

469 calories
0 g fat
108 g sugars

SONIC

In many respects, the fried-and-fatty pitfalls are more dramatic at Sonic than they are at other chains. You have an oversized selection of deep-fried sides, a tempting lineup of frozen sodas, and an expansive catalogue of shakes, malts, and Sonic Blasts. That said, the chain offers most of its indulgences in small portions, making possible a Jr. Burger with Small Tots and Small Slush for 730 calories—a relative bargain considering what you'd suffer elsewhere.

SURVIVAL STRATEGY

Sounds crazy, but corn dogs, 6-inch hot dogs, and Jr. Burgers are your safest options. Just avoid the shakes. Even a 14-ounce cup can stick you with 600 calories.

Eat This
Chicken Strip Sandwich

440 calories
20 g fat (3.5 g saturated)
790 mg sodium

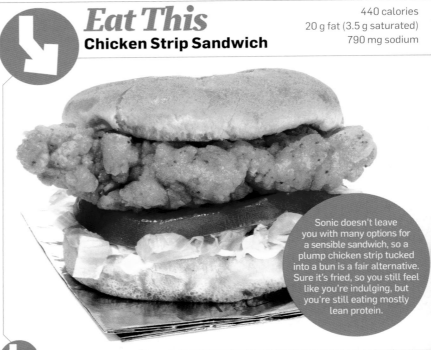

Sonic doesn't leave you with many options for a sensible sandwich, so a plump chicken strip tucked into a bun is a fair alternative. Sure it's fried, so you still feel like you're indulging, but you're still eating mostly lean protein.

Other Picks

Jr. Deluxe Cheeseburger
420 calories
25 g fat
(9 g saturated)
830 mg sodium

Ched 'R' Bites (12)
280 calories
15 g fat
(6 g saturated)
740 mg sodium

Vanilla Cone
250 calories
13 g fat
(9 g saturated)
24 g sugars

690 calories
36 g fat (10 g saturated)
1,540 mg sodium

Not That!
Chicken Club Toaster Sandwich

The dangers here are almost too many to count: thick wedges of Texas toast, melted cheese, mayonnaise, bacon, and a greasy breast of batter-fried chicken. This is one of the worst chicken sandwiches in America.

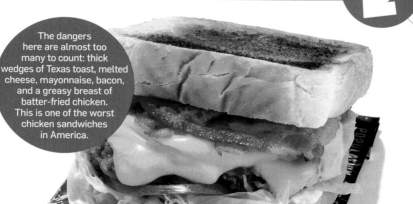

800
CALORIE BOMB
Ultimate Meat & Cheese Breakfast Burrito

56 g fat
(18 g saturated, 1 g trans)
2,030 mg sodium

Anytime a breakfast item has both bacon and sausage, you're asking for trouble. Add eggs, cheese, fried potatoes, and a refined-flour tortilla, and you have one shoddy way to start your day. This is the worst item on Sonic's Breakfast menu.

Guilty Pleasure

Cheese Tots (small)
290 calories
18 g fat (5 g saturated)
890 mg sodium

We never thought the day would come when we'd recommend deep-fried potatoes smothered in cheese, but these cheesy tots have fewer calories than any medium fry order we could find in the country, so we thought they deserved a little recognition.

Other Passes

Vanilla Shake
(small)
540 calories
31 g fat
(23 g saturated)
56 g sugars

Mozzarella Sticks
(5)
440 calories
22 g fat
(9 g saturated, 0.5 g trans)
1,050 mg sodium

Sonic Burger
with Mayonnaise
740 calories
48 g fat
(15 g saturated, 1.5 g trans)
820 mg sodium

STARBUCKS

Once upon a time, Starbucks was a fine place for coffee, but a dangerous place for fancy drinks and food. But recent years have seen the introduction of a solid line of breakfast and lunch sandwiches, wraps, oatmeal, parfaits, and snack plates, making this coffee shop a reliable place to tame a growling stomach on the go. Just ignore the carb-fueled confections. As for the drinks? Unless you keep it simple, they can do some damage.

SURVIVAL STRATEGY

There's no beating a regular cup of joe or unsweetened tea, but if you need a specialty fix, stick with fat-free milk, sugar-free syrup, and no whipped cream. As for food, go with the Perfect Oatmeal or an Egg White, Spinach, and Feta Wrap.

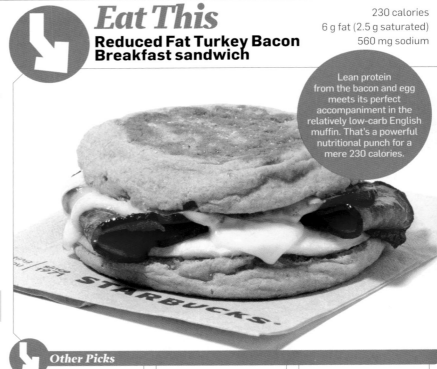

Eat This
Reduced Fat Turkey Bacon Breakfast sandwich

230 calories
6 g fat (2.5 g saturated)
560 mg sodium

Lean protein from the bacon and egg meets its perfect accompaniment in the relatively low-carb English muffin. That's a powerful nutritional punch for a mere 230 calories.

Other Picks

Iced Vanilla Latte
(Grande, 2% milk)

190 calories
4 g fat
(2 g saturated)
28 g sugars

Chicken & Hummus Bistro Box

270 calories
8 g fat
(1 g saturated)
520 mg sodium

Marshmallow Dream Bar

240 calories
5 g fat
(3 g saturated)
23 g sugars

370 calories
20 g fat (4 g saturated)
170 mg sodium

Not That!
Carrot Cake Muffin with Pecans

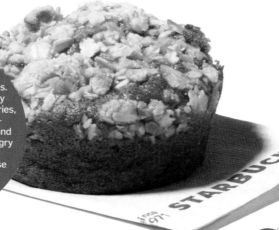

It's time you learned the truth: Muffins are icing-less cupcakes. It doesn't matter what healthy ingredients they boast—blueberries, zucchini, carrots, nuts, bran—they're just flour, eggs, butter, and sugar, and they'll leave you hungry shortly after you eat them. How do we know that? Because this muffin has 20 grams of sugar and not even a full gram of fiber.

Calorie-Cutting Lingo

Hold the whip
Cuts the cream and saves you up to 110 calories

Nonfat
Uses fat-free milk instead of whole or 2%

Sugar-free syrup
Saves up to 150 calories a drink

Skinny
Uses sugar-free syrup and fat-free milk

ESPRESSO DRINK
(Grande, 16 oz)
STACKUP

Espresso
5 calories
0 g sugars

Caffe Americano
15 calories
0 g sugars

Cappuccino
120 calories
10 g sugars

Caffe Latte
190 calories
17 g sugars

Caffe Mocha
260 calories
34 g sugars

Other Passes

Old-Fashioned Glazed Doughnut
480 calories
27 g fat
(13 g saturated)
30 g sugars

Cheese & Fruit Bistro Box
480 calories
28 g fat
(10 g saturated, 0.5 g trans)
470 mg sodium

Iced White Chocolate Mocha
(Grande, 2% Milk, No Whipped Cream)
340 calories
9 g fat
(6 g saturated)
52 g sugars

STEAK 'N SHAKE

For a chain named after two of the most precarious foods on the planet, Steak 'n Shake could be far more dangerous. A single Steakburger with Cheese delivers a modest 330 calories, and not a single salad exceeds 600. Too bad we can't make a similar claim about the shakes. Even the smalls commonly eclipse 600 calories, and at least one—the regular M&M shake—has more sugar than 4 Klondike Bars.

SURVIVAL STRATEGY

Go ahead and order a burger, but keep it simple. If you're feeling extra hungry, add a second steak patty for 110 calories. What you want to avoid are the tricked-out chili dishes. Anything entrée-size will saddle you with 830 to 1,220 calories.

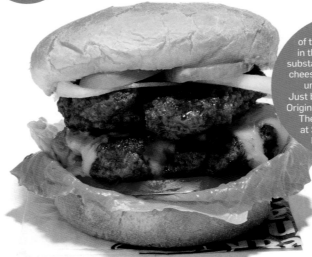

Eat This
Double Steakburger **with Cheese**

440 calories
25 g fat (11 g saturated)
590 mg sodium

This is one of the only drive-thrus in the country where a substantial double-stacked cheeseburger weighs in at under 500 calories. Just be sure to stick to the Original Steakburger menu. The specialty burgers at Steak 'n Shake are less impressive.

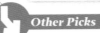

Other Picks

Guacamole Single Steakburger

380 calories
21 g fat
(7 g saturated, 0.5 g trans)
650 mg sodium

Grilled Chicken Salad with Reduced Fat Berry Balsamic Vinaigrette

320 calories
11.5 g fat
(3.5 g saturated)
1,020 mg sodium

Oreo Ice Cream Sandwich

240 calories
10 g fat
(4 g saturated)
19 g sugars

Not That!
Frisco Melt

750 calories
53 g fat (17 g saturated)
1,160 mg sodium

> "Melt" is code for extra cheese and butter-drenched bread, and when you're already dealing with ground beef and cheese, that kind of excess is just plain unnecessary.

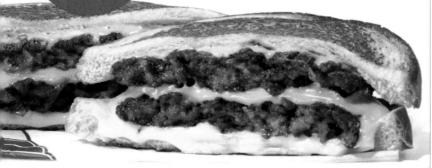

1,220 CALORIE BOMB
Chili Deluxe (bowl)

74 g fat
(39 g saturated,
1.5 g trans)
2,560 mg sodium

At its best, chili is a lean protein- and fiber-packed respite from the fatty offerings on most American menus. But chili is only as lean as the meat that goes into it. Steak 'n Shake must use some ridiculously high-fat beef to produce a cheese-topped chili bowl with the same number of calories and more saturated fat than two (!) Triple Steak-burgers with Cheese.

Other Passes

Cookies 'n Cream Milk Shake (small)

570 calories
18 g fat
(11 g saturated)
74 g sugars

Grilled Chicken Taco Salad
with Ranch Dressing

740 calories
60 g fat
(12.5 g saturated,
0.5 g trans)
2,020 mg sodium

Wisconsin Buttery Steakburger

700 calories
47 g fat
(21 g saturated, 1.5 g trans)
760 mg sodium

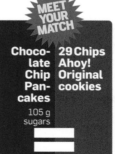

MEET YOUR MATCH

Chocolate Chip Pancakes	29 Chips Ahoy! Original cookies
105 g sugars	

SUBWAY

Subway is the first major fast-food chain to carry avocado (now available at breakfast, too), and all the heart-healthy fats found within, in every one of its 26,688 US stores. And in 2014, the chain removed the creepy plastic dough conditioner azodicarbonamide from its breads, and upped its level of whole grains. If the chain weren't already America's healthiest chain, it certainly is now.

SURVIVAL STRATEGY

Trouble lurks in three areas at Subway: 1) hot subs, 2) footlongs, 3) chips and soda. Stick to 6-inch cold subs made with ham, turkey, roast beef, or chicken. Load up on veggies, and be extra careful about your condiment choices.

Eat This

Steak and Cheese Toasted Sandwich (6") and Veggie Delite Salad with Honey Mustard Dressing

490 calories
12 g fat
(4.5 g saturated)
1,350 mg sodium

Nearly identical sandwiches with one critical difference: The Philly on the opposite page has 120 extra calories and triple the saturated fat. The choice is yours.

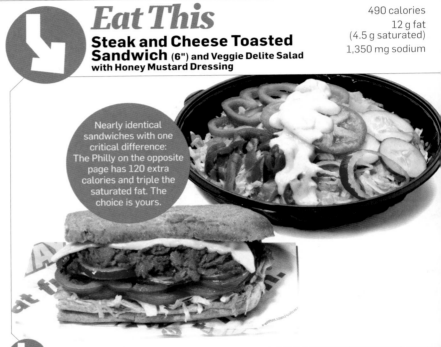

Other Picks

Turkey Breast and Ham (6" with double meat)

280 calories
4 g fat
(1 g saturated)
730 mg sodium

Subway Club with Avocado (6")

370 calories
10 g fat
(2 g saturated)
800 mg sodium

Black Forest Ham, Egg and Cheese Flatbread (2)

400 calories
16 g fat
(5 g saturated)
1,180 mg sodium

770 calories
41 g fat
(12.5 g saturated)
1,760 mg sodium

Not That!
The Big Philly Cheesesteak Toasted Sandwich
(6") and Veggie Delite Salad with Ranch Dressing

Subway does a lot of things better than other sandwich shops, but ranch dressing ain't one of 'em. The salad dressing alone accounts for more than 30 percent of this meal's calories.

12

The number of 6-inch subs with fewer than 350 calories

Other Passes

Sriracha Chicken Melt Salad
(with Ranch Dressing)

880 calories
49 g fat
(10.5 g saturated)
1,470 mg sodium

Chicken & Bacon Ranch Melt

570 calories
28 g fat
(10 g saturated, 0.5 g trans)
1,050 mg sodium

Cold Cut Combo (6")

360 calories
12 g fat
(3.5 g saturated)
1,030 mg sodium

CONDIMENT CATASTROPHE

All Sandwiches

Subway's numbers are good, but the calorie counts don't include condiments. Mayo and ranch will each cost you 110 calories and up to 12 grams of fat. Stick to veggies, mustard, and light mayonnaise.

T.G.I. FRIDAY'S

After much analysis, we've finally figured out the real acronym here: Tremendous-Gut-Inducing Fridays. While Friday's has reintroduced our favorite part of the menu, the small portions option (the Taste & Share menu), it still turns too many healthy-sounding dishes into nutritional nuclear attacks. How does Pan-Seared Flounder break the 1,100-calorie mark? That's more than two Big Macs! But if you're a steak lover who can get along with a healthy side dish, you actually have plenty of options.

SURVIVAL STRATEGY

Danger is waiting in every crack and corner of Friday's menu. Your best bets? The grilled salmon, or perhaps a Black Angus steak (either the Petite Sirloin or the FlatIron).

Eat This
Balsamic-Glazed Chicken Caesar Salad

500 calories
31 g fat
(7 g saturated)
1,340 mg sodium

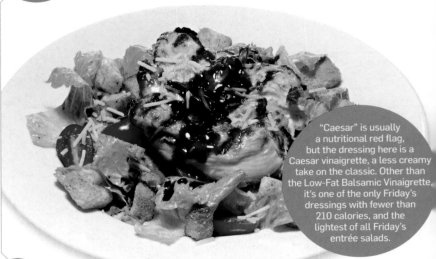

"Caesar" is usually a nutritional red flag, but the dressing here is a Caesar vinaigrette, a less creamy take on the classic. Other than the Low-Fat Balsamic Vinaigrette, it's one of the only Friday's dressings with fewer than 210 calories, and the lightest of all Friday's entrée salads.

 Other Picks

Petite Sirloin with Crispy Shrimp

640 calories
20 g fat (9.5 g saturated)
2,110 mg sodium

Sizzling Chicken and Shrimp

530 calories
14 g fat (3 g saturated)
1,680 mg sodium

Thai Pork Tacos

280 calories
14 g fat (3.5 g saturated)
700 mg sodium

840 calories
60 g fat
(21 g saturated)
1,560 mg sodium

Not That!
Chipotle Yucatan Chicken Salad

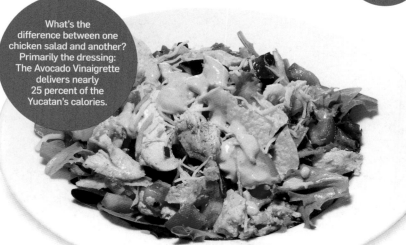

What's the difference between one chicken salad and another? Primarily the dressing: The Avocado Vinaigrette delivers nearly 25 percent of the Yucatan's calories.

STEAK STACKUP

Petite Sirloin
370 calories
23 g fat

Flat Iron
380 calories
27 g fat

Rib-Eye
560 calories
32 g fat

10 oz Sirloin
590 calories
44 g fat

Jack Daniel's Rib-Eye
690 calories
22 g fat

Jack Daniel's Sirloin
720 calories
34 g fat

ALL THIS

- Rib-Eye
- Grilled Lobster Tail
- Sweet Potato Fries
- Tomato Mozzarella Salad
- Triple Berry Smoothie

and
- Oreo Madness

OR THAT!

- Blue Cheese Stacked Burger

2,070 calories

Other Passes

Tuscan Spinach Dip
1,110 calories
71 g fat (15 g saturated)
1,650 mg sodium

Friday's Shrimp
730 calories
48 g fat (15 g sat fat)
2,870 mg sodium

Jack Daniel's Black Angus Rib-Eye & Grilled Shrimp Scampi
1,150 calories
42 g fat (15 g saturated)
2,490 mg sodium

TACO BELL

"Taco Bell breakfast" is sort of like "ax-murderer babysitter." It's an inherently bad idea, proven by the insane products the Bell brought out in its attempt to start charging you money earlier and earlier. Waffle Taco is all we have to say, really. But the Bell wasn't satisfied with ruining all three meals—the chain tried to invent the Fourth Meal, which is something you eat after a late night of doing whatever works up your appetite. Limit yourself to lunch and dinner, and keep the wee hours sacred.

SURVIVAL STRATEGY

Stay away from anything "smothered" or "XXL," and be skeptical of the salads. Instead, order any two of the following: crunchy tacos, bean burritos, or anything on the Fresco menu.

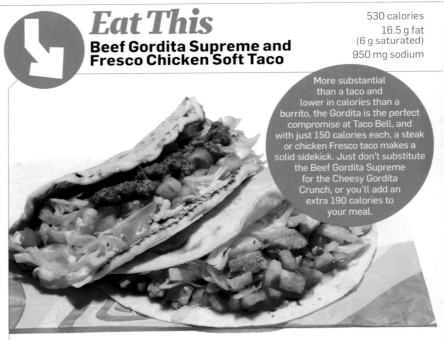

Eat This
Beef Gordita Supreme and Fresco Chicken Soft Taco

530 calories
16.5 g fat
(6 g saturated)
950 mg sodium

More substantial than a taco and lower in calories than a burrito, the Gordita is the perfect compromise at Taco Bell, and with just 150 calories each, a steak or chicken Fresco taco makes a solid sidekick. Just don't substitute the Beef Gordita Supreme for the Cheesy Gordita Crunch, or you'll add an extra 190 calories to your meal.

Other Picks

Chili Cheese Burrito

370 calories
16 g fat
(8 g saturated, 0.5 g trans)
900 mg sodium

Cantina Power Bowl

490 calories
20 g fat
(6 g saturated)
1,270 mg sodium

Cinnamon Twists

170 calories
7 g fat
(0 g saturated)
10 g sugars

580 calories
29 g fat
(10 g saturated, 1 g trans)
1,380 mg sodium

Not That!
Express Taco Salad
with Chips

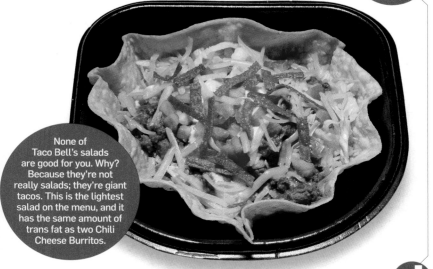

None of Taco Bell's salads are good for you. Why? Because they're not really salads; they're giant tacos. This is the lightest salad on the menu, and it has the same amount of trans fat as two Chili Cheese Burritos.

Other Passes

Caramel Apple Empanada
310 calories
15 g fat
(2.5 g saturated)
13 g sugars

Chicken Quesadilla
510 calories
27 g fat
(12 g saturated, 0.5 g trans)
1,200 mg sodium

Beefy 5-Layer Burrito
510 calories
20 g fat
(8 g saturated)
1,290 mg sodium

ALL THIS
- 1 Beef Soft Taco
- 1 Cheese Roll-Up
- 1 order of Cheesy Fiesta Potatoes

and
- a Brisk Mango Fiesta (16 oz)

OR THAT!
- Fiesta Taco Salad— Chicken

740 calories

TIM HORTONS

When it comes to sandwiches, Tim Hortons trumps the competition. Not a single lunch sandwich tops 600 calories, and its worst breakfast item is a 530-calorie sausage, egg, and cheese bagel. Supplement a lighter sandwich with Tim's oatmeal, yogurt, or soup, and you're golden. The menu still houses a variety of confections and empty carbohydrates, though, so don't let your guard down.

SURVIVAL STRATEGY

More than ever, it's about the quality of your calories instead of quantity. Your best bet at breakfast is the fruit-topped yogurt or maple oatmeal. For lunch, choose either two wraps or one sandwich and a zero-calorie beverage, and you'll be on solid ground.

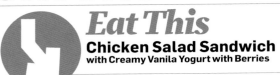

Eat This
Chicken Salad Sandwich
with Creamy Vanila Yogurt with Berries

500 calories
11.5 g fat
(2.5 g saturated)
940 mg sodium

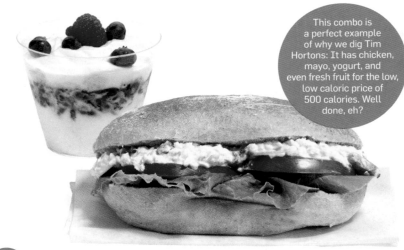

This combo is a perfect example of why we dig Tim Hortons: It has chicken, mayo, yogurt, and even fresh fruit for the low, low caloric price of 500 calories. Well done, eh?

Other Picks

Chocolate Dip Donut

190 calories
7 g fat (2.5 g saturated)
8 g sugars

BBQ Chicken Wrap Snacker and Chicken Noodle Soup (small)

290 calories
8.5 g fat (7.5 g saturated)
1,250 mg sodium

Iced Coffee with Cream and Sugar (medium)

110 calories
6 g fat (3.5 g saturated)
12 g sugars

770 calories
22 g fat
(7.5 g saturated)
1,335 mg sodium

Not That!
Pesto Chicken Panini
and Mixed Berry Yogurt Smoothie (medium)

Ultimate Cinnamon Bowl	5 bowls of Cinnamon Toast Crunch cereal
47 g sugars	

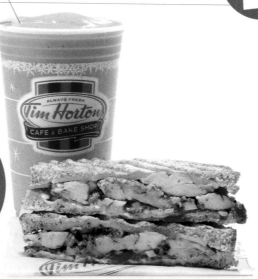

These two lunches share nearly every ingredient, and yet this version packs an extra 270 calories and nearly twice the fat. Make a mistake like this once a day and you'll have an extra 20 pounds to contend with after a year.

BREAKFAST SANDWICH STACKUP

Egg and Cheese Breakfast Wrap
220 calories
12 g fat (3.5 g saturated)
550 mg sodium

Egg and Cheese English Muffin
280 calories
11 g fat (5 g saturated)
650 mg sodium

Egg and Cheese Breakfast Sandwich on a Biscuit
360 calories
18 g fat
(11 g saturated)
930 mg sodium

Egg and Cheese Bagel
420 calories
13 g fat (5 g saturated)
1,010 mg sodium

Other Passes

Iced Cappuccino
with Cream (medium)
430 calories
22 g fat (14 g saturated)
50 g sugars

Bacon, Tomato and Cheese Panini
600 calories
29 g fat (8 g saturated)
1,380 mg sodium

Smile Cookie
300 calories
12 g fat (7 g saturated)
27 g sugars

UNO PIZZERIA & GRILL

Uno strikes a curious (if not altogether healthy) balance between oversized sandwiches and burgers, lean grilled steaks and fish entrées, and one of the world's most calorie-dense foods, deep-dish pizza, which Uno's invented. It may pride itself on its nutrition transparency, but the only thing that's truly transparent is that there are far too many dishes here that pack 1,000 calories or more.

SURVIVAL STRATEGY

Stick with flatbread instead of deep-dish pizzas—this one move could save you close to 1,000 calories at a sitting. Beyond that, turn to the steak and seafood parts of the menu, or else Uno is going to give you an unhealthy dose.

Eat This
Margherita Flatbread Artisan Crust Pizza (½ pie)

445 calories
14.5 g fat
(7.5 g saturated)
750 mg sodium

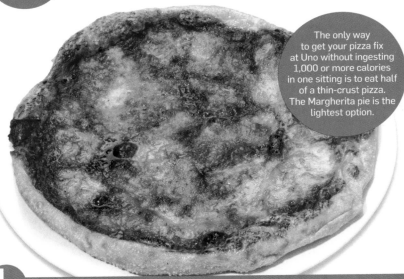

The only way to get your pizza fix at Uno without ingesting 1,000 or more calories in one sitting is to eat half of a thin-crust pizza. The Margherita pie is the lightest option.

Other Picks

Roasted Eggplant, Spinach & Feta
Traditional Flatbread (½ pie)
440 calories
16 g fat
(5.5 g saturated)
815 mg sodium

Baked Spinoccoli Chicken
360 calories
14 g fat
(7 g saturated)
1,440 mg sodium

Red Bliss Mashed Potatoes
270 calories
14 g fat
(3.5 g saturated)
650 mg sodium

1,750 calories
121 g fat
(33 g saturated)
3,010 mg sodium

Not That!
Prima Pepperoni Individual Deep Dish Pizza with Traditional Crust

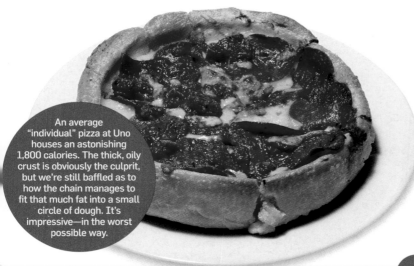

An average "individual" pizza at Uno houses an astonishing 1,800 calories. The thick, oily crust is obviously the culprit, but we're still baffled as to how the chain manages to fit that much fat into a small circle of dough. It's impressive—in the worst possible way.

ATTACK OF THE APPETIZER
Pizza Skins

2,070 calories
140 g fat
(48 g saturated,
1 g trans)
3,050 mg sodium

Uno's pizza crust is already the worst in the country, so we're not surprised that filling it with potatoes, bacon, cheese, and sour cream results in a catastrophe.

HEALTH-FOOD FRAUD

Farmer's Market Individual Pizza
with Nine Grain Crust

1,490 calories
91 g fat (25 g saturated)
1,950 mg sodium

This is the lightest individual pizza on Uno's menu, which is like being the least-wealthy Kardashian sister. The Nine Grain dough has nearly the same amounts of calories and fat as the Traditional deep dish crust. Stay away.

Other Passes

Mediterranean Farro Salad
with Honey Lime Dressing

520 calories
39 g fat
(9 g saturated)
990 mg sodium

Chicken Milanese

850 calories
56 g fat
(12 g saturated)
2,370 mg sodium

Wild Mushroom & White Cheddar
Traditional Flatbread
(½ pie)

640 calories
39.5 g fat
(13.5 g saturated)
1,120 mg sodium

WENDY'S

Scoring a decent meal at Wendy's is just about as easy as scoring a bad one, and that's a big compliment to pay a burger joint. Options such as chili and apple slices offer the side-order variety that's missing from less-evolved fast-food chains. Plus, Wendy's offers a handful of Jr. Burgers that stay below 400 calories. Where Wendy's errs is in the trans fats and the roster of double- and triple-patty burgers. The ongoing bacon obsession doesn't help either.

SURVIVAL STRATEGY

Choose a grilled chicken sandwich or a wrap—they don't exceed 320 calories. Or opt for a small burger and pair it with chili or a side salad.

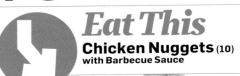

Eat This

Chicken Nuggets (10)
with Barbecue Sauce

450 calories
30 g fat
(7 g saturated)
870 mg sodium

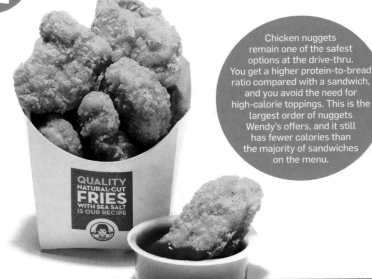

Chicken nuggets remain one of the safest options at the drive-thru. You get a higher protein-to-bread ratio compared with a sandwich, and you avoid the need for high-calorie toppings. This is the largest order of nuggets Wendy's offers, and it still has fewer calories than the majority of sandwiches on the menu.

Other Picks

Double Stack

460 calories
25 g fat
(12 g saturated, 1.5 g trans)
1,280 mg sodium

Ultimate Chicken Grill

370 calories
7 g fat
(1.5 g saturated)
880 mg sodium

Chocolate Frosty
(small)

340 calories
9 g fat
(6 g saturated)
46 g sugars

670 calories
32 g fat
(9 g saturated)
1,610 mg sodium

Not That!
Asiago Ranch Homestyle Chicken Club

Junior Bacon Cheeseburger
370 calories
21g fat (8 g saturated,
0.5 g trans).

Son of Baconator
660 calories
36 g fat (14 g saturated,
1.5 g trans)

Pretzel Bacon Cheeseburger
680 calories
36 g fat (15 g saturated,
1.5 g trans).

Baconator
940 calories
57 g fat (23 g saturated,
2.5 g trans)

Specialty sandwiches are usually tricked out with tons of unnecessary extras. In this case, bacon, cheese, ranch sauce, and a buttered bun combine to make a chicken sandwich with nearly as many calories as a Baconator. Order it with grilled chicken to bring it down to a much more reasonable 580 calories.

HIDDEN DANGER

Trans Fats

Most processed beef contains trace amounts of trans fats, but Wendy's beef is loaded with the stuff. Even a basic Quarter-Pound Cheeseburger has 1.5 grams, nearly as much as the American Heart Association recommends you eat in an entire day.

Other Passes

Chocolate Frosty Shake (small)
540 calories
13 g fat
(8 g saturated, 1 g trans)
98 g sugars

Bacon and Cheese Baked Potato
540 calories
23 g fat
(11 g saturated, 0.5 g trans)
890 mg sodium

Dave's Hot 'N Juicy Quarter Pound Single
580 calories
31 g fat
(13 g saturated, 1.5 g trans)
1,220 mg sodium

Chapter 5

AT THE SUPER-MARKET

Unpack a load of groceries that will boost your health—and trim your waist

Everybody loves food. Everybody loves shopping. And yet, oddly, nobody loves food shopping, despite the fact that we make an average of 1.6 trips a week to buy groceries.

Maybe that's why more and more of our grocery shopping is happening at places other than grocery stores. (Target, Walmart, Walgreens, CVS and Costco are the top non-super-market stops for folks buying their foodstuffs.) And while a recent survey found that alternative grocery stores can be cheaper (up to 20 percent cheaper at a Walmart Supercenter or SuperTarget, compared to Giant or Safeway), the sprawl of groceries is making it harder than ever to find what we're looking for. In one survey, shoppers found only 61 percent of their shopping list for sale at Target. Other "alternative" markets like Trader Joe's and Aldi fared worse, if only because Coca Cola and Charmin are just as important as organic kohlrabi and free-range bison.

Meanwhile, grocery-delivery services like Fresh Direct and Pea Pod are inspiring tons of imitators, and aiming to make the act of pushing a dodgy shopping cart along a strip of buzzing fluorescent lights a thing of the past. But regardless of whether you're ordering groceries online, slipping into the local bodega, or standing behind a line of people who are utterly confused by "self-checkout," a cheat sheet to guide you through the questionable claims and hyperbolic come-ons of modern food packaging is an invaluable resource. So dive in to the following pages and prepare to be amazed. One seemingly insignificant swap—starting your day with Quaker Reduced-Sugar Oatmeal instead of Quaker Granola Oats & Honey—can save you 300 calories every morning. That's enough to save you more than 31 pounds this year alone!

SWEET CEREALS

Eat This

Kellogg's Froot Loops
(1 cup)
110 calories
1 g fat (0.5 g saturated)
135 mg sodium
3 g fiber
12 g sugars

Kellogg's Special K Red Berries (1 cup)
110 calories
0 g fat
190 mg sodium
3 g fiber
9 g sugars

This cereal employs wheat bran to up the fiber count and dried strawberries for sweetness.

General Mills Cinnamon Burst Cheerios (1 cup)
120 calories
2 g fat
(0 g saturated)
125 mg sodium
3 g fiber
9 g sugars

All the cholesterol-busting power of oat bran with just a touch of sweetness.

General Mills Kix (1 cup)
88 calories
1 g fat
(0 g saturated)
144 mg sodium
2.5 g fiber
2.5 g sugars

Kix just might be the safest of all the sweetened kids' cereals. Try it with blueberries.

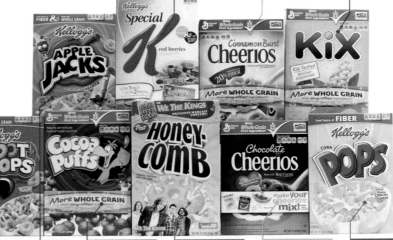

It's still not exactly a health food, but the denigrated Froot Loops has a similar fiber-to-sugar ratio as the health-conscious Kashi, and far fewer calories.

Kellogg's Apple Jacks (1 cup)
110 calories
1 g fat
(0.5 g saturated)
130 mg sodium
3 g fiber
12 g sugars

The whole-grain corn flour adds just enough fiber to offset the sugar.

General Mills Cocoa Puffs (1 cup)
133 calories
2 g fat
(0 g saturated)
200 mg sodium
2.5 g fiber
13.5 g sugars

General Mills has slowly added more whole grains to all of its Big G cereals.

Post Honeycomb (1 cup)
87 calories
0.5 g fat
(0 g saturated)
120 mg sodium
0.5 g fiber
7 g sugars

We'd love more fiber, but at least Post keeps the sugar and calories down.

General Mills Chocolate Cheerios (1 cup)
133 calories
2 g fat
(0 g saturated)
200 mg sodium
2.5 g fiber
12 g sugars

Two of the first five ingredients are whole grains.

Kellogg's Corn Pops (1 cup)
120 calories
0 g fat
105 mg sodium
3 g fiber
9 g sugars

Following General Mills' lead, Kellogg's began bulking up its fiber profile in 2009.

Quaker Life
(1 cup)
160 calories
2 g fat
(0 g saturated)
213 mg sodium
2.5 g fiber
8 g sugars

Life isn't the worst cereal on the shelf, but it does pack in more than three times as much sugar as fiber.

General Mills Cinnamon Chex
(1 cup)
160 calories
3 g fat
(0 g saturated)
240 mg sodium
1 g fiber
11 g sugars

This cereal delivers more than 130 calories of pure carbohydrates.

Post Honey Bunches of Oats with Real Strawberries
(1 cup)
160 calories
2 g fat
(0 g saturated)
167 mg sodium
3 g fiber
11 g sugars

Heavy on the carbs.

Not That!
Kashi Strawberry Fields
(1 cup)
200 calories
0 g fat
190 mg sodium
3 g fiber
11 g sugars

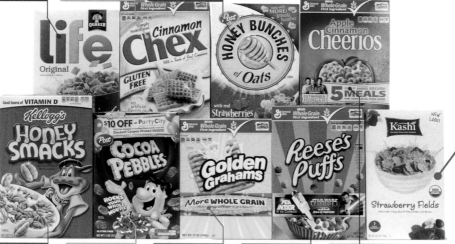

This is one of Kashi's biggest flops. Strawberry Fields features white rice instead of the 7 Whole Grain blend found in many of its cereals.

Kellogg's Honey Smacks
(1 cup)
133 calories
0.5 g fat
(0 g saturated)
53 mg sodium
1.5 g fiber
20 g sugars

This is among the most sugar-loaded boxes in the cereal aisle.

Post Cocoa Pebbles
(1 cup)
160 calories
1 g fat
(1 g saturated)
227 mg sodium
0 g fiber
13 g sugars

Not just devoid of fiber, but also soaked with hydrogenated oils.

General Mills Golden Grahams
(1 cup)
160 calories
1 g fat
(0 g saturated)
320 mg sodium
2.5 g fiber
13.5 g sugars

Loaded with sugar, lacking in fiber, and saturated with sodium.

General Mills Reese's Puffs
(1 cup)
213 calories
4 g fat
(0.5 g saturated)
213 mg sodium
1 g fiber
13.5 g sugars

Oxford researchers rated this the unhealthiest cereal in the supermarket.

General Mills Apple Cinnamon Cheerios
(1 cup)
160 calories
2 g fat
(0 g saturated)
153 mg sodium
2.5 g fiber
13 g sugars

Worse than most junk cereal.

WHOLESOME CEREALS

Eat This

Kellogg's Raisin Bran Cinnamon Almond (1 cup)

160 calories
1 g fat (0 g saturated)
176 mg sodium
4 g fiber
14 g sugars

Cinnamon is a worthwhile addition to any cereal. Studies show that it helps your body manage blood sugar. Most of the sugars here come from the coating on the raisins. Pick some out if you want to reduce your intake.

Kashi GoLean Crunch! (1 cup)
250 calories
4 g fat (0 g saturated)
133 mg sodium
10 g fiber
17 g sugars

Ten grams of fiber goes a long way toward making up for the higher than ideal sugar content.

Post Shredded Wheat Spoon Size Wheat 'n Bran (1 cup)
160 calories
1 g fat (0 g saturated)
0 mg sodium
7 g fiber
0 g sugars

Made with just whole-grain wheat and wheat bran—a pure base crying out for fresh blueberries or bananas.

General Mills Total Raisin Bran (1 cup)
160 calories
1 g fat (0 g saturated)
180 mg sodium
5 g fiber
17 g sugars

Among the many nutrients added to each serving in this box are an entire day's worth of calcium and vitamin E.

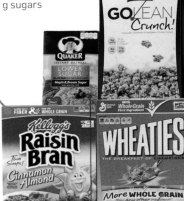

Quaker Instant Oatmeal Lower Sugar Maple & Brown Sugar (1 packet)
120 calories
2 g fat (0 g saturated)
290 mg sodium
3 g fiber
4 g sugars

It has a third of the sugar, but the same great taste. Promise.

General Mills Wheaties (1 cup)
133 calories
1 g fat (0 g saturated)
253 mg sodium
4 g fiber
5 g sugars

Being made with whole grains should be the minimum requirement for a cereal to land on your breakfast table. Anything less should be relegated to dessert.

General Mills Fiber One (1 cup)
120 calories
2 g fat (0 g saturated)
220 mg sodium
28 g fiber
0 g sugars

Sprinkle over Greek yogurt instead of granola for a fiber- and protein-filled start to the day.

Kellog's Special K Multi-Grain (1 cup)
110 calories
0 g fat (0 g saturated)
190 mg sodium
3 g fiber
6 g sugars

The sugar count could be a little lower, but at least it has the fiber to back it up.

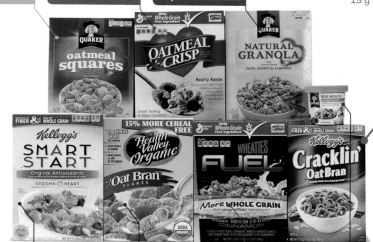

Quaker Cinnamon Oatmeal Squares (1 cup)
210 calories
2.5 g fat (0.5 g saturated)
190 mg sodium
5 g fiber
9 g sugars

Overloaded with sugar and cheap refined carbs like maltodextrin.

General Mills Oatmeal Crisp Hearty Raisin (1 cup)
230 calories
2.5 g fat (0.5 g saturated)
120 mg sodium
5 g fiber
17 g sugars

Each bowl before adding milk has just 10 calories fewer than a McDonald's hamburger.

Quaker Natural Granola Oats & Honey (1 cup)
420 calories
10 g fat (1 g saturated)
60 mg sodium
10 g fiber
26 g sugars

Rumors of granola's healthfulness have been vastly overstated. You'd be wise to keep it far away from your breakfast bowl.

Not That!
Kellogg's Cracklin' Oat Bran (1 cup)
267 calories
9 g fat (4 g saturated)
180 mg sodium
8 g fiber
19 g sugars

Kellogg's Smart Start Strong Heart Original Antioxidants (1 cup)
190 calories
1 g fat (0 g saturated)
210 mg sodium
3 g fiber
14 g sugars

What's so smart about a high-sugar, low-fiber cereal? We still don't know.

Health Valley Organic Oat Bran Flakes (1 cup)
190 calories
1.5 g fat (0.5 g saturated)
190 mg sodium
4 g fiber
11 g sugars

Sugar outnumbers fiber nearly three to one.

General Mills Wheaties Fuel (1 cup)
253 calories
4 g fat (0 g saturated)
187 mg sodium
10.5 g fiber
18.5 g sugars

Confusing this box with regular Wheaties will cost you nearly double the calories and nearly four times the sugar.

Quaker Real Medleys Apple Walnut Oatmeal (1 container)
290 calories
8 g fat (1 g saturated)
270 mg sodium
5 g fiber
22 g sugars

A full 30 percent of these calories come from sugar.

Nearly 20 g of sugar alone make this cereal less than wholesome, but Cracklin' Oat Bran also comes with a massive glut of palm oil that loads this box with fat.

235

BREAKFAST BREADS

Eat This

Thomas' Light Multi-Grain English Muffins
(1 muffin, 57 g)

100 calories
1 g fat (0 g saturated)
180 mg sodium
26 g carbohydrates
8 g fiber

Outside of green vegetables, you'll find very few foods that pack 8 grams of fiber into 100 calories. That makes this an unbeatable foundation for breakfast sandwiches.

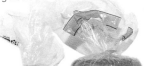
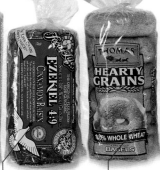
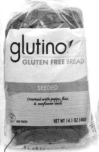
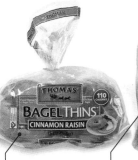
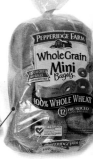

Food for Life Ezekiel 4:9 Sprouted 100% Whole Grain Cinnamon Raisin Bread (1 slice, 34 g)

80 calories
0 g fat
65 mg sodium
18 g carbohydrates
2 g fiber

Barley, millet, and spelt help boost fiber.

Thomas' Hearty Grains 100% Whole Wheat Bagels (1 bagel, 95 g)

240 calories
2 g fat (0.5 g saturated)
400 mg sodium
49 g carbohydrates
7 g fiber

One of the best bagels we've seen. Tons of fiber, plus 10 grams of protein in each serving.

Glutino Seeded Bread (1 slice, 29 g)

80 calories
4.5 g fat (0 g saturated)
120 mg sodium
10 g carbohydrates
1 g fiber

Sunflower, flax and poppy seeds give this bread a decent hit of healthy fats for hardly any calories.

Thomas' Bagel Thins Cinnamon Raisin (1 bagel, 46 g)

110 calories
1 g fat (0 g saturated)
160 mg sodium
25 g carbohydrates
5 g fiber

Switching to these is the best way to wean yourself off bagels. Try a swipe of peanut butter instead of cream cheese for a near-perfect snack.

Pepperidge Farm Whole Grain Mini Bagels 100% Whole Wheat (1 bagel, 40 g)

100 calories
0.5 g fat (0 g saturated)
120 mg sodium
20 g carbohydrates
3 g fiber

The perfect base for a ham and egg breakfast sandwich.

Sara Lee Original Made with Whole Grain English Muffins

(1 muffin, 66 g)

140 calories
1 g fat (0 g saturated)
210 mg sodium
27 g carbohydrates
2 g fiber

The more fiber you work into your breakfast, the more likely you'll be to make it to lunch without experiencing hunger pangs. That means this muffin is a recipe for midmorning cravings.

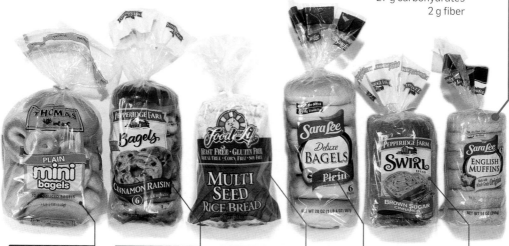

Thomas' Plain Mini Bagels
(1 bagel, 43 g)
120 calories
1 g fat (0 g saturated)
210 mg sodium
24 g carbohydrates
<1 g fiber

Once your palate is accustomed to whole grains, flavorless, nutritionless lumps of refined carbs like this will taste boring.

Pepperidge Farm Bagels Cinnamon Raisin
(1 bagel, 99 g)
270 calories
1 g fat (0 g saturated)
290 mg sodium
57 g carbohydrates
3 g fiber

This bagel belongs on a dessert menu, not a breakfast table.

Food for Life Gluten-Free Multi-Seed Rice Bread (1 slice, 50g)
120 calories
1 g fat (0 g saturated)
170 mg sodium
26 g carbohydrates
1g fiber

What this rice-and-tapioca concoction cuts in gluten it doesn't make up for in whole grains.

Sara Lee Deluxe Bagels Plain
(1 bagel, 95 g)
260 calories
1 g fat (0 g saturated)
400 mg sodium
50 g carbohydrates
2 g fiber

This is a wedge of refined carbohydrates, and as such, it will induce a blood sugar roller coaster that will wreak havoc on your energy reserves.

Pepperidge Farm Brown Sugar Cinnamon Swirl Bread (1 slice, 38 g)
110 calories
2 g fat (0 g saturated)
140 mg sodium
21 g carbohydrates
<1 g fiber

This bread contains five different forms of sugar.

YOGURTS

Eat This
Chobani Vanilla Blended (1 container, 5.3 oz)

120 calories
0 g fat (0 g saturated)
<1 g fiber
13 g sugars
13 g protein

There's a reason why Chobani has become the yogurt of the moment. With nearly three times the protein and just half the sugar, Chobani will keep you feeling full without the carbohydrate crash of most fat-free brands.

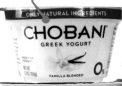

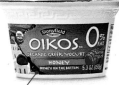

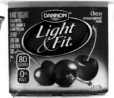

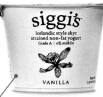

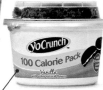

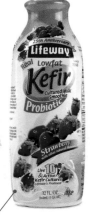

Stonyfield Oikos Organic Greek Yogurt Honey
(1 container, 5.3 oz)
120 calories
0 g fat
0 g fiber
17 g sugars
13 g protein

Oikos uses honey to turn this into a lightly sweetened treat, not a sugary breakfast blunder.

Dannon Light & Fit Cherry
(1 container, 6 oz)
80 calories
0 g fat
0 g fiber
10 g sugars
5 g protein

We prefer a yogurt with more protein, but it's tough to argue against one with just 80 calories per serving.

Siggi's Icelandic Style Skyr Strained Non Fat Yogurt Vanilla
(1 container, 5.3 oz)
100 calories
0 g fat
0 g fiber
9 g sugars
14 g protein

Strained just like Greek yogurt, which makes it creamy and high-protein.

YoCrunch 100 Calorie Vanilla with Chocolate Cookie Pieces
(1 container, 106 g)
100 calories
1 g fat (0 g saturated)
0 g fiber
14 g sugars
3 g protein

Impressively low cal for a cookie-strewn treat.

Lifeway Lowfat Kefir Strawberry
(1 container, 8 oz)
140 calories
2 g fat (1.5 g saturated)
20 g sugars
11 g protein

Kefir is 99 percent lactose free, making it suitable for most intolerant individuals. It also happens to be a stellar source of protein and probiotic bacteria.

Not That!

Yoplait Original 99% Fat Free Harvest Peach (1 container, 6 oz)

170 calories
1.5 g fat (1 g saturated)
0 g fiber
26 g sugars
5 g protein

Yoplait commits the cardinal sin of fruit-flavored yogurts by candying these peaches with more sugar than you'd find in a two-pack of Reese's Peanut Butter Cups. The only yogurts worth eating are those that are unflavored or that can claim to have more fruit than sugar.

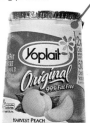

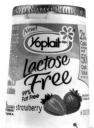
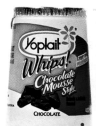
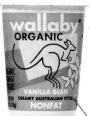
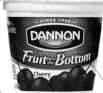
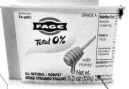

Yoplait Lactose Free Strawberry
(1 container, 6 oz)
170 calories
1.5 g fat (1 g saturated)
26 g sugars
5 g protein

Sure, it's lactose free, but it's also a sugary, low-protein mess.

Yoplait Whips! Chocolate Mousse Style
(1 container, 4 oz)
160 calories
4 g fat (2.5 g saturated)
0 g fiber
22 g sugars
5 g protein

You'd be better off eating a small scoop of Breyers ice cream.

Wallaby Organic Nonfat Yogurt Vanilla Bean
(1 container, 6 oz)
140 calories
0 g fat
0 g fiber
22 g sugars
6 g protein

Organic dairy is worth celebrating, but don't bend your nutritional standards to get it.

Dannon Fruit on the Bottom Cherry
(1 container, 6 oz)
150 calories
1.5 g fat (1 g saturated)
0 g fiber
24 g sugars
6 g protein

"Fruit on the Bottom" means a few cherries muddled with sugar.

Fage Total 0% with Honey
(1 container, 5.3 oz)
170 calories
0 g fat
0 g fiber
29 g sugars
13 g protein

Honey may be better than sugar, but it's not so good that you should eat it by the cupful.

239

CHEESES

Eat This

Kraft Singles 2% Milk Sharp Cheddar
(1 slice, 19 g)

45 calories
2.5 g fat (1.5 g saturated)
250 mg sodium
4 g protein

There may be a few lighter cheeses out there, but they don't taste like cheese. If you're looking for an all-purpose burger or sandwich topper, start here.

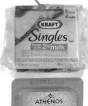
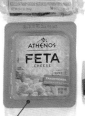

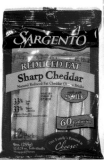
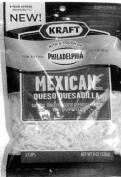
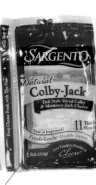

Athenos Traditional Crumbled Feta
(¼ cup, 34 g)
90 calories
7 g fat (4 g saturated)
400 mg sodium
6 g protein

A reasonable fat-to-protein ratio makes feta the most reliable go-to crumbled cheese.

The Laughing Cow Original Creamy Swiss
(1 wedge, 21 g)
50 calories
4 g fat (2.5 g saturated)
190 mg sodium
2 g protein

Spreads every bit as easily as Alouette's, yet it cuts your calorie load by a third.

Cabot 50% Reduced Fat Sharp Cheddar
(1" cube, 28 g)
70 calories
4.5 g fat (3 g saturated)
170 mg sodium
8 g protein

A smart approach: Cut half the fat but leave enough to add a rich, creamy texture.

Sargento Reduced Fat Sharp Cheddar Sticks
(1 stick, 21 g)
60 calories
4.5 g fat (3 g saturated)
135 mg sodium
5 g protein

Portable snacks don't get any better than this.

Kraft Natural Mexican Style Queso Quesadilla with a Touch of Philadelphia
(¼ cup, 28 g)
90 calories
7 g fat (4 g saturated)
160 mg sodium
6 g protein

An unusually low-cal cheese blends.

Sargento Deli Style Sliced Colby & Monterey Jack
(1 slice, 19 g)
70 calories
6 g fat (4 g saturated)
125 mg sodium
4 g protein

Sargento's thinner slices cut calories without sacrificing any flavor.

Not That!
Kraft Deli Deluxe Sharp Cheddar Slices
(1 slice, 19 g)
70 calories
6 g fat (3.5 g saturated)
300 mg sodium
4 g protein

These slices earn three-quarters of their calories from fat. And what does that earn you? Nothing but extra calories.

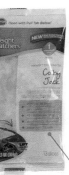

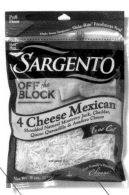

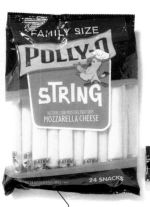

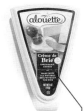

Weight Watchers Colby Jack Slices (1 slice, 28 g)
90 calories
6 g fat (4 g saturated)
200 mg sodium
7 g protein

What makes this a Weight Watchers cheese? We don't know either. It's calorically on par with any other in the deli case.

Sargento Off the Block 4 Cheese Mexican (¼ cup, 28 g)
110 calories
9 g fat (4.5 g saturated)
170 mg sodium
6 g protein

The number of fat calories can vary widely in seemingly similar cheese blends.

Polly-O String Cheese (1 stick, 28 g)
80 calories
6 g fat (3.5 g saturated)
190 mg sodium
7 g protein

The little bird with the hat on the front of the package is hiding more fat than he should.

Kraft Cracker Barrel Extra Sharp Cheddar 2% Milk (28 g)
110 calories
10 g fat (6 g saturated)
170 mg sodium
6 g protein

Switch to Cabot's and you'll cut 20 calories from each ounce of cheese overload.

Alouette Crème de Brie Spreadable (28 g)
100 calories
9 g fat (5 g saturated)
170 mg sodium
5 g protein

If only this had the portion-controlled approach used by the Laughing Cow.

Stella Crumbled Gorgonzola (¼ cup, 28 g)
100 calories
8 g fat (6 g saturated)
380 mg sodium
6 g protein

Even with less cheese in each serving, you still end up with more calories and fat.

DELI MEATS

Eat This

Applegate Organics Smoked Turkey Breast (56 g)

50 calories
0 g fat
360 mg sodium
12 g protein

Applegate Farms eschews antibiotics, producing some of the most pristine, natural meats in the supermarket.

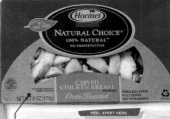

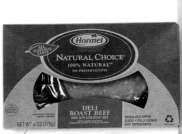

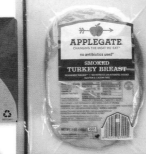

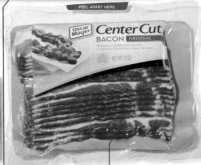

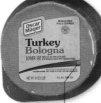

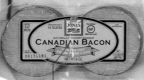

Hormel Natural Choice Deli Roast Beef (56 g)
60 calories
2 g fat (1 g saturated)
520 mg sodium
11 g protein

One of the few deli brands to forgo all nitrites, nitrates, and other preservatives.

Oscar Mayer Turkey Bologna
(1 slice, 28 g)
50 calories
4 g fat (1 g saturated)
270 mg sodium
3 g protein

Turkey doesn't always mean healthier. This time it does.

Jones Naturally Hickory Smoked Canadian Bacon
(51 g)
60 calories
1.5 g fat (0.5 g saturated)
460 mg sodium
11 g protein

The easiest swap in the supermarket; you get twice as much food for half the calories.

Hormel Natural Choice Oven Roasted Carved Chicken Breast
(56 g)
60 calories
1 g fat (0 g saturated)
390 mg sodium
12 g protein

This chicken is almost pure protein.

Oscar Mayer Center Cut Bacon
(2 slices)
60 calories
3.5 g fat (1.5 g saturated)
210 mg sodium
6 g protein

If you want bacon, eat bacon. You won't take in any extra calories and you'll actually cut fat and sodium.

Not That!

Land O'Frost Premium Honey Smoked Turkey Breast (50 g)

Land O'Frost competes with Buddig for the most calorie-dense lunch meat around.

80 calories
5 g fat (1.5 g saturated)
540 mg sodium
8 g protein

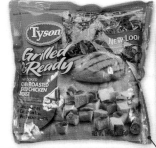

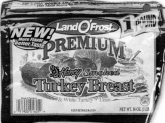

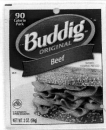

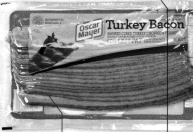

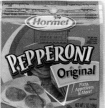

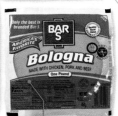

Oscar Mayer Turkey Bacon
(2 slices, 30 g)

70 calories
6 g fat (2 g saturated)
360 mg sodium
4 g protein

More sodium than regular pork bacon, and also more than triple the number of ingredients.

Tyson Grilled & Ready Oven Roasted Diced Chicken Breast
(42 g)

50 calories
1 g fat (0 g saturated)
240 mg sodium
9.5 g protein

The calorie counts are reasonable, but it takes 15 ingredients to make this Franken-Chicken.

Hormel Pepperoni Original (28 g)

140 calories
13 g fat (6 g saturated)
490 mg sodium
5 g protein

Pepperoni is the downfall of far too many pizzas served in America, and the blame rests entirely on its egregious load of fat.

Bar-S Bologna
(1 slice, 32 g)

100 calories
8 g fat (2.5 g saturated)
350 mg sodium
3 g protein

You could eat two slices of Oscar Mayer's Turkey Bologna for the same amount of calories.

Buddig Original Beef (56 g)

90 calories
5 g fat (2 g saturated)
790 mg sodium
9 g protein

Most deli meats fail in one of two ways: too much fat or too much sodium. Buddig's products routinely fail in both ways.

HOT DOGS & SAUSAGES

Eat This

Hebrew National 97% Fat Free Beef Franks

(1 frank, 45 g)
40 calories
1 g fat (0 g saturated)
520 mg sodium
6 g protein

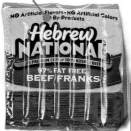

There's no reason to fear hot dogs. A recent study from Kansas State University found that microwave-cooked hot dogs have fewer cancer-causing compounds than even rotisserie chicken. Stick with low-calorie brands and you're never far from a quick, healthy, and protein-packed meal.

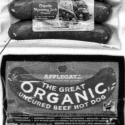

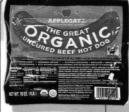

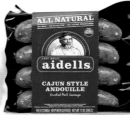

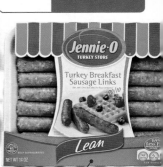

Aidells Cajun Style Andouille
(1 link, 85 g)
160 calories
11 g fat (4 g saturated)
600 mg sodium
15 g protein

Remember Aidells. It's one of the most reliable purveyors in the deli fridge.

Johnsonville Chicken Sausage Chipotle Monterey Jack Cheese
(1 link, 85 g)
150 calories
9 g fat (2.5 g saturated)
650 mg sodium
13 g protein

We're glad to see the sausage behemoth get on board with the chicken variety.

Applegate Farms The Great Organic Uncured Beef Hot Dog (1 frank, 56 g)
110 calories
8 g fat (3 g saturated)
330 mg sodium
7 g protein

It looks and tastes like a classic ballpark frank, but without the dubious waste cuts or antibiotic-heavy meat.

Al Fresco Chipotle Chorizo Chicken Sausage (1 link, 85 g)
140 calories
7 g fat (2 g saturated)
420 mg sodium
15 g protein

Our love for Al Fresco runs deep. No company offers a wider variety of bold-flavored, low-calorie sausages.

Jennie-O Turkey Breakfast Sausage Links Lean
(2 links, 48 g)
65 calories
4 g fat (1 g saturated)
310 mg sodium
8 g protein

Cutting fat doesn't just drop the calorie count, it also makes more space for protein.

Not That!

Oscar Mayer Classic Light Beef Franks
(1 frank, 50 g)
60 calories
3.5 g fat (1.5 g saturated)
380 mg sodium
6 g protein

Hillshire Farm Smoked Bratwurst
(1 link, 66 g)
220 calories
19 g fat (7 g saturated)
520 mg sodium
7 g protein

More than 80 percent of this brat's calories come from fat.

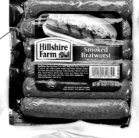

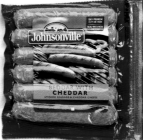

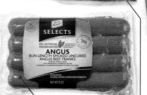

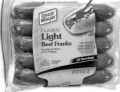

Hot dogs vary widely in terms of fat content, so it's important to flip the package and scan the ingredient statement. Case in point: You could eat three of the Hebrew National dogs on the opposite page and still not reach the fat load of these "light" franks.

Jennie-O Breakfast Lover's Turkey Sausage
(50 g)
90 calories
5 g fat (1.5 g saturated)
550 mg sodium
8 g protein

With "turkey" on the label you should expect more from your breakfast sausage.

Hillshire Farm Polska Kielbasa
(56 g)
180 calories
16 g fat (5 g saturated)
510 mg sodium
7 g protein

Both kielbasa and chorizo are spicy ethnic sausages, but opt for Al Fresco and you double up on protein while cutting calories, fat, and sodium.

Oscar Mayer Selects Angus Beef Franks (1 frank, 50 g)
170 calories
15 g fat (6 g saturated)
370 mg sodium
6 g protein

Applegate provides a more protein-packed dog for fewer calories and less sodium and fat. This is an easy choice.

Johnsonville Beddar with Cheddar (1 link, 66 g)
210 calories
18 g fat (7 g saturated)
630 mg sodium
8 g protein

More calories, less protein, and a hearty dose of MSG.

CONDIMENTS

Eat This

Hellmann's with Olive Oil
(1 Tbsp, 14 g)
60 calories
6 g fat
120 mg sodium
0 g sugars

A study published in the British Journal of Nutrition *suggests that monounsaturated fatty acids might actually facilitate the breakdown of fat. Most mayo makers like Kraft and Hellmann's now offer versions in which some of the soybean oil is replaced with monounsaturated-rich olive oil.*

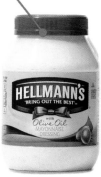

Annie's Naturals Organic Ketchup
(1 Tbsp, 17 g)
15 calories
0 g fat
130 mg sodium
4 g sugars

Go ahead and spring for organic. Research shows that organically raised tomatoes produce nearly twice as much cancer-fighting lycopene.

Ocean Spray Whole Berry Cranberry Sauce
(2 Tbsp, 35 g)
55 calories
0 g fat
5 mg sodium
11 g sugars

Not just for Thanksgiving anymore. Turn to cranberry sauce for a low-calorie, high-antioxidant sandwich companion.

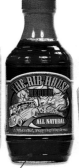

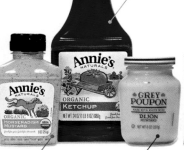

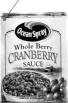

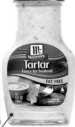

Dinosaur Bar-B-Que Original Sensuous Slathering
(2 Tbsp, 31 g)
28 calories
0 g fat
177 mg sodium
6 g sugars

Two superfoods, tomatoes and yellow mustard, make up the base of this only slightly sweetened sauce. This is as good as barbecue gets.

Annie's Naturals Organic Horseradish Mustard (2 tsp, 10 g)
10 calories
0 g fat
120 mg sodium
0 g sugars

This bottle contains no ingredients that you wouldn't have in your kitchen.

Grey Poupon Classic Dijon
(1 tsp, 5 g)
0 calories
0 g fat
0 mg sodium
0 g sugars

Made mostly from mustard seeds, which are loaded with omega-3 fatty acids.

McCormick Fat Free Tartar Sauce
(2 Tbsp, 32 g)
30 calories
0 g fat
250 mg sodium
5 g sugars

Although by no means a nutritious condiment, this light take on tartar does eliminate more than 100 calories per serving.

Not That!

Hellmann's Real Mayonnaise
(1 Tbsp, 13 g)
90 calories
10 g fat (1.5 g saturated)
90 mg sodium
0 g sugars

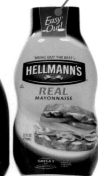

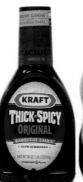

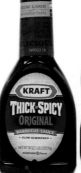

Woeber's Sweet & Tangy Tartar Sauce
(2 Tbsp, 30 g)
140 calories
14 g fat (4 g saturated)
140 mg sodium
2 g sugars

Tartar sauce is little more than mayonnaise with relish stirred in. Go with a light version or switch to cocktail sauce.

Inglehoffer Honey Mustard
(1 Tbsp, 15 g)
45 calories
0 g fat
105 mg sodium
6 g sugars

The first two ingredients are water and sugar, and corn syrup trails close behind.

Woeber's Sandwich Pal Horseradish Sauce
(2 tsp, 10 g)
40 calories
4 g fat (1 g saturated)
60 mg sodium
0 g sugars

As used here, "sauce" means soybean oil and corn syrup.

Kraft Thick 'n Spicy Original Barbecue Sauce
(2 Tbsp, 37 g)
70 calories
0 g fat
340 mg sodium
13 g sugars

High-fructose corn syrup is the primary ingredient, which is why this bottle delivers twice as much sugar as the Rib House sauce.

Aside from pure oil, mayonnaise is the most calorie-dense thing you can put on a sandwich. Every one of its 90 calories comes from low-quality fat. Choosing the olive oil version is one of the best swaps in the supermarket.

BREADS

Eat This

Nature's Own Double Fiber Wheat Bread
(2 slices, 52 g)
200 calories
3 g fat (0 g saturated)
340 mg sodium
42 g carbohydrates
12 g fiber
8 g protein

The high fiber content (40 percent of your daily intake from one sandwich) comes from the addition of inulin, a natural fiber made from chicory.

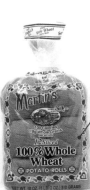

Martin's 100% Whole Wheat Potato Rolls
(1 roll, 42.5 g)
100 calories
1.5 g fat (0 g saturated)
135 mg sodium
26 g carbohydrates
3 g fiber
7 g protein

A perfect hot dog vessel. Whole wheat adds a potent fiber punch.

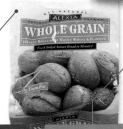

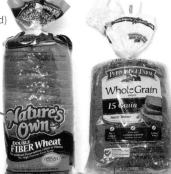

Alexia Whole Grain Hearty Rolls
(1 roll, 43 g)
100 calories
1 g fat (0 g saturated)
200 mg sodium
18 g carbohydrates
1 g fiber
4 g protein

Unless your roll has 100 calories or fewer, it has no place on the dinner table.

Mission Yellow Extra Thin Corn Tortillas
(2 tortillas, 37 g)
80 calories
1 g fat (0 g saturated)
7 mg sodium
16 g carbohydrates
3 g fiber
2 g protein

Fiber-rich corn trumps flour every time in the tortilla battle.

Pepperidge Farm Whole Grain 15 Grain
(2 slices, 86 g)
200 calories
4 g fat (1 g saturated)
230 mg sodium
40 g carbohydrates
8 g fiber
10 g protein

Five grams of protein and 4 grams of fiber per slice? Yes, please!

Arnold Sandwich Thins Flax & Fiber
(1 roll, 43 g)
100 calories
1 g fat (0 g saturated)
170 mg sodium
21 g carbohydrates
5 g fiber
5 g protein

Protein and fiber supply more than a third of these calories.

Flatout Original Flatbread
(1 piece, 57 g)
130 calories
2 g fat (0 g saturated)
310 mg sodium
24 g carbohydrates
3 g fiber
7 g protein

Not one of Flatout's flatbreads has fewer than 3 grams of fiber.

Arnold Potato Hot Dog Rolls
(1 roll, 76 g)
140 calories
1 g fat (0 g saturated)
280 mg sodium
27 g carbohydrates
1 g fiber
5 g protein

Like most rolls, these are just pillows of empty carbs.

Not That!
Arnold's Health Nut
(2 slices, 86 g)
240 calories
4 g fat (0 g saturated)
300 mg sodium
42 g carbohydrates
4 g fiber
10 g protein

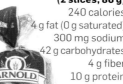

The second, third, and fourth ingredients are enriched flour, water, and sugar, leading to plenty of calories and only a modest amount of fiber.

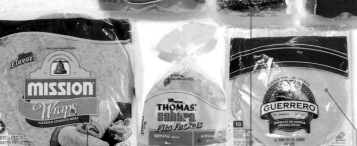

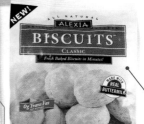

Mission Wraps Garden Spinach Herb (1 wrap, 70 g)
210 calories
5 g fat (2 g saturated)
440 mg sodium
36 g carbohydrates
3 g fiber
6 g protein

The only spinach here is "spinach powder," which accounts for less than 2 percent of each wrap.

Thomas' Sahara Pita Bread White
(1 pita, 57 g)
160 calories
1.5 g fat (0 g saturated)
250 mg sodium
31 g carbohydrates
1 g fiber
6 g protein

Switch to a pita with fewer carbs and use the saved calories to double up on hummus!

Arnold Country Oat Bran
(2 slices, 86 g)
220 calories
3 g fat (0 g saturated)
300 mg sodium
40 g carbohydrates
2 g fiber
6 g protein

Oat bran comes fourth on the ingredients list after refined flour, water, and sugar.

Guerrero Soft Taco Homemade Flour Tortillas
(1 tortilla, 37 g)
130 calories
5 g fat (2.5 g saturated)
260 mg sodium
17 g carbohydrates
1 g fiber
3 g protein

It takes more than 15 ingredients to construct this tortured tortilla.

Alexia Classic Biscuits
(1 biscuit, 50 g)
170 calories
9 g fat (5 g saturated)
450 mg sodium
20 g carbohydrates
<1 g fiber
3 g protein

Traditional biscuits come sodden with fat, and Alexia's are no different.

GRAINS & NOODLES

Eat This

Ronzoni Healthy Harvest Whole Grain Spaghetti (2 oz, 56 g dry)

180 calories
1.5 g fat (0 g saturated)
39 g carbohydrates
5 g fiber

Whole-grain pastas are loaded with fiber, and diets rich in fiber are shown to decrease your odds of developing both diabetes and heart disease. You want about 20 grams per day, and this spaghetti has 30 percent of that.

Near East Rice Pilaf Mix Lentil
(¼ cup, 56 g dry)
180 calories
0.5 g fat (0 g saturated)
650 mg sodium
36 g carbohydrates
8 g fiber

This box contains exactly seven ingredients, and you probably have every one of them in your pantry.

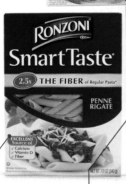

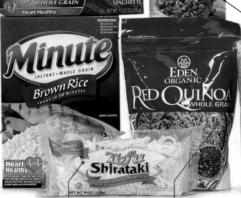

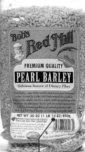

Ronzoni Smart Taste Penne Rigate
(56 g dry)
180 calories
0.5 g fat (0 g saturated)
39 g carbohydrates
5 g fiber

Whole-wheat pasta can be a gritty departure from normal noodles, but Smart Taste combines fiber with the taste of white pasta.

Minute Brown Rice
(½ cup, 43 g dry)
150 calories
1.5 g fat (0 g saturated)
34 g carbohydrates
2 g fiber

Eating healthy doesn't take more time; it just requires being more strategic in the supermarket.

House Foods Tofu Shirataki Spaghetti
(113 g)
20 calories
1 g fat (0 g saturated)
6 g carbohydrates
4 g fiber

These traditional Asian noodles are made from tofu and yam flour. Don't be afraid—they have a neutral flavor that's perfect for dressing up.

Eden Organic Red Quinoa
(¼ cup, 45 g dry)
170 calories
2 g fat (0 g saturated)
32 g carbohydrates
5 g fiber

Quinoa contains every amino acid your body needs from food. That's a claim rice can't make.

Bob's Red Mill Pearl Barley
(¼ cup, 50 g dry)
180 calories
1 g fat (0 g saturated)
39 g carbohydrates
8 g fiber

Perfect for adding nutritional heft to everyday soups. Try using it as a replacement for noodles in minestrone.

This pasta doesn't have the fiber you're looking for. That means it won't keep you full as long, and you'll be pawing through the fridge for snacks in no time.

Not That!

DeBoles All Natural
Artichoke Spaghetti Style Pasta (56 g dry)

210 calories
1 g fat (0 g saturated)
43 g carbohydrates
1 g fiber

Rice-A-Roni Rice Pilaf
(⅓ cup, 70 g dry)
240 calories
1 g fat (0 g saturated)
970 mg sodium
52 g carbohydrates
2 g fiber

The first ingredient is white rice, and shortly after it on the list are monosodium glutamate, hydrolyzed corn protein, and chicken fat.

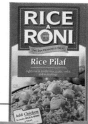

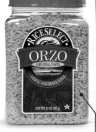

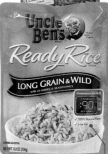

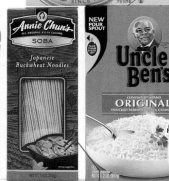

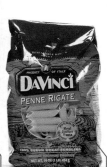

RiceSelect Orzo
(⅓ cup, 56 g dry)
210 calories
2 g fat (0 g saturated)
42 g carbohydrates
2 g fiber

Essentially, these are little nibs of refined pasta. You're far better off using a legitimate whole grain.

Uncle Ben's Ready Rice Long Grain & Wild
(1 cup cooked)
200 calories
0.5 g fat (0 g saturated)
42 g carbohydrates
1 g fiber

This grain performs poorly on the fiber scale, and no rice dish should ever have 650 milligrams of sodium in a serving.

Annie Chun's Soba Noodles
(57 g dry)
200 calories
1 g fat (0 g saturated)
39 g carbohydrates
3 g fiber

Japanese-style soba noodles tend to carry much more salt than Italian pasta noodles. A single serving of these packs 390 milligrams of sodium.

Uncle Ben's Original Rice
(¼ cup, 47 g dry)
170 calories
0 g fat
37 g carbohydrates
0 g fiber

Never eat rice, pasta, or other starchy sides unless they have fiber. Otherwise, they'll spike your blood sugar like a pile of candy.

DaVinci Penne Rigate
(56 g dry)
200 calories
1 g fat (0 g saturated)
41 g carbohydrates
2 g fiber

Healthier noodles are available in all shapes and sizes, so there's never a reason to settle for one that's high in calories and low in fiber, like this one is.

SAUCES

Eat This

La Choy Teriyaki Stir Fry Sauce & Marinade
(1 Tbsp)
10 calories
0 g fat
105 mg sodium
1 g sugars

The typical teriyaki sauce suffers from two blights: too much sodium and too much sugar. This one avoids both, which makes it by far the best teriyaki in the supermarket.

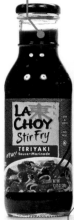

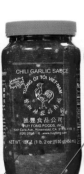

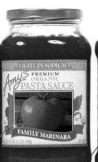

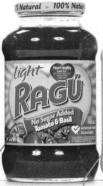

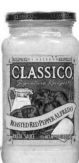

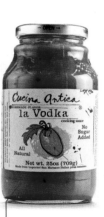

Huy Fong Chili Garlic Sauce
(1 tsp)
0 calories
0 g fat
115 mg sodium
<1 g sugars

Chili pepper is the primary ingredient, and it contains not a single gram of added sugar.

Amy's Light in Sodium Organic Family Marinara
(½ cup)
80 calories
4.5 g fat (0.5 g saturated)
290 mg sodium
5 g sugars

Stick with the low-sodium version. Amy's regular marinara has 290 milligrams more sodium.

Ragú Light No Sugar Added Tomato & Basil
(½ cup)
50 calories
0 g fat (0 g saturated)
320 mg sodium
6 g sugars

Think Italians add sugar to their marinara? Of course not—added sugars mask the naturally sweet flavor of cooked tomatoes.

Classico Roasted Red Pepper Alfredo
(½ cup)
120 calories
8 g fat (5 g saturated)
560 mg sodium
4 g sugars

Smart move: The roasted red peppers in this jar displace a heavy load of fatty cream and cheese calories.

Cucina Antica La Vodka (½ cup)
50 calories
3.5 g fat (2.5 g saturated)
220 mg sodium
2 g sugars

Cucina Antica gets the tomato-to-cream ratio right with this superlative sauce.

Not That!

La Choy Teriyaki Marinade and Sauce
(1 Tbsp)
40 calories
0 g fat
570 mg sodium
8 g sugars

If you end up with 2 tablespoons of this stuff on your plate, you'll be about to take in almost half your day's sodium and more sugar than you'd find in a scoop of Edy's Slow Churned Double Fudge Brownie Ice Cream.

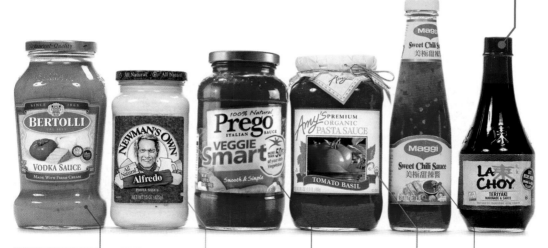

Bertolli Vodka Sauce (½ cup)
150 calories
9 g fat (4.5 g saturated)
700 mg sodium
8 g sugars

It's not the vodka you have to worry about, it's the belt-buckling triad of cream, oil, and sugar.

Newman's Own Alfredo (½ cup)
180 calories
16 g fat (9 g saturated)
820 mg sodium
2 g sugars

Worse Alfredo sauces exist, but that doesn't make Newman's a winner. One serving packs nearly half a day's sodium and saturated fat.

Prego Veggie Smart Smooth and Simple (½ cup)
70 calories
1.5 g fat (0 g saturated)
410 mg sodium
9 g sugars

Nice try, Prego, but the vegetable juice concentrates in this jar do more harm than good. Rule of marinara: Keep it simple.

Amy's Organic Tomato Basil (½ cup)
110 calories
6 g fat (1 g saturated)
580 mg sodium
6 g sugars

We applaud Amy's use of organic tomatoes, but 110 calories is just far too much for a tomato-based pasta sauce.

Maggi Sweet Chili Sauce (1 Tbsp)
35 calories
0 g fat
250 mg sodium
8 g sugars

The first two ingredients are sugar and water. That not only adds unnecessary calories, but also makes this sauce seem less spicy, meaning you'll need more to achieve the desired effect.

SOUPS

Eat This

V8 Tomato Herb
(1 cup)
90 calories
0 g fat
480 mg sodium
19 g carbohydrates
3 g fiber
3 g protein

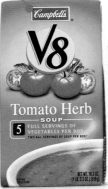

Carrots and red peppers are among the primary ingredients in this carton. That's how each serving earns you nearly half of your daily vitamin A requirement.

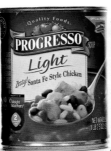

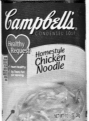

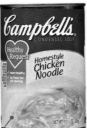

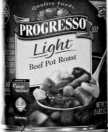

Campbell's Home Style Light Southwestern-Style Vegetable
(1 cup)
60 calories
0 g fat (0 saturated)
650 mg sodium
13 g carbohydrates
3 g fiber
2 g protein

One third of the calories come from fiber.

Progresso Light Zesty! Santa Fe Style Chicken (1 cup)
80 calories
1 g fat (0 g saturated)
460 mg sodium
10 g carbohydrates
2 g fiber
5 g protein

The black beans in this soup bolster the fiber content, plus add a shot of brain-boosting antioxidants.

Campbell's Healthy Request Condensed Homestyle Chicken Noodle
(1 cup prepared)
60 calories
1.5 g fat (0.5 g saturated)
410 mg sodium
10 g carbohydrates
1 g fiber
3 g protein

Low cal, light sodium.

Progresso Light Beef Pot Roast (1 cup)
80 calories
2 g fat (1 g saturated)
470 mg sodium
10 g carbohydrates
2 g fiber
7 g protein

There's a bounty of vegetation in this can, and it includes carrots, green beans, potatoes, tomatoes, celery, and peas.

Campbell's Chunky Grilled Steak Chili with Beans
(1 cup)
200 calories
3 g fat (1 g saturated)
870 mg sodium
27 g carbohydrates
7 g fiber
16 g protein

Campbell's Chunky Chili line is surprisingly lean—not one can tops 240 calories per serving.

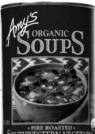

Not That!

Campbell's Slow Kettle Style Soup Tomato & Sweet Basil Bisque

(1 cup)
260 calories
14 g fat (8 g saturated)
750 mg sodium
30 g carbohydrates
3 g fiber
4 g protein

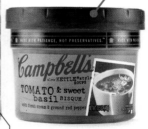

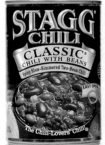

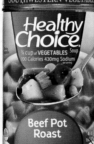

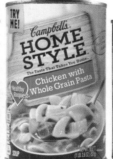

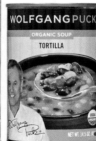

This soup contains as much sugar as 66 Chocolate Teddy Graham cookies.

Stagg Classic Chili with Beans

(1 cup)
330 calories
17 g fat (8 g saturated)
820 mg sodium
28 g carbohydrates
5 g fiber
17 g protein

Stagg should find a new beef purveyor. The meat in one serving packs 40 percent of your daily saturated fat.

Healthy Choice Beef Pot Roast

(1 cup)
100 calories
1 g fat (0 g saturated)
430 mg sodium
18 g carbohydrates
3 g fiber
6 g protein

Switch to Progresso's version and save 20 calories per serving.

Campbell's Homestyle Healthy Request Chicken with Whole Grain Pasta

(1 cup)
100 calories
2 g fat (0.5 g saturated)
410 mg sodium
13 g carbohydrates
1 g fiber
7 g protein

Where's the fiber?

Wolfgang Puck Organic Signature Tortilla Soup

(1 cup)
140 calories
3.5 g fat (1 g saturated)
680 mg sodium
21 g carbohydrates
6 g fiber
5 g protein

Organic, yes, but still loaded with excessive sugar and sodium.

255

BARS

Eat This
KIND Fruit & Nut Delight
(1 bar, 40 g)
200 calories
13 g fat (1.5 g saturated)
17 g carbohydrates
3 g fiber
9 g sugars
6 g protein

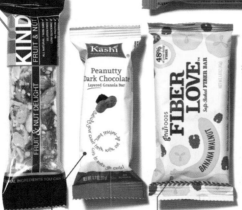

Lärabar Apple Pie
(1 bar, 45 g)
190 calories
10 g fat (1 g saturated)
5 mg sodium
24 g carbohydrates
5 g fiber
18 g sugars
4 g protein

Ordinarily 18 grams is too much sugar, but in Lärabar's case, every single gram comes directly from real fruit.

Here's a great trick for evaluating a bar. Add the fiber and protein grams together. The total should be equal to or greater than the sugar grams. KIND's mix of real fruit, nuts, and not much else makes it worth an extra 10 calories.

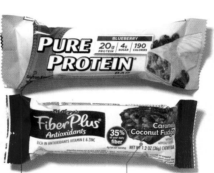

Kashi Layered Granola Bars Peanutty Dark Chocolate
(1 bar, 32 g)
130 calories
4.5 g fat (1 g saturated)
20 g carbohydrates
4 g fiber
7 g sugars
4 g protein

A fiber-and-protein-packed alternative to fix your candy bar cravings.

Gnu Foods Flavor & Fiber Banana Walnut Bar (1 bar, 36 g)
130 calories
4 g fat (3 g saturated)
26 g carbohydrates
9 g fiber
7 g sugars
2 g protein

Gnu builds its fruit-and-nut bars on a base of fiber-rich grains.

Pure Protein Greek Yogurt Blueberry
(1 bar, 50 g)
190 calories
4.5 g fat (2.5 g saturated)
19 g carbohydrates
2 g fiber
4 g sugars
20 g protein

This bar's ratio of protein to sugar is as good as you'll find anywhere in the supermarket.

Kellogg's Fiber Plus Antioxidants Caramel Coconut Fudge
(1 bar, 45 g)
140 calories
4 g fat (0 g saturated)
30 g carbohydrates
12 g fiber
8 g sugars
4 g protein

A hefty dose of fiber to quell your cravings.

Quaker Oatmeal to Go Apples with Cinnamon (1 bar, 60 g)

220 calories
4 g fat (1 g saturated)
200 mg sodium
44 g carbohydrates
5 g fiber
22 g sugars
4 g protein

There's far more sugar, brown sugar, and high-fructose corn syrup than apple.

Not That!

Nature Valley Crunchy Oats 'n Honey (2 bars, 42 g)

190 calories
6 g fat
(0.5 g saturated)
29 g carbohydrates
2 g fiber
12 g sugars
4 g protein

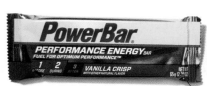

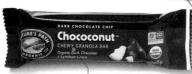

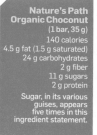

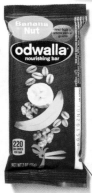

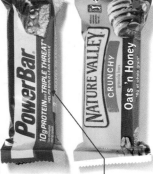

Nature's Path Organic Choconut (1 bar, 35 g)

140 calories
4.5 g fat (1.5 g saturated)
24 g carbohydrates
2 g fiber
11 g sugars
2 g protein

Sugar, in its various guises, appears five times in this ingredient statement.

PowerBar Performance Energy Vanilla Crisp (1 bar, 57 g)

240 calories
3.5 g fat (0.5 g saturated)
45 g carbohydrates
1 g fiber
26 g sugars
8 g protein

Four kinds of sugar make this "performance" bar sweeter than a Kit Kat.

Odwalla Bar Banana Nut (1 bar, 56 g)

220 calories
5 g fat (0.5 g saturated)
39 g carbohydrates
5 g fiber
17 g sugars
4 g protein

Don't be duped by "brown rice syrup," the first ingredient in this bar. It's a euphemism for sugar.

PowerBar Triple Threat Caramel Peanut Fusion (1 bar, 45 g)

230 calories
9 g fat (4.5 g saturated)
31 g carbohydrates
3 g fiber
15 g sugars
10 g protein

The main components of this "Power" bar are caramel and "chocolate coating."

This bar has twice as much sugar as it does fiber and protein combined. That makes it a great example of the sort of snack you want to avoid.

CRACKERS

Eat This

Wheat Thins Fiber Selects Garden Vegetable (15 crackers, 30 g)

120 calories
4 g fat (0 g saturated)
240 mg sodium
21 g carbohydrates
5 g fiber

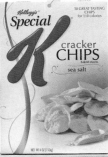

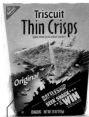

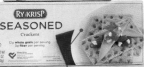

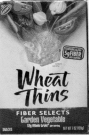

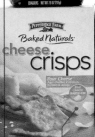

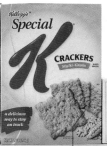

The primary ingredient here is whole-wheat flour, which is precisely what you want. The extra fiber—a form of oat fiber that Nabisco adds to this Fiber Selects line—is just a bonus.

Nabisco Triscuit Thin Crisps Original (15 crackers, 30 g)

130 calories
4.5 g fat (0.5 g saturated)
170 mg sodium
21 g carbohydrates
3 g fiber

You can't beat the purity of this recipe: whole wheat, oil, and salt. Period.

Pepperidge Farm Baked Naturals Cheese Crisps Four Cheese (20 pieces, 30 g)

140 calories
6 g fat (1 g saturated)
270 mg sodium
19 g carbohydrates
1 g fiber

A touch of fiber and real cheese save this cracker.

Special K Multi-Grain Crackers (24 crackers, 30 g)

120 calories
3 g fat (0 g saturated)
220 mg sodium
23 g carbohydrates
3 g fiber

This is as few calories as you can reasonably expect in a serving of whole-grain crackers.

RyKrisp Seasoned Crackers (2 crackers, 14 g)

60 calories
1 g fat (0 g saturated)
90 mg sodium
11 g carbohydrates
3 g fiber

Prevention of gallstones is among the many benefits of foods high in insoluble fiber.

Not That!

Ritz Roasted Vegetable (10 crackers, 32 g)

160 calories
7 g fat (2 g saturated)
300 mg sodium
20 g carbohydrates
0 g fiber

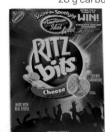

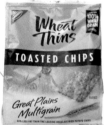

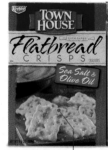

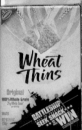

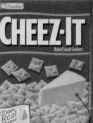

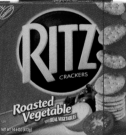

*As the name
suggests, this
box contains
a handful of
dehydrated
vegetables.
The problem
is, the main
ingredient is
still refined
flour, and it's
bogged down
with hydroge-
nated oils and
high-fructose
corn syrup.*

**Keebler Town
House Flatbread
Crisps Sea Salt
& Olive Oil**
(16 crackers, 30 g)
140 calories
4 g fat (0 g saturated)
280 mg sodium
22 g carbohydrates
<1 g fiber

The 4 grams of fat here
come from soybean oil.

**Nabisco Wheat
Thins Original**
(16 crackers, 31 g)
140 calories
5 g fat (1 g saturated)
230 mg sodium
22 g carbohydrates
3 g fiber

Wheat Thins rely heavily
on refined grains, which
means less protein and
fiber in each serving.

**Sunshine
Cheez-It Original**
(27 crackers, 30 g)
150 calories
8 g fat (2 g saturated)
230 mg sodium
17 g carbohydrates
<1 g fiber

Cheez-Its' lack of fiber
prevents these crackers
from having a meaning-
ful impact on hunger.
If you're going to snack,
do so smartly.

**Nabisco
Ritz Bits
Sandwiches
Cheese**
(13 pieces, 31 g)
160 calories
9 g fat (3 g saturated)
160 mg sodium
18 g carbohydrates
0 g fiber

Soiled with sugar and
partially hydrogenated
cottonseed oil.

259

CHIPS

Eat This

Lay's Oven Baked Original Potato Crisps

(18 crisps, 1 oz)
120 calories
2 g fat
(0 g saturated)
135 mg sodium

Snyder's of Hanover Braided Twists Multigrain
(8 twists, 30 g)
120 calories
2 g fat (0 g saturated)
160 mg sodium

The 3 grams of fiber in each serving make this a respectable snack.

Chex Mix Bold Party Blend
(½ cup, 29 g)
120 calories
3.5 g fat (0.5 g saturated)
200 mg sodium

The "bold" blend, surprisingly, is lower in sodium than some of the other Chex mixes.

Popchips Barbeque Potato
(20 chips, 1 oz)
120 calories
4 g fat (0 g saturated)
200 mg sodium

More crunch than a baked chip, yet less fat than a fried chip.

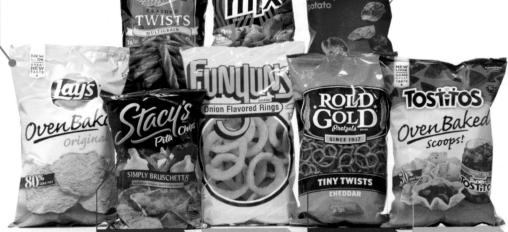

Baked chips don't rely on oil to crisp up, which means they can get by with far less fat. If you eat just one 1-ounce bag a week, you'll shed more than 2 pounds this year by choosing Lay's Baked! instead of Ruffles Reduced Fat.

Stacy's Pita Chips Simply Bruschetta
(9 chips, 1 oz)
130 calories
5 g fat (0.5 g saturated)
190 mg sodium

Delivers a respectable 3 grams of protein per serving.

Funyuns
(13 rings, 1 oz)
130 calories
6 g fat (1 g saturated)
280 mg sodium

Funyuns inflict surprisingly little damage by novelty snack standards.

Rold Gold Tiny Twists Cheddar
(20 pretzels, 1 oz)
110 calories
1 g fat (0 g saturated)
490 mg sodium

We wish Rold Gold would take it easy with the salt, but you won't find a lower-calorie cheese snack in the snack aisle.

Tostitos Oven Baked Scoops!
(16 chips, 1 oz)
120 calories
3 g fat (0.5 g saturated)
140 mg sodium

This is the healthiest salsa-shoveling device on the shelf.

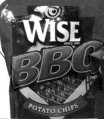
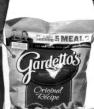
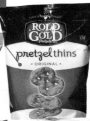

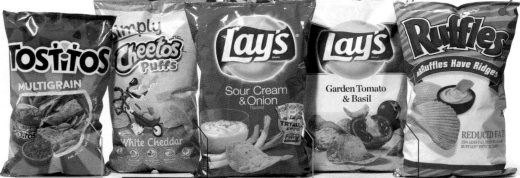

If you could stick Ruffles and its ilk under a hot iron to smooth out the ridges, you'd realize that each chip is actually much bigger than it seems. Avoid the portion distortion by sticking to chips that are already flat.

DIPS & SPREADS

Eat This

Newman's Own Mild Salsa
(2 Tbsp, 32 g)
10 calories
0 g fat
65 mg sodium

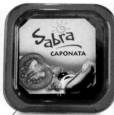

Athenos Hummus Original
(2 Tbsp, 27 g)
50 calories
3 g fat (0 g saturated)
160 mg sodium

Made with real olive oil, which lends an authentic flavor and more heart-healthy fats.

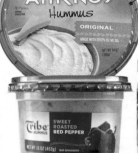

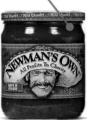

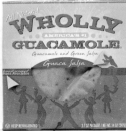

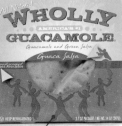

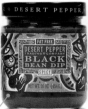

We balked when Ronald Reagan tried to turn ketchup into a vegetable, but if someone did the same for salsa, a legitimate nutritional superpower, we'd throw our support behind it.

Wholly Guacamole Guaca Salsa
(2 Tbsp, 30 g)
35 calories
3 g fat (0 g saturated)
110 mg sodium

Avocados are the first of only seven ingredients, all of which you likely keep stocked in your kitchen.

Tribe Hummus Sweet Roasted Red Peppers
(2 Tbsp, 28 g)
50 calories
3 g fat (0 g saturated)
125 mg sodium

Based on chickpeas and tahini, hummus makes for an incredible vegetable dip and sandwich spread.

Desert Pepper Black Bean Dip Spicy
(2 Tbsp, 31 g)
25 calories
0 g fat
240 mg sodium

This jar contains a trio of nutritional A-listers: black beans, tomatoes, and green bell peppers.

Sabra Caponata
(2 Tbsp, 28 g)
30 calories
2.5 g fat (0 g saturated)
140 mg sodium

Built from potent Mediterranean produce like eggplants and tomatoes, this dip is perfect for dressing up chicken or fish or spreading on a pita.

Sabra Roasted Pine Nut Hummus
(2 Tbsp, 28 g)
80 calories
6 g fat (1 g saturated)
130 mg sodium

Instead of the traditional olive oil, Sabra's ingredient statement lists "soybean and/or canola oil."

Not That!
Herdez Salsa Casera Mild
(2 Tbsp, 31 g)
5 calories
0 g fat
240 mg sodium

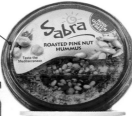

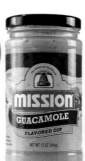

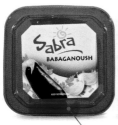

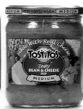

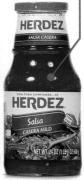

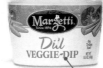

Be on the watch for elevated sodium in salsa. Combined with some salty chips, you could easily approach half a day's sodium intake.

Sabra Babaganoush
(2 Tbsp, 28 g)
70 calories
7 g fat (1 g saturated)
180 mg sodium

Babaganoush traditionally gets its creaminess from tahini and roasted eggplant, but Sabra cheats by loading its version with mayonnaise.

Tostitos Zesty Bean & Cheese Dip Medium
(2 Tbsp, 33 g)
45 calories
2 g fat (0.5 g saturated)
230 mg sodium

Contains more than 25 ingredients, including corn oil, monosodium glutamate, DATEM, and two artificial shades of yellow.

Marzetti Dill Veggie Dip
(2 Tbsp, 30 g)
110 calories
12 g fat (3 g saturated)
170 mg sodium

This dip is mostly sour cream. The veggies you see on the package? You'll have to supply those yourself.

Mission Guacamole Flavored Dip
(2 Tbsp, 32 g)
30 calories
2 g fat (1 g saturated)
130 mg sodium

"Flavored" is the key word. This imposter is made mostly of water, oil, and cornstarch. Oh, and less than 2 percent real avocado.

263

DRESSINGS

Eat This

Bolthouse Farms Yogurt Dressing Chunky Blue Cheese
(2 Tbsp, 30 g)

35 calories
2.5 g fat (1 g saturated)
135 mg sodium

Bolthouse Farms casts yogurt as the star in classic flavors such as ranch, honey mustard, Thousand Island, and blue cheese, allowing you to swap out vegetable oil for worthwhile hits of calcium and probiotic bacteria.

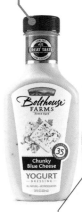

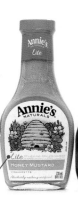

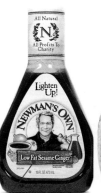

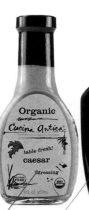

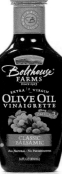

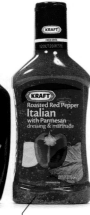

Annie's Naturals Lite Honey Mustard Vinaigrette
(2 Tbsp, 31 g)
40 calories
3 g fat (0 g saturated)
125 mg sodium

After water, mustard is the main ingredient, a surprising rarity among honey mustard dressings.

Newman's Own Lite Low Fat Sesame Ginger
(2 Tbsp, 30 g)
35 calories
1.5 g fat (0 g saturated)
330 mg sodium

Relegates oil to a supporting role so that vinegar, soy sauce, and ginger can drive the flavor.

Cucina Antica Organic Caesar Dressing
(2 Tbsp, 30 g)
80 calories
8 g fat (1 g saturated)
190 mg sodium

A touch of Romano cheese, not an excess of cheap oil, supplies rich flavor for a fraction of the fat.

Bolthouse Farms Classic Balsamic Olive Oil Vinaigrette
(2 Tbsp, 30 g)
30 calories
0 g fat
150 mg sodium

The lightest vinaigrette we've ever come across. Just another reason why Bolthouse is one of our favorite producers.

Kraft Roasted Red Pepper Italian with Parmesan
(2 Tbsp, 32 g)
40 calories
2 g fat (0 g saturated)
349 mg sodium

The bulk of this bottle is filled with vinegar and tomato puree, a huge improvement over the typical oil-based formula.

Kraft Roka Blue Cheese
(2 Tbsp, 29 g)
120 calories
13 g fat (2 g saturated)
290 mg sodium

Virtually every calorie in this bottle comes from soybean oil, which is a common theme in the dressing aisle. Consider them wasted calories; soybean oil doesn't have the same heart-healthy cachet as olive or canola oil.

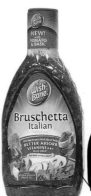
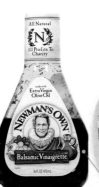
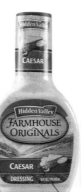
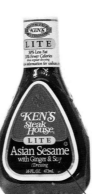
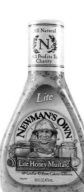
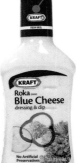

Wish-Bone Bruschetta Italian
(2 Tbsp, 30 ml)
60 calories
5 g fat (1 g saturated)
340 mg sodium

The front label boasts about olive oil, but the ingredient statement reveals that it accounts for less than 2 percent of the recipe.

Newman's Own Balsamic Vinaigrette
(2 Tbsp, 30 g)
90 calories
9 g fat (1 g saturated)
290 mg sodium

Save cash and calories by making your own vinaigrette at home: Mix two parts olive oil with one part balsamic, plus salt and pepper.

Hidden Valley Farmhouse Originals Caesar
(2 Tbsp, 30 ml)
120 calories
11 g fat (1.5 g saturated)
220 mg sodium

Hidden in this valley, you'll find MSG and propylene glycol, an ingredient also found in anti-freeze. We don't remember those from any farm.

Ken's Steak House Lite Asian Sesame with Ginger and Soy
(2 Tbsp, 30 g)
70 calories
4 g fat (0.5 g saturated)
390 mg sodium

After water, sugar is the first ingredient in this bottle, which is why each serving packs 7 grams of the sweet stuff.

Newman's Own Lite Honey Mustard Dressing
(2 Tbsp, 30 g)
70 calories
4 g fat (0.5 g saturated)
280 mg sodium

Keep in mind that "light" is a relative term.

265

COOKIES

Eat This

Newman's Own Newman-Os Chocolate Créme Filled Chocolate
(2 cookies, 27 g)

120 calories
5 g fat (1.5 g saturated)
85 mg sodium
10 g sugars

Compared with Oreo, Newman takes a moderate approach to oil and sugar.

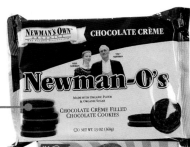

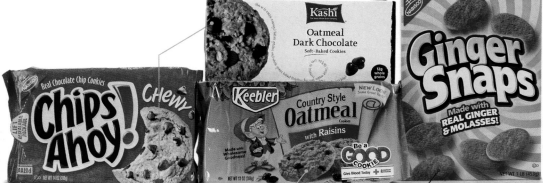

Chips Ahoy! Chewy
(2 cookies, 31 g)
140 calories
6 g fat (3 g saturated)
95 mg sodium
12 g sugars

This cookie is the best of the Chips Ahoy! line, and a surprisingly low-calorie treat for how indulgent it seems.

Kashi Oatmeal Dark Chocolate Soft-Baked Cookies (1 cookie, 30 g)
130 calories
5 g fat (1.5 g saturated)
65 mg sodium
8 g sugars

Thanks to oats, rye, barley, and buckwheat, Kashi's cookie has more fiber (4 grams) than a standard slice of whole-wheat bread.

Keebler Country Style Oatmeal with Raisins
(2 cookies, 28 g)
140 calories
6 g fat (2 g saturated)
100 mg sodium
8 g sugars

Raisins will always trump chocolate chips or candy pieces as a cookie mix-in.

Nabisco Ginger Snaps
(4 cookies, 28 g)
120 calories
2.5 g fat (0 g saturated)
190 mg sodium
11 g sugars

Eating a handful of small cookies instead of one regular cookie is a good strategy—it can help you feel like you're eating more than you actually are.

Not That!

Nabisco Chocolate Crème Oreo
(2 cookies, 29 g)
140 calories
6 g fat (2 g saturated)
100 mg sodium
13 g sugars

Regular Oreos are even worse—they deliver an extra gram of sugar and 20 extra calories per serving.

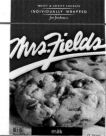

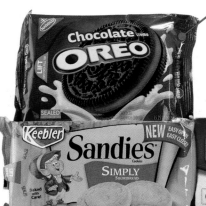

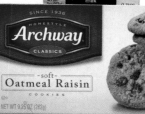

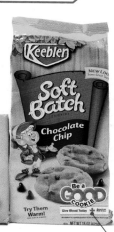

Keebler Sandies Simply Shortbread
(2 cookies, 31 g)
160 calories
9 g fat (4 g saturated)
90 mg sodium
7 g sugars

We love the low sugar count, but not the heavy deposits of soybean and palm oils.

Archway Classics Soft Oatmeal Raisin
(2 cookies, 66 g)
280 calories
9 g fat (4 g saturated)
170 mg sodium
24 g sugars

Add just one of these 140-calorie cookies to your daily diet and you'll gain nearly 15 pounds this year.

Mrs. Fields Milk Chocolate Chip
(1 cookie, 32 g)
140 calories
7 g fat (3.5 g saturated)
125 mg sodium
12 g sugars

The dearth of fiber ensures that this will pass straight through your belly, spike your blood sugar, and convert quickly to flab.

Keebler Soft Batch Chocolate Chip
(2 cookies, 32 g)
150 calories
7 g fat (3 g saturated)
110 mg sodium
12 g sugars

This cookie has more fat, more sodium, and more sugar than the same cookie from Chips Ahoy!

CANDY BARS

Eat This

Pretzel M&M's
(1 bag, 32 g)
150 calories
4.5 g fat (3 g saturated)
17 g sugars

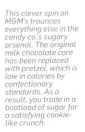

This clever spin on M&M's trounces everything else in the candy co.'s sugary arsenal. The original milk chocolate core has been replaced with pretzel, which is low in calories by confectionary standards. As a result, you trade in a boatload of sugar for a satisfying cookie-like crunch.

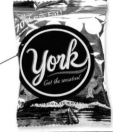

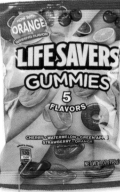

Hershey's Kit Kat
(1 package, 42 g)
210 calories
11 g fat (7 g saturated)
21 g sugars

The wafer core is light and porous, which saves you calories over the denser bars.

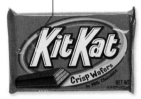

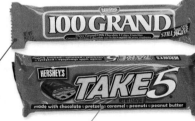

York Peppermint Pattie (1 patty, 39 g)
140 calories
2.5 g fat (1.5 g saturated)
25 g sugars

For a smaller treat, go with York Miniatures. You can have three for about the same number of calories.

Life Savers Gummies
(10 pieces, 42 g)
130 calories
0 g fat
25 g sugars

The secret to the chew: gelatin. Starburst uses the same trick, but spoils it with a strange mix of oils.

Nestlé 100 Grand
(1 package, 43 g)
190 calories
8 g fat (5 g saturated)
22 g sugars

This is an Eat This, Not That! Hall of Famer, routinely beating out more common chocolate bars by 80 or more calories.

Hershey's Take 5
(1 package, 42 g)
210 calories
11 g fat (5 g saturated)
18 g sugars

The pretzel core saves you a boatload of calories.

Nestlé Butterfinger
(1 bar, 60 g)
270 calories
11 g fat (6 g saturated)
29 g sugars

Nobody better lay a finger on this Butterfinger.

Not That!
Milk Chocolate M&M's
(1 bag, 48 g)
240 calories
10 g fat (6 g saturated)
30 g sugars

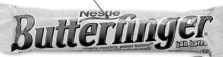

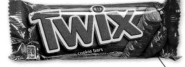

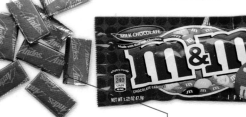

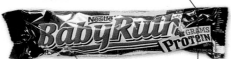

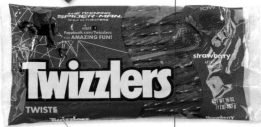

M&M's pack in a lot of sugar even by candy-bar standards. This little bag is loaded with more sweetness than two Little Debbie Chocolate Marshmallow Pies.

Nestlé Baby Ruth
(1 bar, 60 g)
280 calories
14 g fat (8 g saturated)
33 g sugars

Together, saturated fat and sugar account for more than 200 of the calories in this package.

Mars Twix Caramel
(1 package, 51 g)
250 calories
12 g fat (7 g saturated)
24 g sugars

This sticky situation contains nearly as much saturated fat as two Snickers bars.

Twizzlers Twists Strawberry
(4 pieces, 45 g)
160 calories
0.5 g fat (0 g saturated)
19 g sugars

You could have 40 real strawberries for the same number of calories.

Andes Thins Crème de Menthe
(8 pieces, 40 g)
220 calories
14 g fat (13 g saturated)
22 g sugars

This is one of the worst candies in the supermarket. The first two ingredients are sugar and partially hydrogenated oil.

FROZEN BREAKFAST ENTRÉES

Eat This

Jimmy Dean Delights Turkey Sausage Breakfast Bowl (1 bowl, 198 g)

240 calories
8 g fat (3.5 g saturated)
720 mg sodium
19 g carbohydrates
2 g fiber
22 g protein

An ideal breakfast includes a substantial load of protein, and this bowl has that nailed. Protein accounts for 40 percent of the calories, which increases your odds of making it to lunch without snacking.

Amy's Black Beans & Tomatoes Breakfast Burrito
(1 burrito, 170 g)
270 calories
8 g fat (1 g saturated)
540 mg sodium
38 g carbohydrates
6 g fiber
12 g protein

Black beans are one of the healthiest foods on the planet.

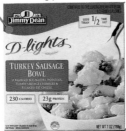

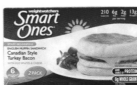

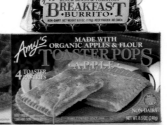

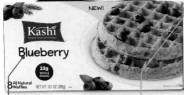

Kashi Blueberry Waffles
(2 waffles, 72 g)
150 calories
5 g fat (0.5 g saturated)
340 mg sodium
25 g carbohydrates
6 g fiber
4 g protein

Blueberries figure prominently in these first-rate waffles, explaining the huge hit of fiber.

Weight Watchers Smart Ones Smart Beginnings Canadian Style Turkey Bacon English Muffin Sandwich
(1 sandwich, 113 g)
210 calories
6 g fat (2.5 g saturated)
510 mg sodium
27 g carbohydrates
2 g fiber
13 g protein

This is a lean protein machine.

Kashi 7 Grain Waffles
(2 waffles, 72 g)
150 calories
5 g fat (0.5 g saturated)
340 mg sodium
25 g carbohydrates
7 g fiber
4 g protein

The most fiber-packed waffles in the freezer.

Amy's Toaster Pops Apple
(1 pastry, 2.11 oz)
160 calories
3.5 g fat (0 g saturated)
110 mg sodium
29 g carbohydrates
2 g fiber
4 g protein

The thinking parent's smarter Pop Tart.

Evol Egg & Potato Burrito (1 burrito, 170 g)
330 calories
13 g fat (5 g saturated)
340 mg sodium
43 g carbohydrates
2 g fiber
11 g protein

Evol makes some decent burritos, but this isn't one of them. It features more potatoes than eggs.

More than 150 of these calories are carbohydrates, which is not how you want to start your day.

Not That!
Lean Pockets Sausage, Egg & Cheese (1 piece, 127 g)
270 calories
9 g fat (4 g saturated)
380 mg sodium
37 g carbohydrates
0 g fiber
11 g protein

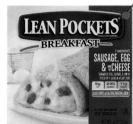

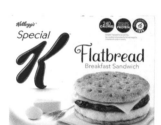

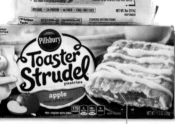

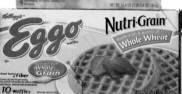

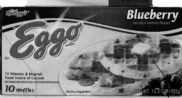

Pillsbury Apple Toaster Strudel (1 pastry, 54 g)
180 calories
7 g fat (3 g saturated)
180 mg sodium
26 g carbohydrates
<1 g fiber
2 g protein

This has half the protein and fiber of Amy's version.

Kellogg's Eggo Nutri-Grain Whole Wheat Waffles (2 waffles, 70 g)
170 calories
6 g fat (1.5 g saturated)
400 mg sodium
26 g carbohydrates
3 g fiber
5 g protein

There are better fiber-rich waffles to be had.

Kellogg's Special K Flatbread Breakfast Sandwich Sausage Egg & Cheese (1 sandwich, 116 g)
240 calories
11 g fat (4 g saturated)
820 mg sodium
20 g carbohydrates
3 g fiber
14 g protein

The ingredients list is a novel.

Kellogg's Eggo Blueberry Waffles (2 waffles, 70 g)
180 calories
6 g fat (1.5 g saturated)
370 mg sodium
29 g carbohydrates
<1 g fiber
4 g protein

Blueberries are the 11th ingredient on the list.

FROZEN PIZZAS

Eat This

Kashi Stone-Fired Thin Crust Pizza Mushroom Trio & Spinach (⅓ pie, 113 g)

150 calories
9 g fat (4.5 g saturated)
660 mg sodium
28 g carbohydrates
4 g fiber
14g protein

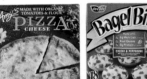

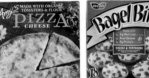

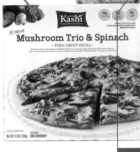

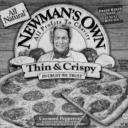

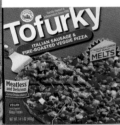

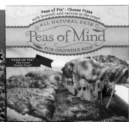

This pie features more pesto than cheese, which means you end up with more mono-unsaturated fat from olive oil than saturated fat from dairy. That's a healthy swap.

Amy's Cheese
(1 pie, 167 g)
420 calories
17 g fat (6 g saturated)
720 mg sodium
49 g carbohydrates
3 g fiber
18 g protein

For the rare times when you allow yourself the privilege of eating a whole pizza, this is exactly where you should turn.

Newman's Own Thin & Crispy Uncured Pepperoni
(⅓ pie, 125 g)
320 calories
16 g fat (6 g saturated)
800 mg sodium
31 g carbohydrates
1 g fiber
15 g protein

Newman's skips the nitrates and nitrites with its pepperoni.

Tofurky Italian Sausage & Fire Roasted Veggie
(⅓ pie, 132 g)
270 calories
6 g fat (1 g saturated)
320 mg sodium
40 g carbohydrates
5 g fiber
13 g protein

Tofurky's lactose-free "cheese" is made using protein, flour, and oils.

Peas of Mind Cheese
(⅓ pie, 109 g)
240 calories
5 g fat (2 g saturated)
510 mg sodium
36 g carbohydrates
2 g fiber
11 g protein

They snuck broccoli and carrots into the crust. Clever devils!

Michelina's Lean Gourmet Pepperoni Pizza Snackers
(11 pieces, 85 g)
200 calories
8 g fat (1.5 g saturated)
290 mg sodium
26 g carbohydrates
2 g fiber
7 g protein

Nitrites and soybean oil, but not much good stuff.

Not That!

Amy's Whole Wheat Crust Cheese & Pesto (⅓ pie, 132 g)
360 calories
18 g fat (4 g saturated)
680 mg sodium
37 g carbohydrates
4 g fiber
13 g protein

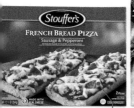

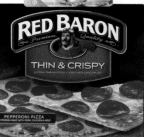

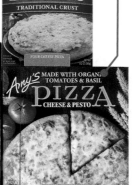

Stouffer's French Bread Sausage & Pepperoni
(2 pieces, 177 g)
460 calories
24 g fat (8 g saturated)
880 mg sodium
43 g carbohydrates
4 g fiber
17 g protein

One contains the saturated fat of 16 Burger King Chicken Tenders.

Amy's Roasted Vegetable No Cheese
(⅓ pie, 113 g)
280 calories
9 g fat (1.5 g saturated)
540 mg sodium
42 g carbohydrates
3 g fiber
7 g protein

For the lactose intolerant, there are options closer to the real thing.

Red Baron Thin & Crispy Pepperoni Pizza
(⅓ pie, 149 g)
400 calories
19 g fat (9 g saturated)
1,020 mg sodium
41 g carbohydrates
2 g fiber
15 g protein

Even the Baron's thin-crust pies pack too much of the bad stuff.

DiGiorno Traditional Crust Four Cheese
(1 pie, 260 g)
350 calories
15 g fat (6 g saturated,)
590 mg sodium
42 g carbohydrates
2 g fiber
13 g protein

These personal pies are undone by thick crusts and excess cheese.

The crust is the least nutritious part of any pie, and unfortunately, Amy's is just a little bit too thick.

FROZEN PASTA ENTRÉES

Eat This

Kashi Chicken Pasta Pomodoro (1 entrée, 283 g)

280 calories
6 g fat (1.5 g saturated)
470 mg sodium
38 g carbohydrates
6 g fiber
19 g protein

Small savings in everyday choices is the key to sustainable weight loss. A simple savings of 20 calories every day adds up to 2 pounds a year. That's 20 pounds over the course of a decade.

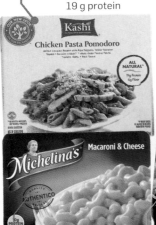

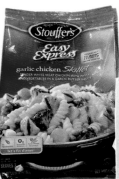

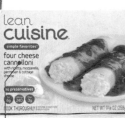

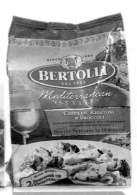

Michelina's Macaroni & Cheese
(1 package, 213 g)
250 calories
6 g fat (2.5 g saturated)
500 mg sodium
38 g carbohydrates
1 g fiber
9 g protein
Diffuse the comfort food's flab-producing potential by opting for this light rendition.

Stouffer's Easy Express Garlic Chicken Skillet
(326 g, ½ package)
330 calories
6 g fat (2.5 g saturated)
990 mg sodium
45 g carbohydrates
5 g fiber
24 g protein
Budding chefs, take note: The more vegetables you use, the less sauce and pasta you'll need.

Lean Cuisine Four Cheese Cannelloni
(1 package, 258 g)
230 calories
6 g fat (3 g saturated)
690 mg sodium
33 g carbohydrates
3 g fiber
11 g protein
Swap out white sauce for red sauce and you'll save a few hundred calories per serving every time.

Bertolli Mediterranean Style Chicken, Rigatoni & Broccoli
(½ package, 340 g)
400 calories
16 g fat (4 g saturated)
860 mg sodium
44 g carbohydrates
4 g fiber
20 g protein
After pasta, the first two ingredients are broccoli and chicken.

Smart Ones Three Cheese Ziti Marinara (1 entrée, 255 g)

300 calories
8 g fat (3 g saturated)
510 mg sodium
45 g carbohydrates
7 g fiber
13 g protein

Marinara is typically the safest of the pasta sauces, but that rule fails to hold as soon as Smart Ones buries the plate under a rubbery quilt of cheese.

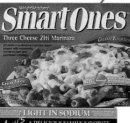

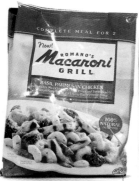

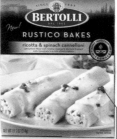

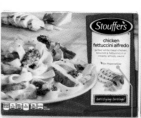

Romano's Macaroni Grill Creamy Basil Parmesan Chicken & Pasta (½ package, 340 g)

470 calories
21 g fat (12 g saturated)
1,040 mg sodium
42 g carbohydrates
4 g fiber
29 g protein

Romano takes a heavy-handed approach with cream, as demonstrated by the exorbitant glut of saturated fat in this dish.

Bertolli Rustico Bakes Ricotta & Spinach Cannelloni (1 meal, 314 g)

500 calories
28 g fat (17 g saturated)
1,290 mg sodium
41 g carbohydrates
5 g fiber
21 g protein

These noodles are stuffed with cheese and covered with cream, plus more than half a day's allotment of salt.

Stouffer's Chicken Fettuccini Alfredo (1 package, 297 g)

570 calories
27 g fat (7 g saturated)
850 mg sodium
55 g carbohydrates
5 g fiber
26 g protein

Alfredo sauce contains any of the following: oil, butter, cheese, cream, and egg yolk. In other words, it's a full-fat assault.

Amy's Light in Sodium Macaroni & Cheese (1 entrée, 255 g)

400 calories
16 g fat (10 g saturated)
290 mg sodium
47 g carbohydrates
3 g fiber
16 g protein

We've seen worse mac out there, but Amy's packages its pasta as a healthy alternative to the normal stuff, and we're just not buying it.

FROZEN FISH ENTRÉES

Eat This

Gorton's Grilled Fillets Cajun Blackened
(1 fillet, 101 g)

90 calories
3 g fat
(0.5 g saturated)
400 mg sodium
15 g protein

The smoky, spicy finesse of a blackening rub can imbue any fillet with massive flavor at no caloric cost. It's easily one of the healthiest ways to prepare meat and fish.

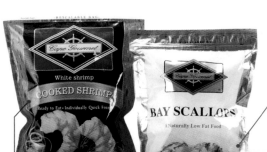

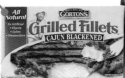
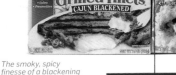

Cape Gourmet Bay Scallops
(4 oz)
150 calories
1 g fat (0 g saturated)
155 mg sodium
29 g protein

Scallops are teeming with the amino acid tryptophan, which bolsters feelings of well-being and helps regulate the sleep cycle.

Cape Gourmet Cooked Shrimp
(3 oz)
50 calories
0.5 g fat
330 mg sodium
10 g protein

Unadulterated shrimp are among the leanest sources of protein on the planet.

Margaritaville Island Lime Shrimp
(6 shrimp, 4 oz)
240 calories
11 g fat (3 g saturated)
330 mg sodium
12 g protein

These shrimp have also been tossed in butter. The difference is quantity; here it's a light bath, but in SeaPak's scampi it's a tidal wave.

SeaPak Salmon Burgers
(1 burger, 91 g)
110 calories
5 g fat (1 g saturated)
340 mg sodium
16 g protein

Toss this on the grill, then sandwich it between a toasted bun with arugula, grilled onions, and Greek yogurt spiked with olive oil, garlic, and fresh dill.

Gourmet Dining Shrimp Stir Fry
(¼ package, 198 g)
200 calories
1 g fat (0 g saturated)
640 mg sodium
12 g protein

American interpretations of Asian cuisine tend to be high in sodium, but this solid blend of fiber and protein more than makes up for it.

Not That!
Van de Kamp's Crunchy Fish Fillets
(2 fillets, 99 g)
230 calories
13 g fat
(4.5 g saturated)
440 mg sodium
8 g protein

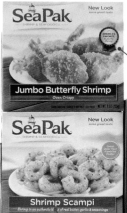

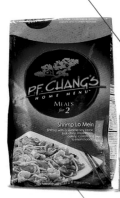

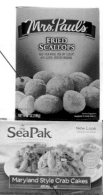

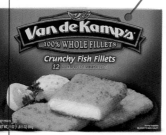

You know what makes the breading crunchy? The same thing that makes it 150 percent more caloric and 267 percent fattier: oil.

P.F. Chang's Home Menu Shrimp Lo Mein
(½ package, 312 g)
390 calories
12 g fat (1.5 g saturated)
740 mg sodium
16 g protein

Chang's sauce is polluted with three kinds of oil.

SeaPak Maryland Style Crab Cakes
(1 crab cake with 1 oz sauce, 113 g)
240 calories
13 g fat (1.5 g saturated)
830 mg sodium
11 g protein

These crab cakes deliver more starchy filler than actual shellfish. Somewhere, a Marylander is shaking his head.

SeaPak Shrimp Scampi
(6 shrimp, 113 g)
340 calories
31 g fat (12 g saturated)
480 mg sodium
12 g protein

Shrimp are essentially pure protein, so it's puzzling to find that protein accounts for just 13 percent of this entrée's calories.

SeaPak Jumbo Butterfly Shrimp
(4 shrimp, 84 g)
230 calories
11 g fat (2 g saturated)
480 mg sodium
10 g protein

Each shrimp delivers more than 50 calories, and nearly half of that comes from unnecessary fats.

FROZEN CHICKEN ENTRÉES

Eat This

Evol Bowls Teriyaki Chicken
(1 bowl, 255 g)
260 calories
3 g fat (0 g saturated)
560 mg sodium
43 g carbohydrates
3 g fiber
14 g protein

Evol's teriyaki bowl is made with brown rice, free-range chicken, and enough produce to meet 90 percent of your day's vitamin A needs.

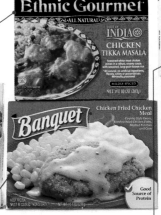

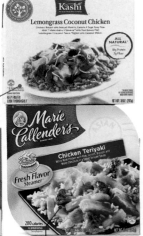

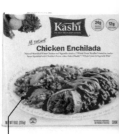

Ethnic Gourmet Chicken Tikka Masala
(1 package, 283 g)
260 calories
6 g fat (2 g saturated)
680 mg sodium
32 g carbohydrates
3 g fiber
19 g protein

The sauce is created with fat-free yogurt, for a low-calorie creaminess.

Banquet Chicken Fried Chicken Meal
(1 entrée, 286 g)
350 calories
17 g fat (4 g saturated)
930 mg sodium
35 g carbohydrates
5 g fiber
12 g protein

Thinner breading and better sides save you 90 calories over Banquet's "premium" version.

Kashi Lemongrass Coconut Chicken
(1 entrée, 283 g)
300 calories
8 g fat (4 g saturated)
680 mg sodium
38 g carbohydrates
7 g fiber
18 g protein

Instead of the standard white rice, this meal rests on a blend of oats, wheat, and quinoa.

Marie Callender's Fresh Flavor Steamer Chicken Teriyaki
(1 meal, 283 g)
280 calories
3.5 g fat (1 g saturated)
890 mg sodium
44 g carbohydrates
3 g fiber
17 g protein

The wealth of veggies keeps the calories low.

Kashi Chicken Enchilada
(1 entrée)
280 calories
9 g fat (2.5 g saturated)
620 mg sodium
6 g fiber
12 g protein

Kashi's blend of whole grains makes these corn tortillas surprisingly healthy.

Not That!

Healthy Choice Pineapple Chicken
(1 entrée, 280 g)

300 calories
5 g fat (1 g saturated)
510 mg sodium
46 g carbohydrates
5 g fiber
18 g protein

This bowl contains more sugar than protein—19 grams of sugar, in fact, more than you'd find in a scoop of Breyers Chocolate Ice Cream.

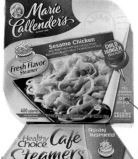

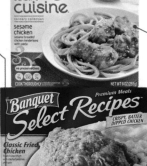

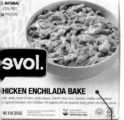

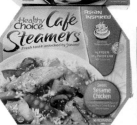

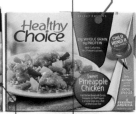

Evol Chicken Enchilada Bake
(1 bowl, 255 g)
380 calories
13 g fat (6 g saturated)
630 mg sodium
46 g carbohydrates
6 g fiber
21 g protein

Make this kind of simple mistake once a day, and that 100 calories adds up to 11 pounds a year.

Healthy Choice Café Steamers Sweet Sesame Chicken
(1 meal, 276 g)
280 calories
7 g fat (1.5 g saturated)
520 mg sodium
31 g carbohydrates
5 g fiber
21 g protein

Packs as much sugar as a two-pack of Twix Peanut Butter.

Marie Callender's Fresh Flavor Steamer Sesame Chicken (1 meal, 291 g)
400 calories
12 g fat (2 g saturated)
710 mg sodium
54 g carbohydrates
5 g fiber
18 g protein

A chicken dish shouldn't be a festival of fat and carbohydrates.

Banquet Select Recipes Classic Fried Chicken Meal
(1 entrée, 228 g)
440 calories
26 g fat (6 g saturated, 1.5 g trans)
1,140 mg sodium
30 g carbohydrates
4 g fiber
22 g protein

Never settle for a frozen dinner with trans fats.

Lean Cuisine Sesame Chicken
(1 package, 255 g)
330 calories
9 g fat (1 g saturated)
650 mg sodium
47 g carbohydrates
2 g fiber
16 g protein

There's nothing lean about breaded chicken tossed with 14 grams of sugar.

FROZEN BEEF ENTRÉES

Eat This

Stouffer's Homestyle Classics
Beef Pot Roast (1 entrée, 251 g)

320 calories
8 g fat (3 g saturated)
1,570 mg sodium
41 g carbohydrates
8 g fiber
20 g protein

In the world of frozen entrées, there's always some sacrifice involved. In this case, we'll take the elevated salt count rather than the trans fats—and double our fiber and protein in the process.

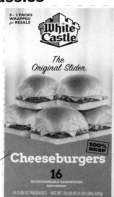

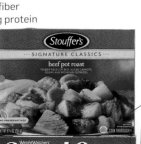

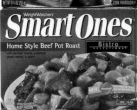

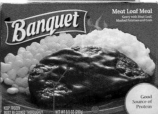

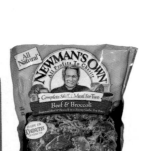

Smart Ones Homestyle Beef Pot Roast
(1 meal, 255 g)
190 calories
6 g fat (2.5 g saturated)
590 mg sodium
18 g carbohydrates
3 g fiber
16 g protein

Most protein bars can't deliver this dose for so few calories. Tack on 3 grams of fiber and you have an amazing 190-calorie package.

White Castle Microwaveable Cheeseburgers
(2 burgers, 104 g)
310 calories
17 g fat (8g saturated)
600 mg sodium
26 g carbohydrates
1 g fiber
14 g protein

With decent at-home nutritionals, Harold and Kumar have less to worry about than ever.

Banquet Meat Loaf Meal
(1 meal, 269 g)
280 calories
13 g fat (5 g saturated)
1,000 mg sodium
28 g carbohydrates
4 g fiber
12 g protein

When it comes to delivering comfort dishes for a reasonable number of calories, Banquet's regular line of entrées is among the best in the freezer.

Newman's Own Beef & Broccoli Complete Skillet Meal
(½ package, 250 g)
250 calories
10 g fat (3 g saturated)
800 mg sodium
22 g carbohydrates
5 g fiber
19 g protein

The first ingredient in this bag is broccoli. In the cost-conscious world of processed foods, that's exceedingly rare.

A potpie crust is essentially an oversized pastry, which is to say lots of carbohydrates glued together with saturated and trans fat.

Not That!

Banquet Beef Pot Pie (1 pie, 198 g)

390 calories
22 g fat (9 g saturated, 0.5 g trans)
1,010 mg sodium
36 g carbohydrates
3 g fiber
12 g protein

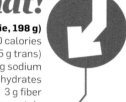

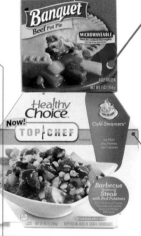

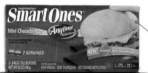

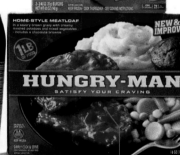

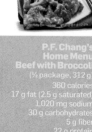

P.F. Chang's Home Menu Beef with Broccoli

(½ package, 312 g)
360 calories
17 g fat (2.5 g saturated)
1,020 mg sodium
30 g carbohydrates
5 g fiber
22 g protein

Chang's bagged meals suffer from the same sodium saturation that plagues its restaurant fare.

Hungry-Man Home-Style Meatloaf

(1 package, 454 g)
660 calories
35 g fat (12 g saturated)
1,660 mg sodium
61 g carbohydrates
5 g fiber
26 g protein

Word of advice to the calorie conscious: Purge Hungry-Man from your freezer for good. This is consistently the worst brand in the frozen-foods aisle.

Smart Ones Smart Anytime Mini Cheeseburgers

(2 mini-burgers, 140 g)
380 calories
16 g fat (6 g saturated)
720 mg sodium
42 g carbohydrates
6 g fiber
18 g protein

There's a lot of bun around these burgers, with nearly twice the carbs as White Castle.

Healthy Choice Café Steamers Barbecue Seasoned Steak with Red Potatoes

(1 meal, 269 g)
260 calories
3.5 g fat (1 g saturated)
470 mg sodium
39 g carbohydrates
6 g fiber
17 g protein

More fat, calories and sugar than the Smart Ones pot roast.

FROZEN SIDES, SNACKS &

Eat This

Ore-Ida Steak Fries (7 fries, 84 g)

110 calories
3 g fat (0.5 g saturated)
290 mg sodium
19 g carbohydrates
2 g protein

A serving of these hulking spuds contains fewer than half the calories you'd find in the average medium order of fast-food fries.

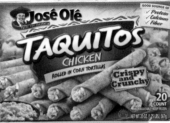

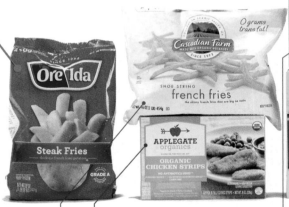

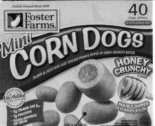

Cascadian Farm Shoe String French Fries
(3 oz, 85 g)
110 calories
5 g fat (1 g saturated)
10 mg sodium
17 g carbohydrates
2 g protein

Cascadian Farm tosses these fries in apple juice, the sugar from which caramelizes into a crisp, golden crust.

Applegate Organics Organic Chicken Strips
(3 strips, 84 g)
170 calories
8 g fat (1 g saturated)
350 mg sodium
12 g carbohydrates
12 g protein

The relatively light breading makes Applegate's strips less fatty than the competition's.

José Olé Chicken Taquitos Rolled in Corn Tortillas
(3 pieces, 85 g)
200 calories
8 g fat (1.5 g saturated)
390 mg sodium
26 g carbohydrates
7 g protein

These taquitos win by virtue of their little corn sleeping bags, which are lower in fat than flour tortillas.

Foster Farms Mini Corn Dogs Honey Crunchy
(4 dogs, 76 g)
210 calories
12 g fat (3.5 g saturated)
490 mg sodium
18 g carbohydrates
7 g protein

At only 53 calories per dog, the damage potential here is relatively low.

APPETIZERS

Not That!

Ore-Ida Sweet Potato Straight Fries (22 fries, 84 g)

A raw sweet potato has more fiber and vitamin A than a raw russet potato, but once the food industry starts plowing fat into the produce, all bets are off.

160 calories
8 g fat (0.5 g saturated)
160 mg sodium
21 g carbohydrates
1 g protein

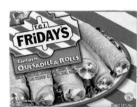

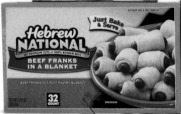

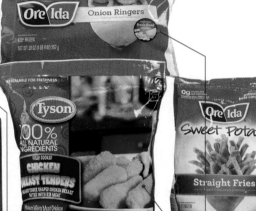

Hebrew National Beef Franks in a Blanket
(5 pieces, 81 g)
300 calories
24 g fat (8 g saturated, 3 g trans)
680 mg sodium
12 g carbohydrates
8 g protein

You shouldn't consume this much trans fat in an entire day, let alone from a snack.

T.G.I. Friday's Chicken Quesadilla Rolls
(2 pieces, 83 g)
230 calories
10 g fat (3 g saturated, 1 g trans)
470 mg sodium
27 g carbohydrates
9 g protein

Frozen flour tortillas are little trans-fat delivery systems.

Tyson Chicken Breast Tenders
(4 pieces, 80 g)
190 calories
12 g fat (2.5 g saturated)
420 mg sodium
12 g carbohydrates
9 g protein

There's a big difference between "organic," a regulated term, and "natural," which means nothing. In this case, that difference is worth an extra dose of fat and sodium.

Ore-Ida Onion Ringers
(3 pieces, 81 g)
180 calories
10 g fat (2 g saturated)
160 mg sodium
21 g carbohydrates
2 g protein

Each ring harbors more than 3 grams of fat. Fries are almost always the better choice.

ICE CREAMS

Eat This

Breyers Black Raspberry Chocolate
(1/2 cup, 67 g)
140 calories
4 g fat (3 g saturated)
16 g sugars

The secret to a low-calorie ice cream is simple: Lead off with something lighter than cream. This one uses regular milk first and cream last.

Häagen-Dazs Chocolate Sorbet
(½ cup, 105 g)
130 calories
0.5 g fat (0 g saturated)
21 g sugars

One of the few Häagen-Dazs products that we can actually stand behind.

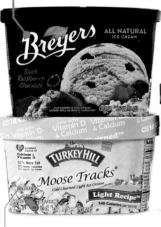

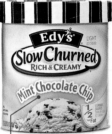

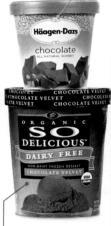

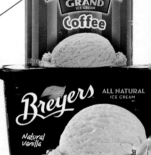

Turkey Hill Light Recipe Moose Tracks
(½ cup, 61 g)
140 calories
6 g fat (2.5 g saturated)
15 g sugars

Swirled ice cream flecked with chocolate peanut butter cups—you won't find a more decadent dessert with fewer calories.

Edy's Slow Churned Mint Chocolate Chip
(½ cup, 60 g)
120 calories
4.5 g fat (3 g saturated)
35 mg sodium
13 g sugars

Edy's Slow Churned line leans more heavily on milk than cream, which keeps the calories in check.

So Delicious Chocolate Velvet
(½ cup, 81 g)
130 calories
3.5 g fat (0.5 g saturated)
14 g sugars

So Delicious cuts the fat without needing to make up for it with an extra hit of sugar.

Edy's Rich & Creamy Grand Coffee
(½ cup, 65 g)
140 calories
7 g fat (4 g saturated)
13 g sugars

Careful—it's made with real coffee, so it's not the best choice right before bed.

Breyers Natural Vanilla
(½ cup, 66 g)
130 calories
7 g fat (4 g saturated)
14 g sugars

Breyers Natural has earned our allegiance for both its low-calorie concoctions and the simplicity of its ingredient statements.

Not That!

Ben & Jerry's FroYo Cherry Garcia Frozen Yogurt
(1/2 cup, 108 g)
200 calories
3 g fat (2 g saturated)
27 g sugars

You buy frozen yogurt thinking you're doing your body a favor, only to find out it's worse than three-quarters of the full-fat ice creams in the freezer. Thanks, Ben & Jerry's.

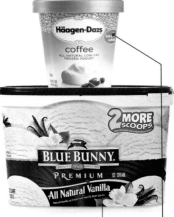
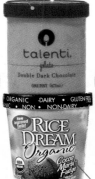
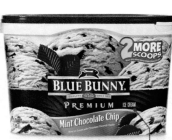
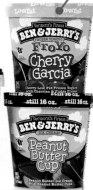

Blue Bunny Premium All Natural Vanilla
(⅓ cup, 69 g)
150 calories
9 g fat (5 g saturated)
16 g sugars

The All Natural line is the worst among the many Blue Bunny vanilla ice creams.

Häagen-Dazs Low Fat Frozen Yogurt Coffee
(⅓ cup, 102 g)
180 calories
2.5 g fat (1 g saturated)
21 g sugars

Leave it to Häagen-Dazs to find a way to mess up frozen yogurt.

Rice Dream Organic Cocoa Marble Fudge
(⅓ cup, 90 g)
170 calories
6 g fat (0.5 g saturated)
17 g sugars

Rice Dream adds vegetable oils to create a high-cal approximation of ice cream.

Blue Bunny Mint Chocolate Chip
(⅓ cup, 67 g)
160 calories
8 g fat (6 g saturated)
15 g sugars

Not terrible, but just north of the calorie and fat counts you want in your ice cream.

Ben & Jerry's Peanut Butter Cup
(⅓ cup, 112 g)
350 calories
24 g fat (13 g saturated)
25 g sugars

Eat two scoops of this and you'll take in more calories than you would with a McDonald's McDouble with a small side of french fries.

FROZEN TREATS

Eat This

Snicker's Ice Cream Bar (1 bar, 49 g)

180 calories
11 g fat (6 g saturated)
15 g sugars

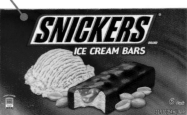

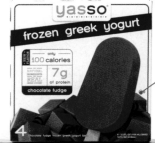

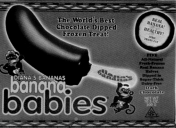

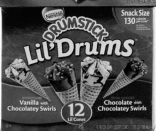

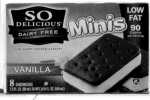

Yasso Frozen Greek Yogurt Chocolate Fudge Bar
(1 bar, 70 g)
100 calories
0 g fat (0 g saturated)
13 g sugars

A classy upgrade to the standard Fudgsicle, this frozen treat delivers 7 grams of belly-filling protein.

As decadent as it may seem, the Snicker's Ice Cream Bar has less fat, sugar, and total calories than an actual Snicker's candy bar.

Nestlé Drumstick Lil' Drums Vanilla with Chocolatey Swirls
(1 cone, 43 g)
110 calories
5 g fat (3.5 g saturated)
10 g sugars

The perfect portion for an after-dinner indulgence.

Diana's Bananas Banana Babies Dark Chocolate
(1 piece, 60 g)
130 calories
6 g fat (3.5 g saturated)
14 g sugars

Banana, chocolate, and peanut oil. You don't find a frozen treat with a simpler recipe.

So Delicious Minis Vanilla
(1 sandwich, 40 g)
90 calories
2 g fat (0.5 g saturated)
8 g sugars

Low in sugar and overall calories, this is a good treat to keep in mind even if you're not lactose intolerant.

Breyers CarbSmart Ice Cream Bar Vanilla
(1 bar, 58 g)
180 calories
14 g fat (10 g saturated)
6 g sugars

Sure it's "carb smart," but it's also sat-fat dumb.

Not That!

Häagen-Dazs Vanilla Milk Chocolate Almond Snack Size (1 bar, 52 g)
195 calories
24.5 g fat (7 g saturated)
11.5 g sugars

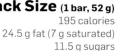

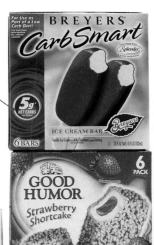

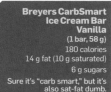

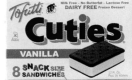

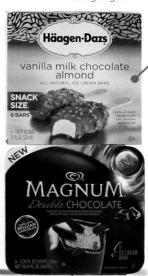

Tofutti Cuties Vanilla
(1 sandwich, 38 g)
130 calories
6 g fat (1 g saturated)
17 g carbohydrates
9 g sugars

Made mostly of sugar, corn syrup solids, and vegetable oils. Tofu plays a mere supporting role.

Good Humor Strawberry Shortcake
(1 bar, 83 g)
230 calories
10 g fat (3.5 g saturated)
17 g sugars

This bar does contain real strawberries, but it contains even more sugar, corn syrup, palm oil and food coloring.

Magnum Double Chocolate
(1 bar, 83 g)
340 calories
21 g fat (15 g saturated)
29 g sugars

If the Magnum is your go-to dessert, you could swap in the Snicker's each night and you'd save more than 16 pounds in a year!

Cream is the first ingredient, which is how it packs 40 percent of your day's saturated fat into each bar.

JUICES

DrinkThis

Lakewood Organic Lemonade
(8 fl oz)

80 calories
0 g fat
16 g sugars

This drink is sweetened with grape juice instead of sugar.

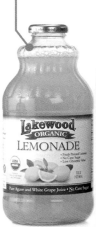

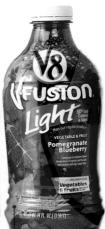

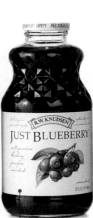

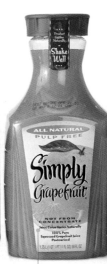

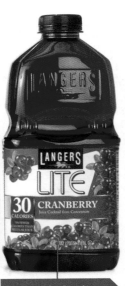

V8 V-Fusion Light Pomegrante Blueberry
(8 fl oz)
50 calories
0 g fat
10 g sugars

Every calorie in this bottle comes from the blend of sweet potatoes, carrots, apples, pomegranates, and blueberries.

R.W. Knudsen Just Blueberry
(8 fl oz)
100 calories
0 g fat
19 g sugars

Blueberries are bursting with brain-boosting antioxidants, and R.W. Knudsen's juice is the only one to give you 100 percent blueberries.

Simply Grapefruit
(8 fl oz)
100 calories
0 g fat
25 g sugars

Grapefruit is the most under-rated juice in the cooler. It's delicious, it's naturally low in sugar, and it delivers a dose of cancer-fighting lycopene.

Langers Lite Cranberry
(8 fl oz)
30 calories
0 g fat
8 g sugars

Cranberries make for a tart juice, which is why you routinely see 15 or more grams of sugar added to each serving. Langers Lite keeps it simple.

Not That!
Simply Lemonade
(8 fl oz)
120 calories
0 g fat
28 g sugars

Contains only 11 percent juice. The rest of the bottle is pure sugar water. Most lemonades follow the same disappointing formula.

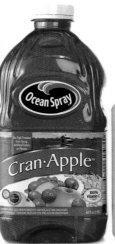

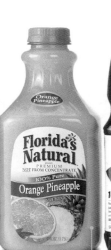

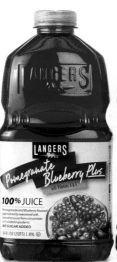

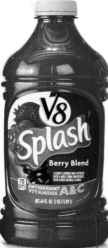

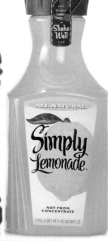

Ocean Spray Cran-Apple
(8 fl oz)
120 calories
0 g fat
31 g sugars

This bottle, like so many in Ocean Spray's lineup, contains only 15 percent juice. Water and sugar are the first two ingredients.

Florida's Natural 100% Pure Orange Pineapple
(8 fl oz)
130 calories
0 g fat
30 g sugars

It's hard to find fault with 100-percent juice products, but blends like this tend to pack in too much sugar.

Langers Pomegranate Blueberry Plus
(8 fl oz)
140 calories
0 g fat
30 g sugars

There's more sugar in this bottle than there are blueberries or pomegranates.

V8 Splash Berry Blend
(8 fl oz)
70 calories
0 g fat
16 g sugars

Splash is unfit to carry the V8 brand name. It's made with artificial colors, high-fructose corn syrup, and a pathetic 5 percent juice.

TEAS & FLAVORED WATERS

DrinkThis

Honest Tea
Community Green Tea
(16 fl oz)
34 calories
0 g fat
10 g sugars

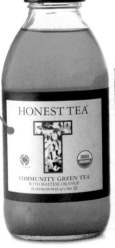

High in antioxidants and low in sugar, Honest Tea is one of the most reliable brands in any cooler.

HONEST TEA

COMMUNITY GREEN TEA
WITH MALTESE ORANGE
16 FLUID OUNCES 475 mL

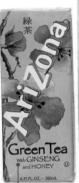

緑茶

AriZona

Green Tea
with GINSENG
and HONEY

6.75 FL. OZ. • 200mL

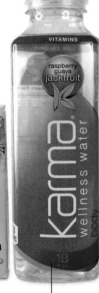

VITAMINS

raspberry
guava
jackfruit

karma
wellness water
body

18
fl oz

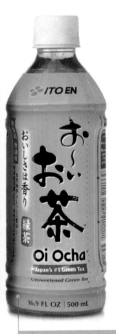

ITO EN

お～いお茶

おいしさは香り

緑茶

Oi Ocha

Japan's #1 Green Tea

Unsweetened Green Tea

16.9 FL OZ | 500 mL

AriZona Green Tea with Ginseng and Honey
(8 fl oz)
70 calories
0 g fat
17 g sugars
This is one of the few AriZona drinks worth purchasing. The generous size and better ingredients list gives it the narrow edge over Ssips.

Karma Wellness Water Raspberry Guava Jackfruit
(18 fl oz)
20 calories
0 g fat
2 g sugars
Pushing the cap releases a vitamin powder lightly sweetened with stevia and cane sugar. Makers claim this mixing method ensures potency. We just like the low sugar count.

ITO EN Oi Ocha Unsweetened Green Tea
(16.9 fl oz)
0 calories
0 g fat
0 g sugars
Researchers believe green tea plays a prominent role in the long life spans of the Japanese. ITO EN is the most popular tea in Japan.

Not That!

Tazo Organic Iced Green Tea

(14 fl oz)

120 calories
0 g fat
30 g sugars

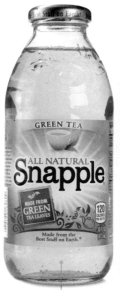

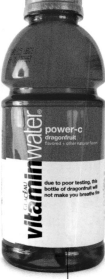

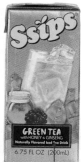

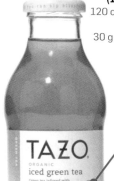

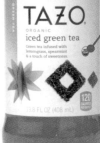

A lot of things that are organic aren't necessarily good for you, and sugar is one of them.

Snapple Green Tea

(16 fl oz)
120 calories
0 g fat
30 g sugars

Catechins found in green tea can boost metabolism, but whatever metabolic boost you find in this bottle is more than offset by the sugar rush.

Vitaminwater Power-C Dragonfruit Flavored

(20 fl oz)
120 calories
0 g fat
31 g sugars

Getting your daily dose of vitamin C shouldn't cost you the sugar equivalent of 13 Jolly Ranchers.

Ssips Green Tea with Honey & Ginseng

(6.75 fl oz)
60 calories
0 g fat
12 g sugars

The honey in the name is just a diversionary tactic. Much of the sweetness here comes from high-fructose corn syrup, which is the second ingredient on the list. Either way, skip it.

MIXERS

Drink This

Stirrings Simple Cosmopolitan Mix
(3 fl oz)
60 calories
0 g fat
16 g sugars

Made with real cranberry and key lime juices—a rarity in the world of mixers.

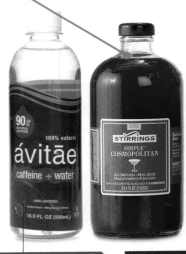

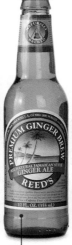

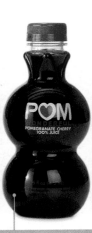

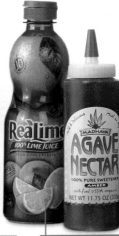

Ávitae Caffeine + Water
(16.9 fl oz)
0 calories
0 g fat
0 g sugars

This club soda will give you the caffeine boost of Red Bull, just without all the sugar.

Reed's Premium
Ginger Brew
(12 fl oz)
145 calories
0 g fat
37.4 g sugars

Ginger beer is made with a larger dose of ginger than ginger ale, which means more of a kick and more of ginger's anti-inflammatory properties.

Pom Wonderful
100% Juice
Pomegranate Cherry
(4 fl oz)
75 calories
0 g fat
14.5 g sugars

These are natural sugars, which means you get nutrients, too.

ReaLime 100% Lime
Juice (3 Tbsp)
Madhava Agave Nectar
(1 Tbsp)
60 calories
0 g fat
15 g sugars

This is how real margaritas are made, with fresh lime juice and a hint of sugar.

Not That!

Mr and Mrs T Strawberry Daiquiri-Margarita Mix

Mostly high-fructose corn syrup and food coloring—enough to spoil any good drink.

(4 fl oz)
190 calories
0 g fat
44 g sugars

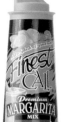

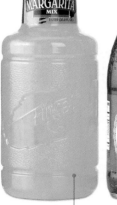

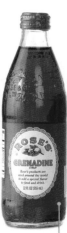

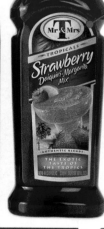

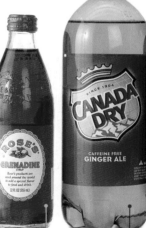

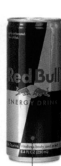

Finest Call Premium Margarita Mix
(4 fl oz)
160 calories
0 g fat
38 g sugars

Real margaritas don't contain corn-based sweeteners or artificial colors. Consider this the crutch of the amateur.

Rose's Grenadine
(2 Tbsp)
80 calories
0 g fat
20 g sugars

Looks fruity. Tastes fruity. Yet in truth, there's not a shred of fruit in this syrupy cocktail staple.

Canada Dry Ginger Ale
(12 fl oz)
138 calories
0 g fat
36 g sugars

Better for you than 7Up or Sprite because Canada Dry also contains real ginger. Still, we prefer the stronger stuff.

Red Bull
(8.4 fl oz)
110 calories
0 g fat
27 g sugars

Be cautious when mixing alcohol with energy drinks. Research has shown people drinking both tend to underestimate their level of intoxication.

293

BEERS

Drink This
Guinness Draught
(11.2 fl oz)
125 calories
10 g carbs
4% alcohol

For our money, Guinness Draught has the best flavor-to-calorie ratio in the cooler.

Keystone Premium
(12 fl oz)
111 calories
5.8 g carbs
4.4% alcohol

Make this swap with a six-pack a week and you'll save more than 3 pounds a year.

Amstel Light
(12 fl oz)
95 calories
5 g carbs
3.5% alcohol

One of our favorite light beers, precisely because it doesn't taste like one.

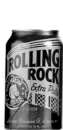
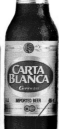
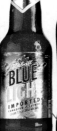
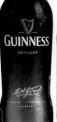
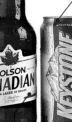
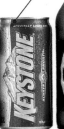
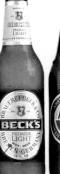
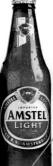
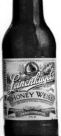

Rolling Rock
(12 fl oz)
130 calories
9.8 g carbs
4.5% alcohol

A first-rate session beer: crisp, refreshing, and surprisingly gentle in the calorie and carb departments.

Carta Blanca
(12 fl oz)
128 calories
11 g carbs
4% alcohol

Perfect for a Michelada, one of Mexico's most popular drinks: Combine in a glass with a squeeze of lime, a dash of Worcestershire, and a few hits of hot sauce.

Labatt Blue Light
(11.5 fl oz)
108 calories
8 g carbs
4% alcohol

Both Labatt and Michelob deliver more robustly flavored light beers. Labatt just does so for fewer calories.

Molson Canadian
(12 fl oz)
148 calories
11 g carbs
5% alcohol

In the North American showdown, Canada wins out by a 45-calorie margin.

Beck's Premier Light
(12 fl oz)
64 calories
3.9 g carbs
3.2% alcohol

Among the lightest beers in the world, Beck's surprises by actually tasting like, well, beer.

Leinenkugel's Honey Weiss
(12 fl oz)
149 calories
12 g carbs
4.9% alcohol

Honey- and fruit-based beers tend to come with high calorie counts, so choose your weapon wisely.

Bass
(12 fl oz)
156 calories
12 g carbs
5.1% alcohol

English-style ales tend to pack on the calories, and Bass, among the most famous of all ales, is no exception.

Pabst Blue Ribbon
(12 fl oz)
144 calories
13 g carbs
4.7% alcohol

PBR has become a throwback favorite of the hipster crowd in recent years, which doesn't bode well for the bellies of America's young drinkers.

Not That!
Guinness Extra Stout
(12 fl oz)
176 calories
14 g carbs
6% alcohol

Mix up these two popular Guinness varieties and it could cost you 10 pounds or more over the course of a year if you drink just one a day.

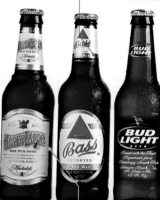
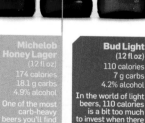
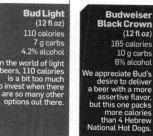
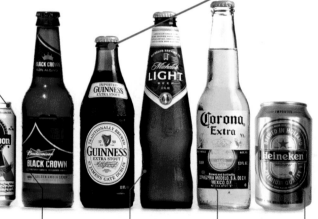

Michelob Honey Lager
(12 fl oz)
174 calories
18.1 g carbs
4.9% alcohol

One of the most carb-heavy beers you'll find in the cooler.

Bud Light
(12 fl oz)
110 calories
7 g carbs
4.2% alcohol

In the world of light beers, 110 calories is a bit too much to invest when there are so many other options out there.

Budweiser Black Crown
(12 fl oz)
165 calories
10 g carbs
6% alcohol

We appreciate Bud's desire to deliver a beer with a more assertive flavor, but this one packs more calories than 4 Hebrew National Hot Dogs.

Michelob Light
(12 fl oz)
123 calories
9 g carbs
4.1% alcohol

The heaviest light beer in the cooler. A bottle of Guinness Draught has just 2 calories more.

Corona Extra
(12 fl oz)
148 calories
14 g carbs
4.6% alcohol

For a beer that doesn't taste like much, it sure comes with plenty of calories.

Heineken
(12 fl oz)
135 calories
10 g carbs
5% alcohol

It's one of the world's best-selling beers, but for 135 calories a can, we'd expect a lot more flavor.

Chapter 6

LITTLE KIDS VERSUS BIG FOOD

Our children are the targets of a junk-food campaign. Arm them to fight back!

Let's say a new toy store opened in town, and it had a marvelous array of fascinating gadgets and gizmos that dazzled your eye and that of your towheaded toddler at prices that fit comfortably within your family budget. Sounds great, right?

Now, what if it turned out that more than one in every three toys you bought there was completely broken? The Rock 'Em Sock 'Em Robots couldn't rock or sock, the Mr. Potato Heads were total lemons, and the Barbies all came with Lady Gaga's wardrobe. You'd never shop there again.

Well, when it comes to feeding our children, your local supermarket and fast-food joint have track records that are just as awful. More than a third of the foods our kids are consuming are utterly broken and useless. One study found that nearly 40 percent of the calories eaten by kids are empty calories. For a 9-year-old boy consuming 1,400 calories a day, that's equivalent to 19 Starburst candies every single day of the week.

Now, getting kids to eat anything remotely nutritious is often a tug-of-war, and not one you can win through will and force alone. Indeed, the best thing to do is not to fight at all. Instead, do what the smartest parents do: cheat, dupe, deceive, dissemble, falsify, beguile, fabricate, prevaricate, exaggerate, and if that doesn't work, then just lie. Trix may be for kids, but tricks are for parents. Use these tactics to fool your kids into eating right, and you'll set them up for a lifetime of health and happiness.

Get 'Em Early

Half of all obese children became overweight when they were still in preschool, according to a 2014 study in the *New England Journal of Medicine*. In fact, by the time they enter kindergarten, 12.4 percent of American children are already obese, and another 14.9 percent are overweight. Childhood obesity is associated with an increased risk of diabetes, hypertension, heart disease, and liver disease, and by the time they enter adolescence, kids with higher body mass indexes (BMIs) experience a 30 percent higher rate of death as young or middle-aged adults.

Play Psychologist with Your Kid

Nowadays, kids avoid vegetables like they're out-of-style sneakers; only one in five of them actually eats enough plant matter. If you want to reverse that trend, a little scheming can go a long way. Research out of England found that using "exposure therapy"—giving children a taste of a new vegetable daily for two weeks—increased their enjoyment and consumption of that food. And give them a little personal power: Simply letting your children choose their vegetables can lead to an 80 percent increase in their consumption.

Never Skip Breakfast. Ever.

"Don't skip breakfast" is the persistent platitude heard 'round the world. Which may explain why so few pay attention—especially children. Yet studies show that kids skipped breakfast more than any other meal despite its reign as the king of meals. The effects of this epidemic are by now well known. Test after test shows that breakfast-eating students score higher on short-term memory and verbal fluency, among many other academic benefits.

Maybe breakfast's most important contribution, however, is found not in its own nutritional value, but in its impact on the rest of the day's eating habits. Research says children eating a meal in the morning will themselves choose less soda and fewer fries while opting for more vegetables and milk throughout the rest of the day.

We know time can be an issue in the chaos of the early-morning hours. But a nutritious bowl of cereal, cup of yogurt, or even microwaveable breakfast is never more than a few minutes away. Check out the dozens of smart swaps in the coming pages.

Ground the Helicopter, Parents

Whether it's a Clean Plate Club membership drive or castigations about starving Africans, efforts by parents to get their children to eat healthy foods can backfire. In a 2013 study published in the journal *Pediatrics*, researchers found that between 30 and 40 percent of parents encourage their kids to continue eating even after they are full, while up to 60 percent say they require their child to eat all of the food on their plate at a meal. The researchers advise that pressuring your child to eat more takes away from his or her ability to respond to internal signals of hunger and satiety, leading to overeating later in life.

Shrink Your Silverware

According to a study from Cornell, portion size is the most powerful predictor of how much preschool-age children eat. And with the typical manufacturers' snack package being 2.5 times bigger than the appropriate amount for young kids, health-conscious parents fight an uphill battle.

Control what you can. Splitting a dish with a sibling is never a bad idea (as long as you ask for two toys). At home, use smaller bowls, plates, and utensils. Jedi mind trick or not, there's plenty of evidence that kids will consume fewer calories when you downsize the dishes.

Set an Example (Especially You, Dad)

The portion of America's food dollars spent on meals out increased from 34 percent to 48 percent between 1974 and 2012. Parents' increasing penchant for restaurant food can translate to nutritionally unsound decisions by kids. One recent study laid the heaviest blame on fathers. Researchers at Texas A&M University say dads carry the most influence largely because when they take their kids to Mickey D's, it's often as a treat or some sort of celebration. This enforces the idea that unhealthy eating is positive. Mothers, on the other hand, often choose fast food due to time constraints, so the food doesn't hold as much psychological sway.

Feed Them Like Grown-Ups

No, we don't mean giving them steak knives and red wine. But more and more it seems like food companies are being reckless when it comes to the health of our children. Yale researchers reported recently that child-targeted cereals have 57 percent more sugar and 52 percent less fiber than cereals marketed to adults. And restaurant kids' meals are often fattier and more caloric by weight than adult portions (as you'll see in the coming pages). In many cases, you're better off giving them a small portion of your own meal than ordering them one of their own.

Turn Off the Tube

Since 1970, the number of television ads aimed at children has doubled to 40,000 per year, and several studies suggest that the amount of time kids watch television is a strong predictor of how often they request specific foods. This spells big trouble for one reason: Half of all TV ads directed at children promote junk food.

The solution is simple: Shove your kids outside. Surprise them with a bike, a soccer ball, a Chihuahua dog—anything to get them moving. More time spent outdoors means less time being exposed to television marketing. Of course, the larger benefit is that they get more exercise, which decreases the risk of a lot of bad stuff: obesity, diabetes, heart disease, even boredom.

Linger at the Table

We've become so trained to snarf down our food quickly that we forget to celebrate the simple act of eating together. And the consequences of that are measureable. In a 2014 study from *Pediatrics*, researchers found that families with healthy-weight children spent about 18 minutes, on average, eating dinner each night. Families of overweight kids, on the other hand, spent just 13.5 minutes together at the table.

And healthy eating is like real estate: location, location, location. Eighty percent of healthy-weight kids typically ate dinner with their parents at the kitchen table, compared to just 55 percent of overweight kids. More families of overweight children tended to eat in the family room, office, or bedroom.

20 WORST FOODS FOR CHILDREN

The world can be a scary place for a kid.

You've got bogeymen hiding in the closet, overbearing teachers pelting you with homework, and mean girls telling the world you've got cooties. But nothing is quite as frightening as what's going on in the supermarket aisles and on the kids' menus of our favorite restaurants. All across the food landscape, there are cartoon cavemen and creepy, redheaded clowns trying to tell your kids what to eat. Good thing you're there to stick up for them. Seize control of your child's diet today, and when they finally grow up to know better, they'll be thankful. Here are 20 smart swaps that will set your child on the path to better health.

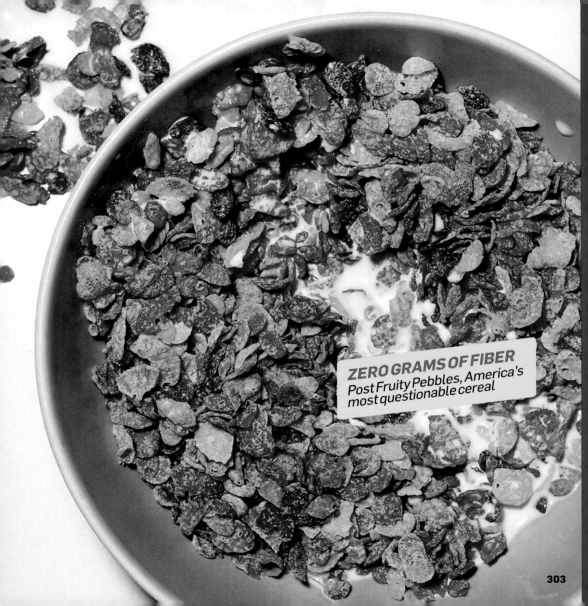

ZERO GRAMS OF FIBER
Post Fruity Pebbles, America's most questionable cereal

20
WORST BREAKFAST CEREAL

Post Fruity Pebbles
(1 cup)

213 calories
1.3 g fat (1 g saturated)
20 g sugars
0 g fiber

Here's how Post describes its product: "Fruity Pebbles is a wholesome, sweetened rice cereal. It is low in fat, cholesterol free, and provides 10 essential vitamins and minerals." Here's the truth: "Fruity Pebbles is a heavily manipulated, egregiously sweetened rice cereal. It is low in nutrients, fiber free, and the second and third ingredients are sugar and hydrogenated vegetable oil." If you plan to feed this to your kids when they wake up, you may as well let them keep sleeping.

Eat This Instead!

General Mills Kix
(1 cup)

110 calories
1 g fat (0 g saturated)
3 g sugars
3 g fiber

19
WORST SIDE DISH

Denny's Kids' French Fries

510 calories
28 g fat (5 g saturated)
59 g carbohydrates

As important as it is for your kids to choose healthy entrées, a bad side can bring down even the leanest dinner centerpiece. These fries (disturbingly, the exact same portion as the adult version) alone pack as many calories and grams of fat as a child should consume in an entire meal.

Eat This Instead!

Kids' Apple Dunkers

140 calories
0 g fat
30 g carbohydrates

18
WORST FROZEN KIDS' MEAL

Kid Cuisine All American Fried Chicken (286 g, 1 meal)

530 calories
22 g fat (5 g saturated, 1 g trans)
800 mg sodium

Despite its cutesy packaging, this Kid Cuisine entrée sports not just excessive amounts of calories and fat, but also a dose of trans fats derived from partially hydrogenated oil—the last thing a growing body needs. While icy blocks of meat and vegetables can never stack up to a fresh, home-cooked meal, there are plenty of solid options out there. Just by switching from Kid Cuisine to Banquet, you'll cut calories and fat nearly in half.

Eat This Instead!

Banquet Chicken Nuggets and Fries (142 g, 1 meal)

280 calories
13 g fat (2.5 g saturated)
560 mg sodium

17
WORST PIZZA

California Pizza Kitchen Kids BBQ Chicken Pizza

560 calories
9 g fat (4.5 g saturated)
1,470 mg sodium
89 g carbohydrates

The sad truth is that we could have picked any of the kids' pizzas for this list. Even the cheese pizza has 560 calories, and the other options go up from there. Thank the thick dough and heavy-handed cheese application. The little ones could eat two slices of Original BBQ Chicken pizza from a six-slice adult pie and save more than 300 calories.

Eat This Instead!
Kids Grilled Chicken
with Broccoli

240 calories
6 g fat (1.5 g saturated)
210 mg sodium
9 g carbohydrates

16
WORST PB&J

Atlanta Bread Company Kids' Peanut Butter & Jelly

580 calories
15 g fat (3.5 g saturated)
89 g carbohydrates

It's hard to lose with the sturdy alliance of peanut butter and jelly—that is, unless you let your kid order it at Atlanta Bread Company. It would be easy to blame it on an excess of peanut butter, but sugary

jelly is equally to blame here. Listed first on the sandwich's ingredients list, it accounts for a significant portion of the 89 grams of carbohydrates and helps to make this sandwich more caloric than the chain's grilled cheese.

Eat This Instead!
Kids' Grilled Cheese

390 calories
15 g fat (9 g saturated)
46 g carbohydrates

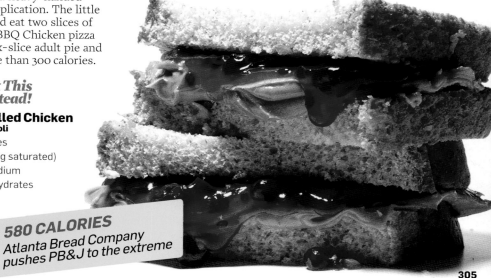

580 CALORIES
Atlanta Bread Company pushes PB&J to the extreme

15

WORST CHINESE ENTRÉE

P.F. Chang's Kid's Chicken Fried Rice

580 calories
10 fat (2 g saturated)
1,120 mg sodium

Chang's tries to shroud its nutrition numbers by breaking meals into multiple servings. Don't be fooled. The restaurant continues its usual sodium assault on its new kids' menu. There you find a dish whose potential (chicken and rice, what could possibly go wrong?) is outweighed only by the surplus of salt saturating every last greasy grain of rice.

 Eat This Instead!

Kid's Stir-Fried Baby Buddha's Feast

60 calories
0 g fat
50 mg sodium

14

WORST FISH MEAL

Long John Silver's Popcorn Shrimp Kid's Meal
(one hush puppy, green beans) with Pepsi

589 calories
18.5 g fat (5 g saturated)
1,102 mg sodium

While we applaud Long John Silver's for doing away with trans fats, they haven't gotten the memo about monosodium glutamate (MSG). In fact, these little poppers are doused with the stuff and similar chemical-based flavor enhancers. Then these poor shrimp hit the vat of frying oil and meet a chemical called dimethylpolysiloxane, a silicone-based anti-foaming agent that's also an ingredient in Silly Putty.

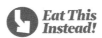 *Eat This Instead!*

Garlic Shrimp Scampi
with Ice Water

200 calories
13 g fat (2.5 g saturated)
650 mg sodium

13

WORST FAST-FOOD CHICKEN MEAL

KFC Extra-Crispy Chicken Tender, Mac-n-Cheese,
Capri Sun, and Gogo Squeeze

610 calories
32 g fat (6.5 g saturated)
2,085 mg sodium

Fried chicken is almost always trouble, but the Mac-n-Cheese constitutes this meal's biggest calorie portion. And its most dangerous. Empty carbs and cheese sauce may make kids salivate, but this meal also packs adult-sized numbers. The sodium alone is more than most grown-ups should consume in one day, let alone one meal.

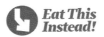 *Eat This Instead!*

Kids Meal with Grilled Chicken Drumstick, Mashed Potatoes
(with Gravy), Capri Sun, and Gogo Squeeze

300 calories
8 g fat (2 g saturated)
835 mg sodium

12
WORST GRILLED CHEESE

Ruby Tuesday Kids Grilled Cheese

660 calories
29 g fat
1,525 sodium

How hard is it to create a sensible grilled cheese for your kids' menu? For Ruby Tuesday, kinda hard. It has six "kid" items coming in at more than 500 calories (the Turkey "Minis" are more than 700). It's just bread and cheese, yet this sandwich packs a caloric wallop and has enough sodium to make a hypertensive adult nervous. So why feed it to a child?

 Eat This Instead!

Kids Chicken Breast

335 calories
14 g fat
895 mg sodium

11
WORST "HEALTHY" MENU CHOICE

Outback Steakhouse Kids Live Well Sirloin Medallions with Apple Juice

714 calories
11 g fat (3 g saturated)
594 mg sodium

Look at Outback's "Joey" menu (that's a baby kangaroo, get it?) and you'll see a bunch of sensible entrees kids will love in sensible portions. But wait. You'll also see a series of "Kids Live Well" meals that suggest that they are extra-healthy. Great, right? Wrong. Compare this "Live Well" steak meal at 714 calories to the regular Joey sirloin, which has...212. What gives? Well, the calories from fat for both dishes are identical at 95 grams, so your baby kangaroo is getting 500 calories of insulin-spiking apple juice (or orange, you choose!). That's crikey on any continent.

 Eat This Instead!

Joey Sirloin

212 calories
11 g fat (4 g saturated)
188 mg sodium

10
WORST FAST-FOOD BURGER MEAL

McDonald's Mighty Kids Meal with Double Cheeseburger, Fries (small), and Fat-Free Chocolate Milk Jug

730 calories
28 g fat (9 g saturated, 1 g trans)
1,100 mg sodium

The Golden Arches should be commended for increasing the number of healthy options in recent years. In particular, its Apple Dippers have inspired other large chains to offer alternatives to fried potatoes. Unfortunately, it's still easier to construct a lousy meal at McDonald's than it is a good one. This combo chews through more than a half day's worth of calories, fat, and sodium. And no toy in the bottom of the box can make that better.

 Eat This Instead!

Happy Meal with Hamburger, Yoplait Go-Gurt Strawberry Yogurt, Kids Fries, and Apple Juice Box

490 calories
14 g fat (4 g saturated, 0 g trans)
590 mg sodium

9

WORST SIT-DOWN BURGER

Applebee's Kids Mini Cheeseburgers (2)

760 calories
50 g fat
(18 g saturated, 2 g trans)
1,600 mg sodium

Just another sad example of Restaurant Law 172A, the Mini-Burger Paradox (MBP). The MBP states that the more diminutive the burger, the more potential it possesses for nutritional mayhem (see: Ruby Tuesday, Chili's, et al.). If restaurants stopped with one mini, you'd be fine, but these baby burgers normally come in groups of two or more—so you end up with two buns, two slices of cheese, two sets of condiments. The result is a total package with more calories, fat, and sodium than you'd find in one normal-size burger.

 Eat This Instead!

Kids Corn Dog

220 calories
12 g fat (3 g saturated)
590 mg sodium

8

WORST BREAKFAST

Bob Evans Kids Plenty-o-Pancakes
with Chocolate Chips

766 calories
22 g fat (13 g saturated fat)
1,281 mg sodium
137 g carbohydrates

As if five saucer-size pancakes studded with chocolate weren't bad enough, scoops of whipped cream top each piece. The result is a load of refined carbohydrates that will have your kid bouncing in the booth (and crashing on the way home). And Bob's nutrition information doesn't even include the sugar dump found in the syrup or the additional fat and calories in the bacon or sausage that comes on the side.

Eat This Instead!

Kids Fruit Dippers

222 calories
1 g fat (0 g saturated)
62 mg sodium
51 g carbohydrates

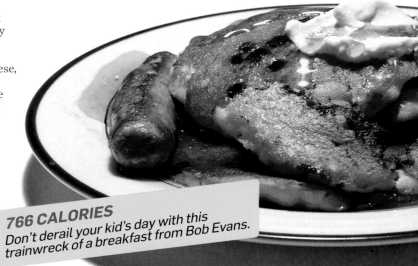

766 CALORIES
Don't derail your kid's day with this trainwreck of a breakfast from Bob Evans.

7
WORST DRINK
Applebee's Kids Oreo Cookie Shake

770 calories
39 g fat (22 g saturated, 1.5 trans)
97 g carbohydrates
450 mg sodium

Though Applebee's doesn't list the ingredients in its nutrition guide, we have a sneaking suspicion that nearly all of those 97 grams of carbohydrates are pure sugar. That's an insulin spike that would make diabetes specialists cringe (not to mention dentists). Your child would have to eat 15 Oreos to match this shake's caloric heft. Better off going with chocolate milk— or a scoop of ice cream.

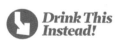

Drink This Instead!
Kids Chocolate Milk

150 calories
2.5 g fat (0 g trans)
45 g carbohydrates
200 mg sodium

6
WORST NACHOS
On the Border Kid's Bean & Cheese Nachos

770 calories
45 g fat (25 g saturated)
1,380 mg sodium

On the Border has scaled back this dish since *Eat This, Not That!* last attacked it, but the changes don't even come close to reining in this time bomb. The only thing worse than the 25 grams of saturated fat— nearly twice as much as an 8-year-old kid should consume in an entire day—is the fact that these nachos come with a complimentary sundae, pushing the meal total north of 1,100 calories.

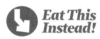

Eat This Instead!
Kid's Grilled Chicken
with Black Beans

260 calories
2.5 g fat (1 g saturated)
630 mg sodium

5
WORST MACARONI AND CHEESE
California Pizza Kitchen Kids Curly Mac n' Cheese
with Edamame

770 calories
46 g fat (28 g saturated)
780 mg sodium

Whereas most kid favorites— chicken fingers, cheeseburgers, even hot dogs—offer some redeeming nutritional value, macaroni and cheese brings nothing but cheese, cream, and refined carbohydrates to the table. CPK appears willing to solve that problem with the inclusion of protein- and fiber-rich edamame in its mac, but instead it stuffs its kiddie bowls to the brim with one of the most calorie-dense pastas we've ever seen. Another good opportunity squandered by the restaurant industry's penchant for excess.

Eat This Instead!
Kids Fusilli **with Tomato Sauce**

400 calories
8 g fat (1 g saturated)
680 mg sodium

4
WORST CHICKEN MEAL
T.G.I. Friday's Chicken Fingers
with Seasoned Fries

790 calories
55 g fat (14.5 g saturated)
2,140 mg sodium

One of the big dangers of this meal, as with the others on this list, is the frightening number of calories consumed in a short amount of time. A kids' portion of chicken fingers with a side of fries at Friday's delivers nearly 800 calories and a shaker of salt, and you just know that plate will be clean inside of 10 minutes. Even scarier: Pair this meal with a sweetened drink like soda or chocolate milk and the calorie count rockets past a cool grand, just like that.

 Eat This Instead!

Chicken Skewers Grilled Pita
with Fruit Cup

370 calories
11 g fat (2 g saturated)
655 mg sodium

3
WORST SALAD
Friendly's Dippin' Chicken
Fried with Carrot and Celery Sticks

810 calories
44 g fat (8 g saturated)
2,570 mg sodium

It's an incredible thing to get a child excited about eating a salad. Just not this one. First off, this isn't so much a salad as a fried chicken dish with a few token veggies packed into a cone. Friendly's just doesn't know when to stop. On the side of the deep fried meat are bowls filled with croutons, cheese, and a honey mustard dipping sauce, which itself has 15 grams of fat. You end up with a "salad" that has more fat than three Snickers bars.

 Eat This Instead!

Grilled Cheese Sandwich
with Mandarin Oranges

430 calories
18 g fat (9 g saturated)
1,050 mg sodium

2
WORST CHICKEN FINGERS
Perkins Kid's Chicken Strips

1,000 calories
68 g fat (13 g saturated)
1,900 mg sodium

These fingers would be criminally caloric even if they were intended for adults. In fact, to match this four-digit calorie count, a kid would need to eat 22 McDonald's Chicken McNuggets. The road to nutritional safety with Perkins' kids' menu is pocked with potholes, so either order the mac and cheese or keep on driving.

 Eat This Instead!

Kid's Mac & Cheese

300 calories
9 g fat (2.5 g saturated)
580 mg sodium

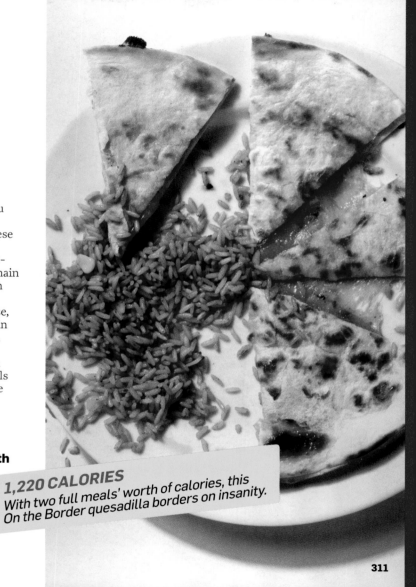

1
WORST KIDS' MEAL

On the Border Kid's Cheese Quesadilla
with Mexican Rice

1,220 calories
75 g fat (31 g saturated)
1,930 mg sodium

On the Border's kids' menu mostly offers reasonable Mexican fare, but this cheese quesadilla, along with the nachos, stands out as a disturbing outlier. How the chain veers so far off course with this item, we don't know. Is it overloaded with cheese, or is the chicken poached in butter? Whatever the case, this quesadilla and rice provide more calories than should be in two kids' meals and enough sodium to cure a whole hog.

 Eat This Instead!

Kid's Mexican Plate with Crispy Chicken Taco
(with Rice, Without Beans)

430 calories
15 g fat (5 g saturated)
930 mg sodium

1,220 CALORIES
With two full meals' worth of calories, this On the Border quesadilla borders on insanity.

Chapter 7

COOK THIS, NOT THAT!
A PERFECT FOOD WEEK

Use these simple recipes to whip up a week's worth of fat-melting, tonsil-exciting meals

It's time to stand up for yourself. All the restaurant swa
in the world won't make a difference if you're still putti
yourself at the mercy of short-order cooks and corporat
food marketers. No matter how smartly you swap one
food for another, you can never know for sure that what
you're eating is the healthiest possible choice. The only
way to do that is to take control, by cooking more at hor

Consider this: thanks to our restaurant-and-prepared-food culture,
the average American woman now eats 1,858 calories a day; the average
American man, about 2,697. That's far more than we need to maintain ou
weight (women should be at or under 1,800, while guys shouldn't top 2,20
And remember, that's to maintain. If you want to lose weight, and you're
not signed up for the Boston Marathon, then you need to cut from there.

Does that mean skipping meals? Subsisting only on rice cakes and wat
No, but it may mean learning how to wield a spatula. On the following pa
we've created a series of mix-n-match recipes that can combine for any
number of all-day meal plans. A breakfast-lunch-and-dinner combinatic
from these pages will cost you between 990 and 1,240 calories. Add in a
couple of Eat This! snacks (say, a LaraBar for 190 calories and a Dairy Qu
sundae for 300 calories) and you're still somewhere between 1,480 and
1,730 calories—enough of a savings for the average woman to lose up to
33 pounds this year, and the average man up to 75 pounds. And that make
the kitchen a lot more appealing, and effective, than the gym.

VANILLA-BOURBON FRENCH TOAST

...ast is called pain perdu—"lost bread," a nod to the fact that the dish works ...d. More important, pain perdu isn't served at breakfast, but rather as a dessert, ... dish is traditionally soaked in sugar and cream. This version forgoes cream for ...f sugar for vanilla and a slug of bourbon. It's still a pretty decadent way to start ...t you won't need a nap afterward.

How to Make It:

• *Preheat the oven to 225°F.*

• *Combine the eggs, milk, bourbon, vanilla, sugar, and nutmeg in a shallow baking dish and whisk to combine. Soak each slice of bread for 30 seconds, turning once, before cooking.*

• *Heat a large cast-iron skillet or nonstick pan over medium heat. Melt a small pat of butter in the pan, enough to coat the surface. Add 2 to 4 slices of the soaked bread and cook for about 3 minutes, until a deep brown crust forms. Flip the bread and continue cooking for another 2 to 3 minutes, until golden brown and firm to the touch. Keep the cooked French toast in the oven while you work through the rest of the batch.*

• *Serve with warm syrup and a dusting of powdered sugar, if you like.*

MAKES 4 SERVINGS

y bread,
heat,

for serving

erving
40

alories
g saturated)
carbs

NUTRITIONAL

Upgrade

While we've managed to take most of the sting out of the French toast, it's still by definition a carb-heavy breakfast. But by increasing your fiber intake, you can blunt the impact on your blood sugar levels. Try replacing the syrup with any of the following:

• Sliced bananas, either raw or caramelized in a pan over medium heat for a few minutes

• Raw strawberries with powdered sugar

• Blueberries cooked for 15 minutes with a spoonful of water and sugar

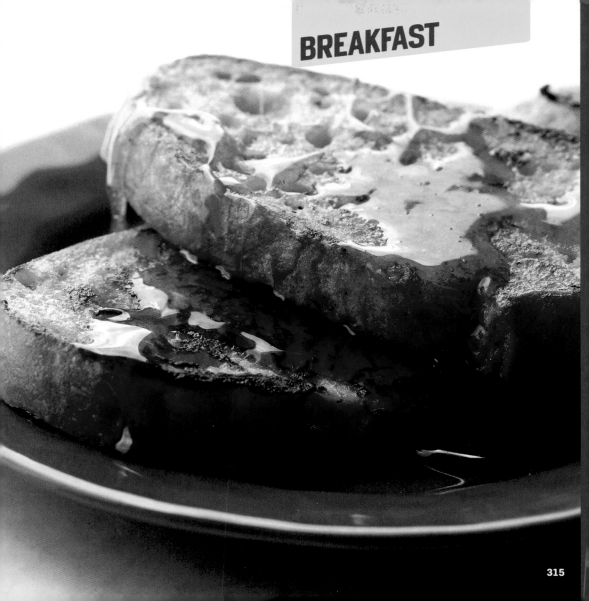

Cook This
MILE-HIGH OMELETS

The classic diner omelet is an oversize envelope of eggs soaked in cheap oil and bulging with fatty fillers. The damage, with toast and hash browns: about 1,400 calories and 70 grams of fat. Our ode to Denver doesn't cut the cheese or the meat or even turn to Egg Beaters. No, this is just honest cooking with good ingredients in reasonable portions, exactly what an omelet should be.

You'll Need:

- ½ Tbsp olive oil, plus more for cooking the omelets
- 1 green bell pepper, diced
- 4 oz cremini or button mushrooms, sliced
- 1 small onion, diced
- 4 oz smoked ham, cubed or sliced into thin strips
- Salt and black pepper to taste
- 8 eggs
- 2 Tbsp 2% milk
- ½ cup shredded sharp Cheddar

How to Make It:

- *Heat the olive oil in a medium sauté pan over medium heat. Add the bell pepper, mushrooms, and onions and cook for about 7 minutes, until the vegetables are soft and lightly browned. Add the ham, cook for 1 minute more, then season with salt and pepper.*

- *Combine the eggs and milk and whisk until fully blended. Season with a few pinches of salt.*

- *Heat a small nonstick pan over medium heat. Swirl with just enough olive oil to coat. Ladle in one-quarter of the eggs and as soon as they begin to set, use a wooden spoon to scrape the egg from the bottom, working from one side of the pan to the other (like you were scrambling eggs). Stop scraping just before the egg is fully cooked, then spread one-quarter of the cheese and one-quarter of the vegetable mixture across the omelet. Use a spatula to carefully fold the egg over on itself. Slide the omelet out onto a warm plate. Repeat to make 4 omelets.*

MAKES 4 SERVINGS

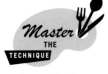

Master
THE
TECHNIQUE

Super-Fluffy Omelets

Achieve a soufflé-like texture with any omelet with one simple move. Combine the eggs and a splash of milk in a blender as you heat up your pan. Blend for 20 seconds, then add the eggs directly to the pan. The action from the blender helps whip air into the eggs, creating a tender curd and pillowy texture as the eggs cook.

Per Serving
$1.84
280 calories
19 g fat (7 g saturated)
740 mg sodium

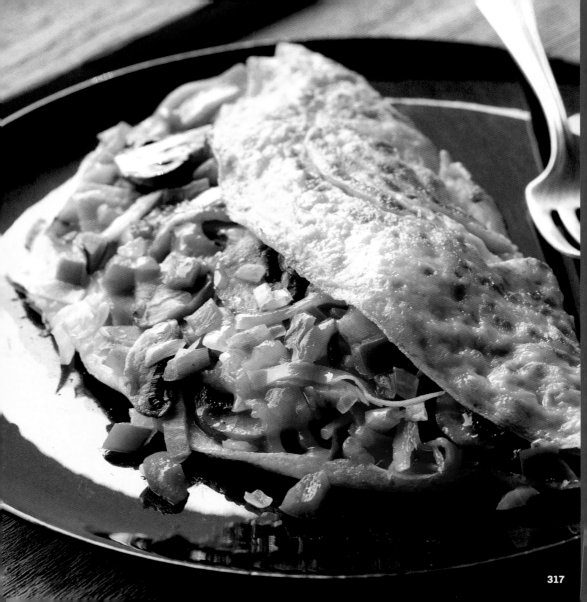

SHIITAKE, SPINACH & GOAT CHEESE SCRAMBLE

Skillfully scrambled eggs are a joy on their own, but by taking the next step and folding in a few supporting players, you accomplish two goals: First, you make a simple breakfast suddenly taste and feel like something special. But also, most additions you can introduce to a sauté pan will further boost the nutritional profile of the heroic egg. For soft, extra-creamy scrambled eggs, make sure to turn the heat down and stir the eggs constantly.

You'll Need:

1½ Tbsp butter

1 cup sliced shiitake mushrooms

1 cup frozen spinach, thawed

Salt and black pepper to taste

8 eggs

2 Tbsp 2% milk

½ cup fresh goat cheese

Per Serving
$1.98
240 calories
17 g fat (5 g saturated)
640 mg sodium

How to Make It:

• *Heat 1 tablespoon of the butter in a large nonstick pan over medium heat. When bubbling, add the shiitakes and cook for about 5 minutes, until lightly browned. Remove and reserve on a plate.*

• *In the same pan, sauté the spinach until heated all the way through. Season with salt and pepper. Transfer to a colander and squeeze out any excess water.*

• *Combine the eggs and the milk in a large bowl. Season with salt and whisk thoroughly. Add the remaining ½ tablespoon butter to the pan, turn the heat to low, and add the eggs. Use a wooden spoon to stir the eggs constantly, scraping the bottom of the pan to create small, delicate curds. Continue stirring in this manner for about 5 minutes, until the eggs are still very soft and loose. Add the mushrooms, spinach, and goat cheese and cook for about 2 minutes longer. Season to taste with black pepper.*

MAKES 4 SERVINGS

MEAL MULTIPLIER

Other ways to bolster a breakfast scramble:

- Asparagus, feta, and cherry tomatoes
- Baby shrimp, garlic, and scallions
- Chicken sausage, mushrooms, scallions, and sharp Cheddar

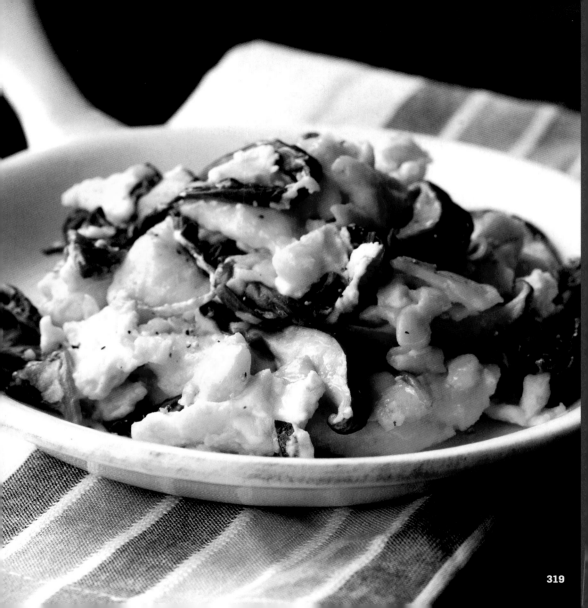

ULTIMATE CLUB SANDWICH WITH SUPER MAYO

There are many people who believe that you can judge the quality of a hotel by its club sandwich. The reason being that it's the one item you will find on nearly all room service menus, and a place that puts love into the sandwich is likely putting love into the other small things that make a hotel great. We think our version—ham, turkey, bacon, and a souped-up mayo—would win over any guest, with the added bonus of containing half the calories of the club sandwiches that normally show up on the room service cart.

You'll Need:

2 Tbsp olive oil mayonnaise

1 Tbsp Dijon mustard

1 clove garlic, finely minced (or grated on a microplane)

1 tsp dried oregano

6 sandwich rolls, split and lightly toasted (12 pieces total; see Secret Weapon, right)

2 cups shredded romaine

8 slices tomato

8 strips cooked bacon

4 oz ham in 8 slices

4 oz turkey in 8 slices

How to Make It:

• *In a mixing bowl combine the mayonnaise, mustard, garlic, and oregano.*

• *Spread the mayo mixture on 8 pieces of the toasted sandwich rolls. Top each piece with shredded romaine, a slice of tomato, and a strip of bacon. Top 4 of the pieces with ham and the other 4 with turkey.*

• *Build each sandwich with a turkey half, a ham half, and top with a final piece of sandwich roll for a tri-level sandwich.*

MAKES 4 SERVINGS

Per Serving
$2.68
330 calories
12 g fat
(2.5 g saturated)
980 mg sodium

SECRET WEAPON

Sandwich Thins

Most club sandwiches are more refined carbs than meat or produce—the extra layer of bread adding nothing but excess calories to the mix. Our version is built on sandwich rolls (aka sandwich thins), great low-calorie, high-fiber bread now widely available throughout North America. Both Oroweat and Nature's Own make varieties that contain just 100 calories and pack 5 grams of fiber per roll—more fiber and fewer calories than you'd get with two slices of whole-wheat bread. Make these your go-to sandwich vessels.

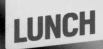

Cook This
CHINESE CHICKEN SALAD

This salad is one of the world's ultimate fusion foods. It's an Eastern-inspired dish popularized by an Austrian chef (Wolfgang Puck) in Beverly Hills (at his restaurant Spago back in the 1980s). Whatever its disparate origins, it's undeniably one of the most popular salads in America, sharing space on menus in four-star restaurants and Wendy's alike. Too bad most versions are nutritional disasters, bogged down by too much dressing and too many fried noodles. This lighter version is true to Wolfgang's original creation.

You'll Need:

1 head napa cabbage

½ head red cabbage

½ Tbsp sugar

2 cups chopped or shredded cooked chicken (freshly grilled or from a store-bought rotisserie chicken)

⅓ cup Asian-style dressing, like Annie's Shiitake and Sesame Vinaigrette

1 cup fresh cilantro leaves

1 cup canned mandarin oranges, drained

¼ cup sliced almonds, toasted

Salt and black pepper to taste

How to Make It:

• Slice the cabbages in half lengthwise and remove the cores. Slice the cabbage into thin strips. Toss with the sugar in a large bowl.

• If the chicken is cold, toss with a few tablespoons of vinaigrette and heat in a microwave at 50% power. Add to the cabbage, along with the cilantro, mandarins, almonds, and the remaining vinaigrette. Toss to combine. Season with salt and pepper.

MAKES 4 SERVINGS

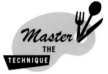

Master **THE TECHNIQUE**

Properly dressing salads

Most salads end up overdressed, which compromises the flavor and the inherent nutritional value of the creation. For a properly dressed salad, add the dressing a few tablespoons at a time immediately before serving (otherwise the lettuce will wilt) and use a pair of tongs to thoroughly distribute each new addition. Pluck a leaf and taste; it should have a light sheen, not a heavy coat, of dressing.

Per Serving
$3.30
380 calories
21 g fat (3.5 saturated)
23 g carbs

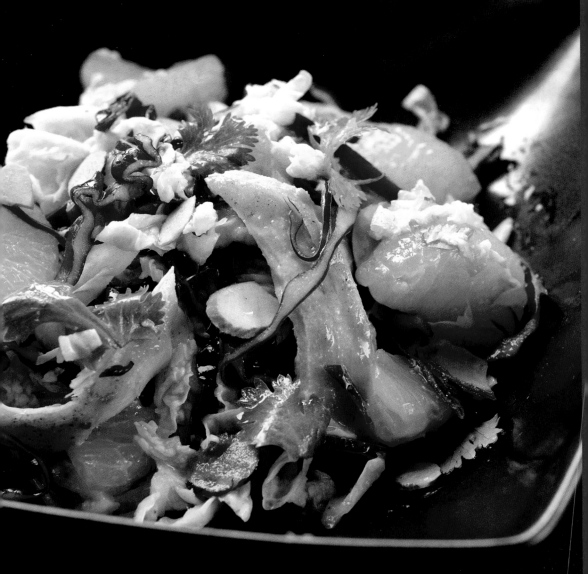

GRILLED CHEESE & TOMATO SOUP

An oozing grilled cheese and a cup of warm tomato soup constitute one of the great one-two combos of the comfort food world. Our grilled cheese is a play on that gooey Southern staple, pimento cheese, which diffuses the calories of the cheese with healthy additions like roasted peppers and Greek yogurt. The soup? Pure tomato intensity, thanks to the oven roasting, which concentrates the natural sugars of the tomatoes.

GRILLED PIMENTO CHEESE SANDWICH

You'll Need:

- 1¼ cups finely shredded sharp Cheddar cheese
- 1 jar (4 oz) diced pimentos
- 1 jalapeño pepper, seeded and minced
- ¼ cup finely sliced scallions
- ¼ cup 2% Greek yogurt
- 1 Tbsp olive-oil mayonnaise
- Few shakes Tabasco
- 8 slices bread
- Butter

How to Make It:

- *Combine the cheese, pimentos, jalapeño, scallions, yogurt, mayonnaise, and a few shakes of Tabasco in a mixing bowl. Divide among 4 slices of bread and top with the remaining slices.*

- *Heat a bit of butter in a cast-iron skillet or nonstick pan over medium heat. Cook the sandwiches, turning once, for about 10 minutes, until golden brown on both sides and the cheese is melted (have patience—an extra minute or two means everything with good grilled cheese!).*

Per Serving
$1.46

320 calories
17 g fat
(8 g saturated)
490 mg sodium

MAKES 4 SERVINGS

ROASTED TOMATO SOUP

You'll Need:

- 3 lbs Roma tomatoes, halved lengthwise
- 2 Tbsp olive oil, plus more for drizzling
- 4 cloves garlic, peeled
- 3 cups low-sodium chicken stock
- Salt and black pepper to taste

How to Make It:

- *Preheat the oven to 425°F. Place the tomatoes cut side up on a baking sheet and drizzle with olive oil. Place the garlic cloves in the center of a sheet of aluminum foil, drizzle with olive oil, and fold to create an enclosed packet.*

- *Roast the tomatoes and the garlic for about 40 minutes, until both are very soft. Transfer the tomatoes and garlic to a blender, add the olive oil, and puree. Transfer to a pot, stir in the chicken stock, and simmer for 15 minutes. Season with salt and black pepper.*

Per Serving
$1.67

130 calories
7 g fat (1 g saturated)
370 mg sodium

MAKES 4 SERVINGS

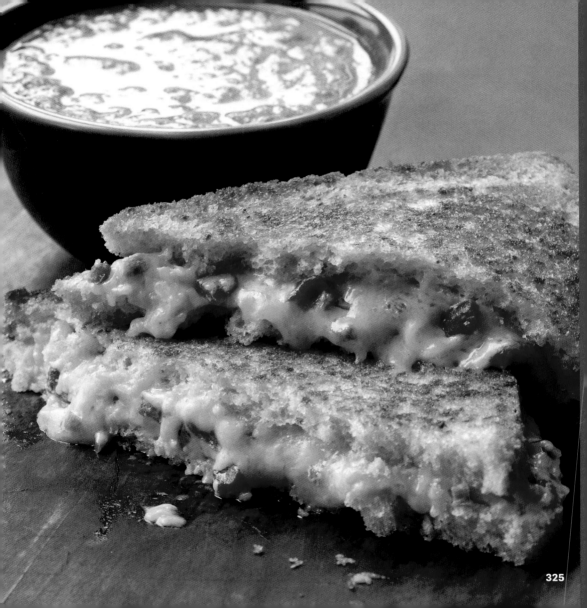

COWBOY BURGERS

We're not afraid to admit when a fast-food joint has a good idea. The inspiration for this burger comes from a Carl's Jr. classic, the Western Bacon Cheeseburger, a how-can-it-not-be-delicious comingling of beef, barbecue sauce, and fried onions. Problem is, the small version of Carl's burger packs 740 calories and a full day's worth of saturated fat. This version uses naturally lean bison and replaces the breaded onion rings with sweet grilled ones.

You'll Need:

1 lb ground bison or beef sirloin

1 medium red onion, sliced into ¼"-thick rings and skewered with toothpicks

½ Tbsp finely ground coffee

1 tsp chipotle or ancho chile powder

Salt and black pepper to taste

4 slices sharp Cheddar

4 sesame seed buns, lightly toasted

6 strips bacon, cooked until crisp and halved

4 Tbsp barbeque sauce

How to Make It:

• Gently form the meat into 4 patties, being careful not to overwork the meat. Let the patties rest for 15 minutes.

• Preheat the grill or grill pan over medium heat. Grill the onion slices, turning, for about 10 minutes, until soft and lightly charred. Just before cooking the patties, season them on both sides with the coffee, chile powder, and salt and pepper. Grill the patties alongside the onions for about 4 minutes, until nicely browned. Flip, top with the cheese, and continue grilling for 3 to 4 minutes longer, until the centers of the patties are firm but gently yielding to the touch and an instant-read thermometer inserted into the thickest part of a burger registers 135°F.

• Place the burgers on the bun bottoms, and top with onions, bacon, and barbecue sauce.

MAKES 4 SERVINGS

Per Serving:
$2.62

460 calories
22 g fat
(11 g saturated)
850 mg sodium

We have no idea if cowboys actually eat burgers, but if they did, they would taste an awful lot like this one.

Normally we're not huge fans of heavily spiced burgers, but the coffee here adds a roasted depth to the burger that pairs beautifully with the barbecue sauce and bacon.

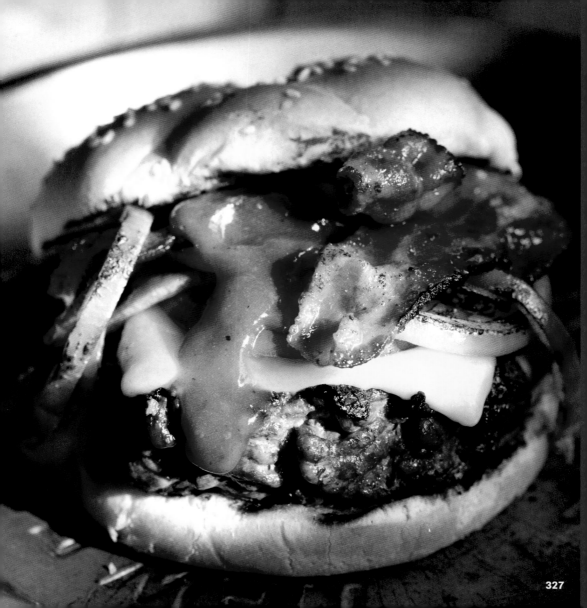

SPINACH-ARTICHOKE MANICOTTI WITH SPICY TOMATO SAUCE

There are a thousand ways to stuff a piece of pasta—from three-cheese ravioli to a meaty, saucy tower of lasagna—but the one common denominator is a deluge of calories and an abundance of sodium. To deliver the creature comforts of red-sauce Italian food, we keep the cheesy stuffing, but to make it something you can feel good about eating, we use low-fat ricotta and cottage cheese cut with plenty of sautéed spinach and artichoke hearts.

You'll Need:

1 Tbsp olive oil

3 cloves garlic, minced

1 jar (6 oz) marinated artichoke hearts

1 bag (10 oz) frozen spinach, thawed

Salt and black pepper to taste

1 small onion, minced

½ tsp red pepper flakes

1 can (28 oz) crushed tomatoes

12 manicotti tubes

½ cup low-fat ricotta cheese

¼ cup low-fat cottage cheese

¼ cup grated Parmesan

½ cup shredded mozzarella

How to Make It:

• Preheat the oven to 350°F.

• Heat half the olive oil in a medium sauté pan over medium heat. Add one-third of the garlic and sauté for about 1 minute, until soft and light brown. Add the artichoke hearts and spinach. Cook for about 3 minutes, until the vegetables are warmed through. Drain any water that collects in the bottom of the pan. Season with salt and black pepper.

• Heat the remaining olive oil in a medium saucepan over medium heat. Add the remaining garlic, the onions, and red pepper flakes and cook for about 3 minutes, until the onion is soft. Add the tomatoes and simmer for 10 minutes. Season with salt and pepper.

• While the sauce simmers, cook the manicotti in a large pot of boiling water for about 7 minutes, until soft but short of al dente. Drain.

• Combine the artichoke-spinach mixture with the ricotta, cottage cheese, and Parmesan. Use a small spoon to carefully stuff each manicotti with the cheese mixture.

• Spoon half of the tomato sauce on the bottom of a 13" x 9" baking dish. Top with the manicotti, then cover with the remaining sauce. Sprinkle the mozzarella all over. Bake for about 20 minutes, until the cheese is melted and the sauce is bubbling.

MAKES 4 SERVINGS

Per Serving
$2.63

450 calories
11 g fat (4 g saturated)
810 mg sodium

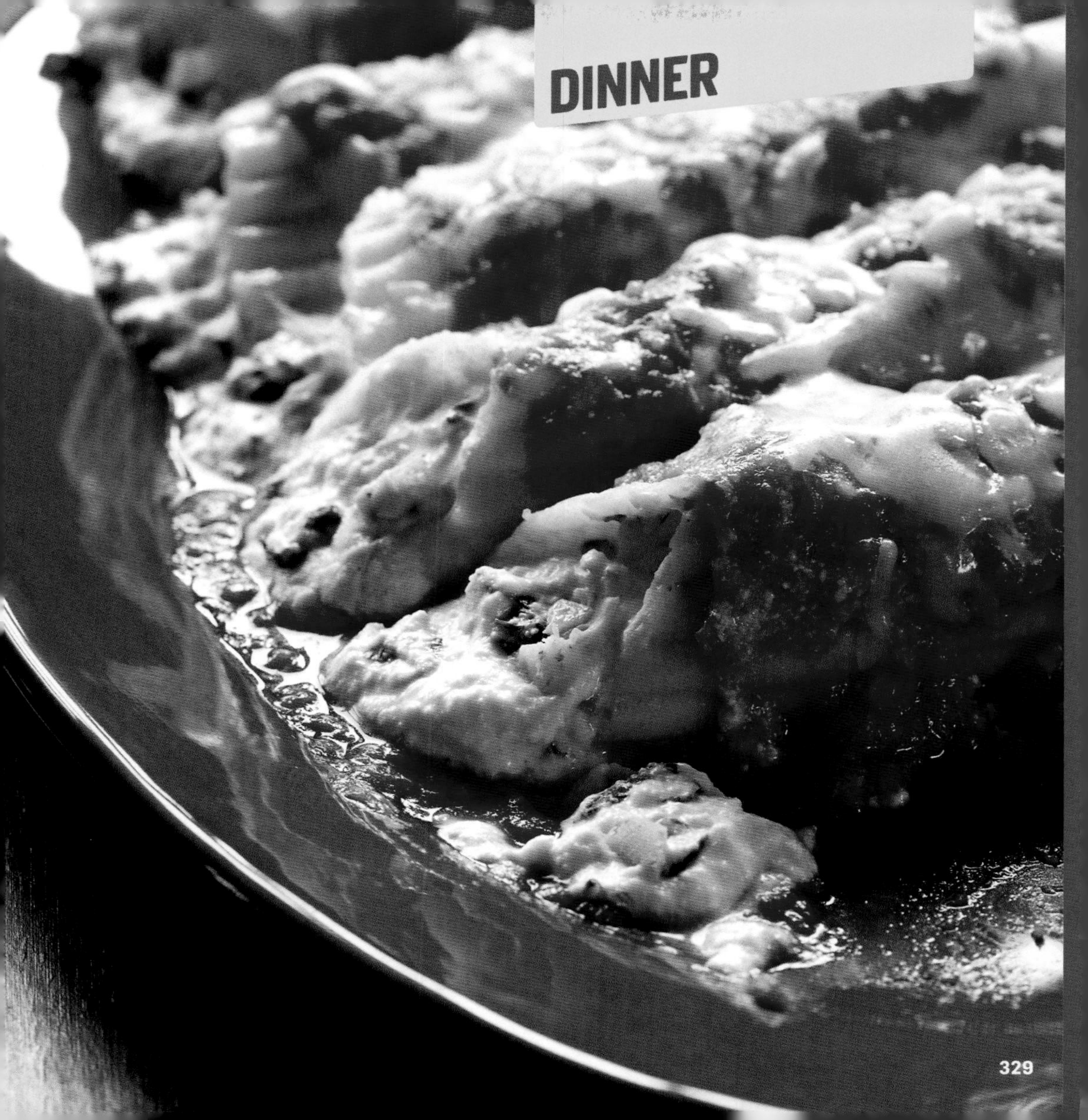

DINNER

Cook This
CHICKEN & DUMPLINGS

This is the kind of food Mom makes when the sniffles set in. It has many of the same magical powers and core flavors of chicken noodle soup—root vegetables, savory broth, shredded chicken—but is made more substantial by the addition of a roux to thicken the soup base and, of course, fluffy dumplings. Of course, the real magic is in those pillows of rosemary-scented joy, which soak up the hearty liquid and, when combined with the juicy chicken, make for one of the most satisfying, savory bites imaginable.

You'll Need:

2 Tbsp butter

4 medium carrots, diced

1 medium onion, diced

3 Tbsp plus ⅔ cup flour

½ tsp dried thyme

4 cups low-sodium chicken stock

1 lb boneless, skinless chicken thighs

Salt and black pepper to taste

1½ tsp baking powder

1 tsp chopped fresh rosemary

½ cup 2% milk

½ cup frozen peas

How to Make It:

• Heat the butter in a pot or large saucepan over medium heat. Add the carrots and onions and cook for about 5 minutes, until softened. Add the 3 tablespoons flour and the thyme, stirring so that the vegetables are evenly coated. Slowly add the stock, whisking to prevent lumps from forming. Bring to a gentle simmer.

• Season the chicken thighs with salt and black pepper and add to the pot, submerging them in the stock. Poach the chicken for about 8 minutes, until just cooked through. Remove to a cutting board to rest.

• Combine the remaining ⅔ cup flour with the baking powder, rosemary, ¼ teaspoon salt, and lots of black pepper. Add the milk and gently stir until the dough just comes together. Form loosely into 8 dumplings and drop them directly into the soup. Cover the pot and cook over low heat for 10 minutes, until the dumplings have firmed up.

• Shred the reserved chicken. Add to the pot, along with the peas, stirring carefully so as not to break up the dumplings. Heat through for 1 minute before serving.

MAKES 4 SERVINGS

Per Serving
$1.83

380 calories
12 g fat
(5 g saturated)
810 mg sodium

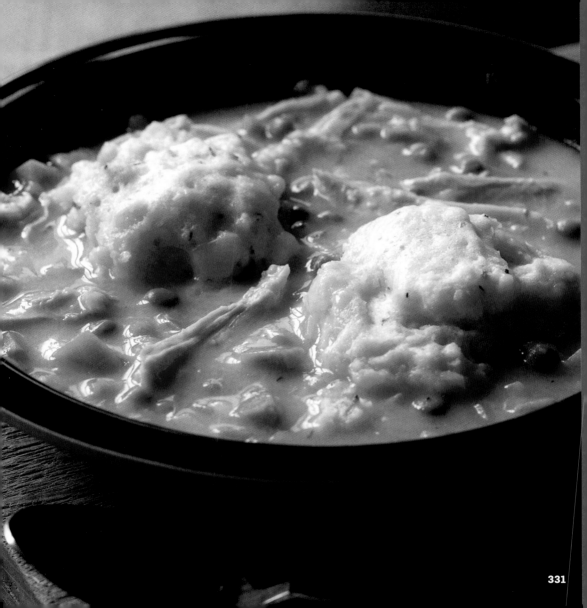

Cook This
JAMBALAYA

No city or region in America lays claim to a richer, more influential lineup of culinary creations than New Orleans and the surrounding Creole country. Gumbo, étouffée, beignets, po'boys—all are part of Louisiana's incomparable culinary heritage. No dish, though, is more famous than jambalaya, the rice-based hodgepodge of meat, seafood, and vegetables not unlike the Spanish paella. By decreasing the rice ratio and increasing the produce and protein, this recipe cuts the calories and carbs dramatically. But it still has enough soul to satisfy the most discerning Creole critics.

You'll Need:

1 tsp olive or canola oil

1 cup diced turkey kielbasa

1 medium onion, diced

1 medium green bell pepper, diced

2 cloves garlic, minced

8 oz boneless, skinless chicken breast, cut into ½" cubes

1 cup long-grain rice

2¼ cups low-sodium chicken stock

1 can (14 oz) diced tomatoes

1 Tbsp tomato paste

⅛ tsp cayenne

2 bay leaves

8 oz medium shrimp, peeled and deveined

Salt and black pepper to taste

Frank's RedHot, Tabasco, or other hot sauce

Chopped scallions (optional)

How to Make It:

• Heat the oil in a large skillet or saute pan over medium heat. Add the kielbasa and cook for about 3 minutes, until lightly browned. Add the onion, bell pepper, and garlic and cook, stirring occasionally, for 4 to 5 minutes, until the vegetables have softened.

• Push the vegetables and kielbasa to the perimeter, making a well in the center of the pan. Add the chicken and sauté until lightly browned but not cooked through, about 3 minutes. Stir in the rice, stock, tomatoes, tomato paste, cayenne, and bay leaves. Turn the heat to low, cover, and simmer for 17 minutes, until nearly all of the liquid has been absorbed by the rice. Uncover, add the shrimp, and cook for 2 to 3 minutes, until the rice is tender and the shrimp is cooked through. Discard the bay leaves. Season with salt, black pepper, and hot sauce and garnish with the scallions, if using.

MAKES 4 SERVINGS

Per Serving
$4.15

380 calories
15 g fat
(4.5 g saturated)
1,070 mg sodium

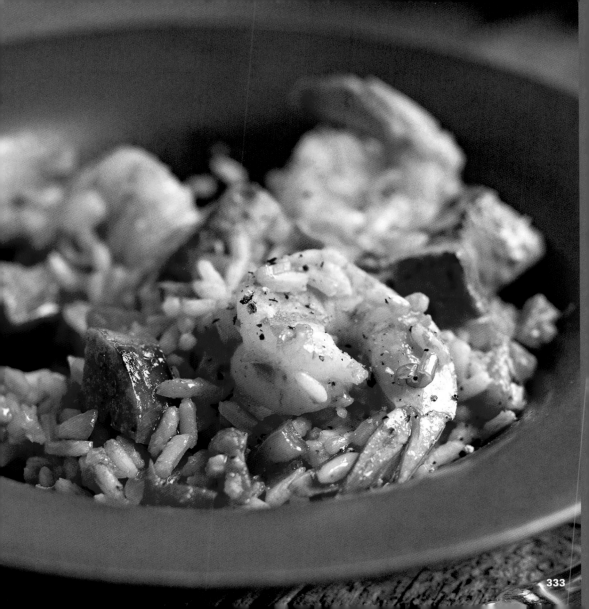

INDEX

Boldface page references indicate photographs.

A

A&W food, 114–115, **114–115**
Abominations 46–49
Additives, food, 6, 19, 40, 59, 61, 133
Affordable Care Act, 17
Alcohol
  beer, 294–295, **294–295**
  mixers, 292–293, **292–293**
American Journal of Clinical Nutrition,
  10, 12, 219
American Journal of Health Promotion,
  55
Antibiotics in meat, 242
Appetizers. *See also* Snacks
  at Thai restaurant, 108
  frozen, 282–283, **282–283**
  restaurant
    Baja Fresh, <u>65</u>
    Chili's, 147
    On the Border, 184
    Outback Steakhouse, 186-187
Applebee's
  and *Eat This, Not That!*, 14
  excess calories, 5
  food, 116–117, **116–117**
  full disclosure, 15, 16
  "special occasion mentality", 113
  worst, desserts, 35, **35**
  worst, fish, 88, **88**
  worst, kids, 307, 309
Apples with skin on, **9**, 11
Apple fritter, 177, **177**

Apricots, 58
Arby's food, 118–119, **118–119**
  "special occasion mentality", 113
Archives of Internal Medicine study, xvii
Artificial flavor, 43, 54
Arugula, 276
Asparagus
  at Outback, 166, **166**
  Shiitake, Spinach & Goat Cheese
    Scramble, 318, **319**
Atlanta Bread Company food, 305, **305**
Au Bon Pain food, 120–121, **120–121**

B

Bacon
  burger, 87
  health-food fraud, worst, 83, **83**
  homemade recipe
    Cowboy Burgers, 326, **327**
  restaurant
    A& W, 114
    Arby's, 118
    Burger King, 134
    Bob Evans, 130
    Chick-fil-A, 142
    Denny's, 154
    Domino's, 156
    Five Guys, 160
    Hardee's, 165
    IHOP, 166
    Jack in the Box, 16, 48, 170, 171
    McDonalds, 180, 181

    Panera Bread, 191
    Perkins, 194
    Subway, 32
    Popeyes, 200
    Quiznos, 32
    Romano's Macaroni Grill, 207
    Sonic, 213
    Starbucks, 214
    Subway, 219
    Tim Hortons, 225
    Wendy's, 229
  supermarket
    deli meats, 242–243, **242–243**
    frozen breakfast, 270
    supermarket, 188–89, **188–89**
  worst, eggs, 85, **85**
  worst, fast-food burger, 78, **78**
  worst, fries 76, **76**
  worst, salad, 77, **77**
Bagels
  breakfast breads, 236–237, **236–237**
  frozen pizzas, 272, **272**
  at Dunkin' Donuts, 159, **159**
  at McDonald's, 181
  at Panera Bread, 191
Baja Fresh food, 122–123, **122–123**
  worst, burrito 85, **85**
Balsamic vinegar
  Dressings, 264, **264**
Bananas, 57
Barbecue sauce
  Cowboy Burgers, 326, **327**
  condiments, 246, **246**
Bareburger, 45
Barley, 250, **250**
Baskin-Robbins
  changes in, 16
  food, 124–125, **124–125**
  worst, milkshake, 81, **81**
Beans
  dips and spreads, 262
  frozen breakfast, 270
  gluten free, 68

paleo, 70
Beef. *See also* Burgers
    frozen entrées, 280–281, **280–281**
    homemade recipe
        Cowboy Burgers, 326, **327**
    paleo, 70
    restaurant
        Applebees, 116–117
        Arby's, 118–119, **118**
        Au Bon Pain, 121–122
        Baja Fresh, 122–123
        Blimpie, 128–129, **128–129**
        Bob Evans, 130
        Boston Market, 133
        California Pizza Kitchen, 137
        Chili's, 144, **144**
        Chipotle, 146
        Denny's, 154–155
        On the Border, 184–185
        Outback Steakhouse, 186, **186**
        Panera Bread, 190, **190**
        Perkins, 194, **194**
        Ruby Tuesday, 208–209, **208–209**
        Subway, 218–219, **218–219**
        T.G.I. Friday's, **221**
        Taco Bell, 222–223, **222–223**
Beer, 294–295, **294–295**
Ben & Jerry's
    ice cream
        in store, 126–127, **126–127**
        supermarket, 285
Berries
    frozen yogurt, 105
    Jamba Juice smoothies, 34, **34**
    vitamin C, 58
Beverages. *See* Drinks; *specific type*
Bhatia, Tasneem, M.D., 40
Biscuits
    Perkins, 195
    supermarket, 249, **249**
    worst, eggs, 84, **84**
Bisquick, 65, **65**

Blimpie food, 128–129, **128-129**
BluePrint, 66
Bob Evans food, 130–131, **130–131**
    worst, kids, 308, **308**
Bob's Red Mill, 65, **65**
Body fat, 18, 20, 57
Body mass index (BMI), 300
Bolthouse Farms, 66
Boston Market food, 132–133, **132–133**
Breads. *See also* Sandwiches
    breakfast, 236–237, **236–237**
    homemade recipes
        Cowboy Burgers, 326, **327**
        Vanilla-Bourbon French Toast, 314, **315**
        Grilled Cheese & Tomato Soup, 324, **325**
        Ultimate Club Sandwich, 320, **321**
    supermarket, 248–249, **248–249**
    whole grain, 7, 60, 68
    vegan, 111
Breakfast. *See also specific food*
    burritos, 26, **26**, 139, 213, 270
    eggs, 11, 56, 84
    kids
        worst breakfast, 308, **308**
        worst cereal, 304, **304**
    restaurant
        Au Bon Pain, 120
        Blimpie, 128
        Bob Evans, 130–131, **130–131**
        Burger King, 134, **135**
        Carl's Jr., 138
        Così, 150
        The Cheesecake Factory, 51, **51**
        Denny's, 154, **154**, 155
        Dunkin' Donuts, 158–159, **158–159**
        Friendly's, 162
        Hardee's, 164–165
        IHOP, 166–67, **166–167**
        Jack in the Box, 170–171, **170–171**
        Jamba Juice, 172–173
        McDonald's, 180–181

        Panera Bread, 190–191
        Perkins, 194–195
        Sonic, 213
        Krispy Kreme, 118–19, **118–19**
        Perkins, 42, **42**
        Starbucks, 214–215, **214–215**
        Tim Hortons, 225
    supermarket
        breakfast breads, 236–237, **236–237**
        frozen breakfast entrées, 270–271, **244–245**
        sausages, 244–245, **244–245**
        wholesome cereals, 234–235, **234–235**
        yogurts, 238–239, **238–239**
    skipping, 48, 298
    worst, 93, **93**
    worst, pastry, 33, **33**
British Journal of Psychiatry,56
Brownies
    at Cold Stone Creamery 149, **149**
    worst, dessert, 79, **79**
Brussels sprouts, 58, 60
Burger King
    burrito, 26, **26**
    chicken, 134
    decline of, 17
    food, 134–135, **134–135**
Burgers
    abominations, 46
    food swap, 25, **25**
    homemade recipe
        Cowboy Burgers, 298, **299**
    restaurant
        A&W, 114–115, **114–115**
        Bareburger, 45
        Burger King, 134–135, **134–135**
        Carl's Jr., 138–139, **138–139**
        The Cheesecake Factory, 140, **140**
        Chili's, 145, **145**
        Dairy Queen, 152–153
        Elevation Burger, 45

Five Guys, 25, **25**, 160–161, **160–161**
Friendly's, 162–163 **162–163**
Hardee's, 164–165, **164–165**
In-N-Out Burger, 168–169, **168–169**
Jack in the Box, 170–171
McDonald's, 180–181
Outback Steakhouse, 187, **187**
Ruby Tuesday, 209
Sonic, 212–213
Steak 'n Shake, 216–217, **216–217**
T.G.I. Friday's, 221
Wendy's, 228–229
supermarket
cheeseburgers, 280
salmon, 276
veggie, 111
worst, kids, 307
Burritos
breakfast, 26, **26,** 139, 165, 171, 213, 270–271, **270–271**
food swap, 26, **26**
frozen, 216–17, **216–17**
Menu Decoder, 98
restaurant
Baja Fresh, 86, **86,** 123
Burger King, 26, **26**
Chick-fil-A, 26, **26**
Chipotle Mexican Grill, 71, **71,** 146–147, **147**
Taco Bell, 222–223
worst, 86, **86**
B vitamins, 11

C

Cabbage
Chinese Chicken Salad, 322, **323**
California Pizza Kitchen
food, 136–137, **136–137,** 273
food swap, 29
worst, kids, 306, 310
Calories
belly fat, 19, 20
intake, 6, 22

nutrition versus, 4
restaurants and inaccurate count of, 4
Candy bars
supermarket, 268–269, **268–269**
Capri Sun, 16
Carl's Jr.
changes in, 17
food, 138–139, **138–139**
Cereals
awards, 43
oatmeal, 57
sweet, 232–233, **232–233**
wholesome, 234–235, **234–235,** 299, 300
worst, kids, **303,** 304
Cheese
homemade recipes
Mile-High Omelets, 316, **317**
Shiitake, Spinach & Goat Cheese Scramble, 318, **319**
Grilled Cheese & Tomato Soup, 324, **325**
Cowboy Burgers, 326, **327**
Spinach-Artichoke Manicotti, 328, **329**
supermarket, 240–241, **240–241**
The Cheesecake Factory
calories, 5
food, 140–141, **140–141**
worst, breakfast, 93, **93**
worst, health-food fraud, 83, **83**
worst, pasta, 91, **91**
Chevys Fresh Mex food, 30, **30**
Chia seeds, 10
Chick-fil-A
food swap, 26, **26**
food, 142–143, **142–143**
Chicken
abomination, 48
food swap, 26, **26** 29, **29,** 30, **30**
homemade recipes
Chinese Chicken Salad, 322, **323**
Chicken & Dumplings, 330, **331**
Jambalaya, 332, **333**
paleo, 71
restaurant
A&W, 114–115
Applebee's, 116–117, **116–117**

Arby's, 118, **118**
Au Bon Pain, 120–121, **120**
Baja Fresh, , 86, **86,** 123
Blimpie, 128
Bob Evans, 130–131
Boston Market, 132–133, **133**
Burger King, 134–135
California Pizza Kitchen, 29, **29,** 136–137, **136–137**
Carl's Jr., 138–139
The Cheesecake Factory, 80, **80,** 141, **141**
Chevys, 30, **30**
Chick-fil-A, 142–143, **142–143**
Chili's, 30, **30,** 144–145
Chipotle, 146–147
Così, 150–151, **150–151**
Dairy Queen, 152–153
Domino's, 156–157, **156–157**
Five Guys, 161
Friendly's, 89, **89,** 162–163, **162–163,** 310
Hardee's, 164–165
IHOP, 77, **77,** 166–167
Jack in the Box, 170–171, **170–171**
KFC, 174–175, **174–175,** 306
Long John Silver's, 179
McDonald's, 180–181, **180–181**
Olive Garden, 182–183, **182–183**
On the Border, 184–185, **184–185**
Outback Steakhouse, 187
Panda Express, 188–189, **188–189**
Panera Bread, 190–191, **191**
Papa John's, 192, **192**
Perkins, 81, **81,** 195, 310
P.F. Chang's, 196–197, 306
Pizza Hut, 198, **198,** 199
Popeyes, 200–201, **200**
Quiznos, 77, **79,** 202–203, **202–203**
Romano's Macaroni Grill, 206–207, **206–207**
Ruby Tuesday, 29, **29,** 208–209
Sonic, 212–213, **212–213**
Starbucks, 214
Steak 'n Shake, 216–217

Subway, 218–219
T.G.I. Friday's, 220–221, **220–221**, 310
Taco Bell, 222–223, **222**
Tim Hortons, 224–225, **224–225**
Uno Pizzeria & Grill, 226–227
Wendy's, 228–229, **228–229**
rotisserie, 3
supermarket
deli meats, 242–243, **242–243**
frozen entrées, 278–279, **278–279**
worst foods, featuring chicken
burrito, 86, **86**
chicken, 89, **89**
eggs, 81, **81**
grilled entrée, 91, **91**
health-food fraud, 81, **81**
pasta, 92, **92**
salad, 17, **17**
sub, 79, **79**
worst, kids, 304, 306, 310
Children's food. See Kids' food
Chili powder
Cowboy Burgers, 326, **327**
Chili sauces, 252–253, **252–253**
Chili's
chips & dip, worst, 82, **82**
food, 144–145, **144–145**
food swap, 30, **30**
grilled entrée, worst, 92, **92**
worst, burger, 87, **87**
Chinese food. See specific restaurant
name
Chipotle Mexican Grill
customizable, 98
fast casual, 39
food, 148–149, **148–149**
paleo diet, 71, **71**
Chipotle pepper
homemade recipe
Cowboy Burgers, 326, **327**
Chips,
& dip, worst, 82, **82**
labels, 41
supermarket, 260–261, **260–261**
Cholesterol, 10, 19, 56, 63, 73, 89, 100
Cilantro
Chinese Chicken Salad, 322, **323**

Cinnabon
worst, pastry 75, **75**
Cinnamon, **9**, 12
Coca-Cola, 17, 39
Coconut Oil, 10, 19
Coffee
Cowboy Burgers, 326, **327**
creamer, 48
Dunkin' Donuts iced, 158, **158**, 159
Krispy Kreme, iced, 176
Menu Decoder, 95–97
nutrition facts, 18, 53
Starbucks, iced, 214–215
Turkish, 109
Cold Stone Creamery
food, 148–149, **148–149**
Condiments, 246–247, **246–247**
Cookies
Blimpie, 128–129
Chick-fil-A, 143
Cold Stone Creamery, 148
Dunkin' Donuts, 158–159
KFC, 174–175
Panda Express, 188–189
Perkins, 194
Tim Hortons, 225
supermarket, 266–267, **266–267**
Così food, 150–151, **150–151**
Crackers, 258–259, **258–259**
Cucumbers
Grilled Vietnamese Steak, 292, **293**

D

Dairy Queen
smaller sizes, 17
food, 152–153, **152–153**
Dark chocolate, 19, 56
DeeBee's, 44, **44**
Deli meats, 242–243, **242–243**
Denny's
food, 154–155, **154–155**
kids, worst side dish, 304
Desserts. See also Cookies, Ice cream,
Frozen Yogurt
abomination, 47

brownies, 83, **83**, 149, **149**
cakes, 35, **35**, 175, 205, 207
food swap, 35, **35**
restaurant
Applebee's, 35, **35**
Blimpie, 128–129
Chick-fil-A, **143**
Cold Stone Creamery, 148, 149, **149**
Dunkin' Donuts, 158, 159
Jack in the Box, 35, **35**
KFC, 174, 175
Panda Express, 188, 189
Perkins, 194
Outback Steakhouse, 83
Red Lobster, 205
Romano's Macaroni Grill, 207
Tim Hortons, 225
supermarket, 266–267, **266–267**,
268–269, **268–269**, 284–285,
284–285, 286–287, **286–287**
worst, 83, **83**
Dietary fats
coconut oil, 19
healthy fats, 108, 197, 218, 236, 262
saturated, 63
trans fats, 48, 55, 57, 64, 88, 115, 122,
158, 178, 180, 201, 228, 261, 279,
280, 304, 306
unsaturated, 59
Diet industry secrets, 62–71
Diet soda, 54
Dijon mustard
supermarket, 246, 247
Ultimate Club Sandwich, 320, **321**
Dimethylpolysiloxane, 306
Dinner. See Entrées
Dips
babaganoush, 108
supermarket, 262–263, **262–263**
worst, chips &, 82, **82**
Djokovic, Novak, 68
Domino's food
food, 156–157, **156–157**
food swap, 28, **28**
Doughnuts
decoder, 177
Dunkin' Donuts, 158–159, **158**

Krispy Kreme, 176, **176**, 177
Starbucks, 215
Dressings, 264–265, **264–265**
Drinks. *See also* Coffee, Smoothies
    energy drinks, 53
    supermarket
        juices, 288–289, **288–289**
        teas, 290–291, **290–291**
        mixers, 292–293, **292–293**
        beers, 294–295, **294–295**
    Vitaminwater, 15
    worst, milk shake, 39, **39**
Dr Pepper Snapple Group, 17
Dunkin' Donuts
    food, 158–159, **158–159**

E

Eating habits
    blast belly fat, 18–19
    for kids and parents, 297–301
Eatthis.com, 17
Eat This, Not That! Awards, 42–44
Eggs
    & cheese, 96
    food swap, 26
    Happy Egg Company, 44
    homemade recipes
        Vanilla Bourbon French Toast, 314,
            315
        Mile High Omelets, 316, **317**
        Shiitake, Spinach and Goat Cheese
            Scramble, 318, **319**
    restaurant
        Au Bon Pain, 120
        Blimpie, 128
        Bob Evans, 130–131, **130–131**
        Burger King, 134–135
        Carl's Jr., 139
        Chick-fil-A, 142–143
        Denny's, 154, **154**
        Friendly's, 162
        Hardee's, 165
        IHOP, 166–167, **166–167**
        McDonald's, 180–181

Panera Bread, 191
Perkins, 195
Sonic, 213
Starbucks, 214
Tim Hortons, 224
substitute, 56
superfood, **9**, 11
supermarket, 270–271
VitaEgg Flatbread Sandwiches, 43
worst, 84, **84**
Energy bars, 256–257, **265–257**
Enjoy Life, 69, **69**
Entrées. *See also specific food and
        restaurant name*
    food swap, 29
    frozen
        beef, 280–281, **280–281**
        breakfast, 270–271, **270–271**
        chicken, 278–279, **278–279**
        fish, 276–277, **276–277**
        pasta, 274–275, **274–275**
    homemade recipes
        Chicken & Dumplings, 330, **331**
        Chinese Chicken Salad, 322, **323**
        Cowboy Burgers, 326, **327**
        Grilled Cheese & Tomato Soup,
            324, **325**
        Jambalaya, 332, **333**
        Mile-High Omelets, 316, **317**
        Shiitake, Spinach & Goat Cheese
            Scramble, 318, **319**
        Spinach-Artichoke Manicotti, 328, **329**
        Ultimate Club Sandwich, 320, **321**
        Vanilla-Bourbon French Toast, 314,
            315
    worst, grilled, 92, **92**
Evolution Fresh, 67, **67**

F

Fast food, *See specific restaurant name*
FDA, 16, 17, 38, 55
Fiber, 7, 11, 13, 19, 41, 43, 44, 63, 66, 68,
    98, 101, 108, 300, 314
Fish
    frozen entrées, 276–277, **276–277**
    restaurant
        Applebee's, 87, **87**

The Cheesecake Factory, 140–141
Friendly's, 162
Long John Silver's, 178–179,
    178–179
Olive Garden, 182–183
On the Border, 185
Outback Steakhouse, 186–187
P.F. Chang's, 196–197, **196–197**
Red Lobster, 204–205, **204–205**
worst, 87, **87**
Five Guys
    food swap, 25, **25**
    food, 160–161, **160–161**
Flavonoids, 19, 60
Flax seeds, 10
Food. *See also* Food industry; Food labels;
        Food swaps; Nutrition facts; *specific
        type*
    and *Eat This, Not That!*, 14–17
    food abominations 46–49
    food delivery, 1, 3
    food myths busted, 50–61
    food shopping, 3
    food trucks, 2
    frozen
        beef entrées, 280–281, **280–281**
        breakfast entrées, 270–271,
            270–271
        chicken entrées, 278–279, **278–279**
        fish entrées, 276–277, **276–277**
        ice cream, 284–285, **284–285**
        pasta entrées, 274–275, **274–275**
        pizza, 272–273, **272–273**
        sides, snacks & appetizers, 282–
            283, **282–283**
        treats, 286–287, **286–287**
    future of food, 1–7
    photography of, 4
    portions, 299
    prepared foods, 3
    processed, 57, 59, 64, 78, 229, 280
    reader poll, **2–7**
    superfoods, 8–13, **9**
    worst
        appetizer, 90, **90**
        breakfast, 88, **88**
        burrito, 86, **86**

chicken, 89, **89**
chips & dip, 84, **84**
dessert, 83, **83**
eggs, 81, **81**
fast-food burger, 78, **78**
fish, 87, **87**
frankenfood, 74, **74**
fries, 76, **76**
grilled entrée, 91, **91**
health-food fraud, 80, **80**
milkshake, 85, **85**
pasta dish, 92, **92**
pastry, 75, **75**, 75, **75**
pizza, 93, **93**
salad, 77, **77**
sit-down burger, 82, **82**
sub, 79, **79**
Food additives, 6, 40, 59, 61, 133
Food industry. *See also specific restaurant name*; Supermarket food
    changes in, 14–17
Food labels, 6, 7, 41
Food swaps
    breakfast burritos, 26, **26**
    burgers, 25, **25**
    chicken entrées, 29, **29**
    dessert, 35, **35**
    kids' meal, 33, **33**
    pasta, 27, **27**
    pizza, 28, **28**
    ribs, 31, **31**
    salads, 30, **30**
    sub, 32, **32**
    smoothies, 34, **34**
    weight loss and, 24
French fries
    "natural cut," 15
    restaurant
        A&W, 115
        Carl's Jr., 139
        Chili's, 144
        Elevation Burger, 45
        Dairy Queen, 153
        Five Guys, 161, **161**
        Hardee's, 165
        In-And-Out, 168–169, **169**

McDonald's, 180
Outback Steakhouse, 187
Popeye's, 200
Ruby Tuesday, 209
T.G.I. Fridays, 221
Wendy's, 15
    supermarket, 282–283, **282–283**
    worst, 76, **76**, 87, **87**, 89, **89**, 91, **91**
    worst, kids, 304, 309
Friendly's
    food, 162–163 **162–163**
    kids, worst salad, 310
Frozen food
    beef entrées, 280–281, **280–281**
    breakfast entrées, 270–271, **270–271**
    chicken entrées, 278–279, **278–279**
    fish entrées, 276–277, **276–277**
    ice cream, 284–285, **284–285**
    pasta entrées, 274–275, **274–275**
    pizza, 272–273, **272–273**
    sides, snacks & appetizers, 282–283, **282–283**
    treats, 286–287, **286–287**
Frozen yogurt
    Menu Decoder, 104–105
    restaurant
        Baskin Robbins, 124
        Ben & Jerry's, 126–127, **126**
        Cold Stone Creamery, 148, **148**
    supermarket
        Baskin Robbins, 124
        Ben & Jerry's, 284–285, **284–285**, 286–287, **286–287**
Fruits. *See also specific type*
    benefits of, 11, 19, 44, 57–58, 70
    as topping, 105

G

Gatorade, 17
Gelatin, 268
Gluten-free, 45, 68
GMOs, 6, 37, 38, 43, 44
Google, 40
Grains
    supermarket, 250–251, **250–251**
    whole grains, 18, 19, 60, 70, 218, 256, 278
Granola bars, 256

Greek yogurt
    Grilled Cheese & Tomato soup, 324
    supermarkets, 238–239, **238–239**
Green tea, 18
Grilled entrées
    homemade recipes
        Chinese Chicken Salad, 322, **323**
        Grilled Cheese & Tomato Soup, 324, **325**
        Cowboy Burgers, 326, **327**
    restaurants
        Chevys, 30
        Ruby Tuesday, 29, **29**
        Zoë's Kitchen, 45
    worst, 92, **92**
GrubHub, 1, 3

H

Ham
    homemade recipes
        Mile High Omelets, 316, **317**
        Ultimate Club Sandwich, 320, **321**
    restaurants
        Arby's, 119
        The Cheesecake Factory, 141
        Domino's, 157
        Hardee's, 184
        IHOP, 166
        Perkins, 195
Hardee's
    and *Eat This, Not That!*, 17
    food, 184–185, **184–185**
    worst, fast food burger, 78, **78**
Harmless Harvest, 43, **43**
Harvest Soul, 44
Health-Food Fraud
    Applebee's Oriental Chicken Salad, 117
    Baskin-Robbins Mango Banana Smoothie, 125
    Hardee's Low Carb Breakfast Bowl, 165
    McDonald's Mango Pineapple Smoothie, 181
    Quiznos Pesto Caesar Sub, 203

Ruby Tuesday Avocado Grilled Chicken Sandwich, 209
Uno Chicago Grill Farmer's Market Individual Pizza, 227
worst, 83, **83**
High-fructose corn syrup (HFCS), 39, 44, 52, 56
Horton, Tony, 38
Homemade food
calorie savings, 313
recipes
Chicken & Dumplings, 330, **331**
Chinese Chicken Salad, 322, **322**
Cowboy Burgers, 326, **327**
Grilled Cheese & Tomato Soup, 324, **324**
Jambalaya, 332, **333**
Mile-High Omelets, 316, **317**
Shiitake, Spinach and Goat Cheese Scramble, 318, **319**
Spinach-Artichoke Manicotti, 328, **329**
Ultimate Club Sandwich, 320, **321**
Vanilla Bourbon French Toast, 314, **315**
Horizon, 43, **43**
Hors d'oeuvres. See Appetizers; Snacks
Horseradish sauce, 246–247, **246–247**
Hot dogs
buns, 249, **249**
Five Guys, 160
Hardee's, 107
Sonic, 212ˣ
supermarket, 244–245, **244–245**
Hummus, **9**, 13, 108, 137, 214, 262–263, **262–263**
Hunt's Ketchup, 17
Hypertension, 10

I
Ice cream
abomination, 49
restaurant
A&W, 115
Baskin-Robbins, 124–125, **124–125**
Ben & Jerry's, 126–127, **126–127**
Cold Stone Creamery, 148–149, **148–149**

Dairy Queen, 152–153, **152–153**
supermarket, 284–285, **284–285,** 286–287, **286–287**
toppings, 149
worst, dessert, 79, **79**
IHOP
food, 166–167, **166–167**
nutritional information, 17
worst, salad, 80, **80**
In-N-Out Burger food, 168–169, **168–169**
Instagram, 4

J
Jack in the Box
abomination, 48
changes in, 16
food, 170–171, **170–171**
food swap, 35, **35**
Jamba Juice
award winner, 34
changes in, 16
food swap, 34, **34**
smoothies, 172–173, **172–173**
Journal of the American Medical Association (JAMA) study, 4, 73
Juices
cleanse, 66, **67**
cold-pressed, 39
Evolution, 67, **67**
Harvest Soul, 44
Naked, 67, **67**
supermarket, 288–289, **288–289**, 292, **292**

K
Kale, 13, 52
Kellog's, 43, **43**
Kentucky Fried Chicken food. See KFC
Ketchup
changes in, 17
condiments, 246–247, **246–247**
KFC
food, 174–175, **174–175**
for kids, worst, 307
Kids' food
calories in, 297

food swap, 33, **33**
sweet cereals, 300, **303**, 304
tips for healthy eating
breakfast, skipping, 298
"clean your plate," 299
exposure therapy, 298
family eating, 301
obesity, 298
portion size, 299
role models, 300
television and, 301
worst foods, 302–311, **302–311**
Applebee's Kids Mini Cheeseburgers, 307
Applebee's Kids Oreo Cookie Shake, 309
Atlanta Bread Company Kids' Peanut Butter & Jelly, 305, **305**
Bob Evans Kids Plenty-o-Pancakes with Chocolate Chips, 308, **308**
California Pizza Kitchen Kids BBQ Chicken Pizza, 306
California Pizza Kitchen Kids Curly Mac n' Cheese with Edamame, 310
Denny's Kids' French Fries, 304
Friendly's Dippin' Chicken, 310
KFC Extra-Crispy Chicken Tender, Mac-n-Cheese, 307
Kid Cuisine All American Fried Chicken, 304
Long John Silver's Popcorn Shrimp Kid's Meal with Pepsi, 306
McDonald's Mighty Kids Meal with Double Cheeseburger, Fries, and Fat-Free Chocolate Milk Jug, 307
On the Border Kid's Bean & Cheese Nachos, 308
On the Border Kid's Cheese Quesadilla with Mexican Rice, 311
Outback Steakhouse Kids Live Well Sirloin Medallions, 309
Perkins Kid's Chicken Strips, 310
P.F. Chang's Kid's Chicken Fried Rice, 305
Post Fruit Pebbles, **303**, 304
Ruby Tuesday Kids Grilled Cheese, 306
T.G.I. Friday's Chicken Fingers, 309
Krispy Kreme food, 176–177, **176–177**

L

Lamb, 103, 109
LDL cholesterol, 10, 63
Lemonade, 288–289, **288–289**
Lettuce. *See also* Salads
    superfood, **9**, 13, 52
"Light" or "lite" label, 7
Lobster, 121, 196, **196**, 206, 221
Local food, 2
Long John Silver's
    food, 178–179, **178–179**
    worst, kids, 306
Lunch. *See* Entrées
Luvo, 43, **43**
LYFE Kitchen, 45

M

Macaroni and cheese, 121, 133, 274–275,
    274–275
    worst, kids, 310
Marinara sauce, 252, **252**
MasterChef, 7
Mayonnaise, 246–247, **246–247**
    Grilled Cheese & Tomato Soup,
        324–325
McDonald's food
    abomination, 46
    decline of, 17, 39
    food, 180–181, **180–181**
    lose weight, 23
    oatmeal, 57
    worst, kids, 307
Meal planning, 312
Meat. *See also specific type*
    deli, 242–243, **242–243**
    vegan, 41
Menu Decoders
    coffee shop, 96–97
    mexican, 98–99
    sushi, 100–101
    tapas, 102–103
    yogurt, 104–105
    thai, 106–107
    middle eastern, 108–109
    vegan, 110–111

Mexican food. *See specific restaurant name*
    Menu Decoder, 98-99
Michele's, 44, **44**
Milk shake, worst, 81, **81**
Minerals. *See* Salt
Mixers, drink, 238–39, **238–39**
Mold, 66
Morningstar Farms, 64
Movie theaters
    calorie count, 17, 38
    popcorn, 18
Muffins
    Menu Decoder, 97
    restaurants
        Au Bon Pain, 121
        Burger King, 134
        Denny's, 154, **154**
        Krispy Kreme, 119, **119**
        Perkins, 195
        Starbucks, 215, **215**
        Tim Hortons, 225
    supermarket, 236–237, **236–237**
Mushrooms
    homemade recipes
        Mile-High Omelets, 316, **317**
        Shiitake, Spinach and Goat Cheese
           Scramble, 318, **319**
Mustard, 246–247, **246–247**
    Ultimate Club Sandwich, 320, **321**

N

Nachos
    Menu Decoder, 99
    worst, burrito, 95, **95**
    worst, kids, 308
Naked Juice, 67, **67**
"Natural" label, 7, 41, 55
Nature Valley, 43, **43**
Nestle, 16
New England Journal of Medicine, 55
Noodles. *See also* Pasta
    supermarket, 250–251, **250–251,**
        274–275, **274–275**
Nutritional claims, false, 16, 38, 41, 55, 64
    bananas, 57
    comfort food, 59

dark chocolate, 56
diet soda, 54
egg substitutes, 56
energy drinks, 53
high-fructose corn syrup (HFCS), 52
junk food, 56
kale, 52
low-fat foods, 55
"multi-grain," 60
nutrition bars, 61
oatmeal, 57
oranges, 58
peanut butter, 58
potatoes, 60
salt, 53
sugar, 52
"trans-fat free," 55
wraps, 60
yogurt, 54
Nutrition Journal, 12
Nuts, 48, 59

O

Oatmeal, 57
Obesity, 13
Obesity, 33, 54, 298, 301
Ocean Spray, 44
Olive Garden
    and *Eat This, Not That!*, 15
    food, 182–183, **182–183**
    food swap, 27
    worst, frankenfood, 74, **74**
Omega-3, 7, 10, 13, 43, 100, 105, 178,
    197, 246
Omega-6, 10, 13, 178, 261
On the Border food, 184–185, **184–185**
    worst, kids, 308, 311, **311**
OpenTable, 5
Oranges, 58
Organic food, 6
Orzo, 251, **251**
Outback Steakhouse
    and *Eat This, Not That!*, 15
    Bloomin' Onion, 22, 89, **89**
    food, 186–187, **186–187**
    nutrition information, 16

worst, appetizer, 89, **89**
worst, dessert 79, **79**
worst, kids 309

P

P90X, 38
Paleo diet, 70, **71**
Pancakes
    abominations, 48
    mix, 65, **65**
    restaurant
        Bob Evans, 130, 308, **308**
        Denny's, 155
        IHOP, 166–167, **166–167**
    worst, kids, 308, **308**
Panda Express food, 188–189, **188–189**
Panera Bread
    food, 190–191, **190–191**
    "healthy," 7
    save calories, 23
    sugar, 63–64
    worst, kids, 308, **308**
Papa John's food,
    abomination, 49
    food, 192–193, **192–193**
Partially hydrogenated oil, 48, 55, 64,
        170, 269, 304
Pasta
    food swap, 27, **27**
    frozen entrées, 220–21, **220–21**
    gluten free, 68
    restaurant
        Applebee's, 116–117, **117**
        The Cheesecake Factory, 141
        Domino's, 157
        Olive Garden, 182–183, **182–183**
        Romano's Macaroni Grill, 206, **206**
        Ruby Tuesday, 151, **151**
    supermarket, 250–251, **250–251**
    worst, 92, **92**
    worst, kids, 277, **277**
Pastry. See also Doughnuts
    scones, 97
    restaurants
        Au Bon Pain, 120–121
        Cinnabon, 75, **75**

Jamba Juice, 173
supermarket, 270–271, **270–271**
worst, 75, **75**
Peanut butter
    healthy, 58, 59
    reduced fat, 55
Peanut butter and jelly sandwich for kids,
        worst, 305, **305**
Pea Pod, 40
PepsiCo, 17
Perkins food
    calories, 5
    food, 194–195, **194–195**
    worst, eggs, 84, **84**
    worst, kids, 310
Perdue University, 13
P.F. Chang's food
    changes in, 17
    food, 196–197, **196–197**
    worst, kids, 306
Pizza
    food swap, 28, **28**, 33, **33**
    frozen, 272–273, **272–273**
    restaurant
        California Pizza Kitchen, 136–137, **136**
        Così, 151, **151**
        Domino's, 28, **28,** 98–99, **98–99**
        Papa John's, 49, **49**, 192–193,
            192–193
        Pizza Hut, 28, **28**, 198–199, **199**
        Pizzeria Locale, 45
        Uno Pizzeria & Grill, 48, **48**, 226–227,
            226–227
    worst, 93, **93**
    worst, kids, 305
Pizza Hut
    food swap, 28
    pizza, 198–199, **198–199**
Pizzeria Locale, 45
Popeyes food, 200–201, **200–201**
Popcorn, 19
Portions, 17, 299
Potatoes. See also French fries
    carbs, 60
    patatas bravas, 103
Poultry. See specific type
Power bars, 61, 256–257, **256–257**

Produce. See Fruits; Vegetables
Protein, 13, 42, 44, 101, 107, 111
Public Health Nutrition, 6

Q

Quesadilla
    Menu Decoder, 98
    worst, kids, 311
Quinoa, 19, 39, 111, 250, **250**
Quiznos food
    food, 202–203, **202–203**
    food swap, 32
    worst, sub, 79, **79**

R

Red Lobster
    and *Eat This, Not That!*, 15
    food, 204–205, **204–205**
    worst, sub, 79, **79**
Restaurant food. See also specific
            restaurant name
    abominations, 46–49
    and *Eat This, Not That!*, 14–17
    future of, 1
    Menu Decoders, 94–111
    new, 45
    restaurants, 112–229
    worst, 72–93, **72–93**
    Year in Food, 36–41
Ribs
    food swap, 31, **31**
    worst, grilled entrée, 91, **91**
Rice
    Jambalaya, 332, **332**
    supermarket, 250–251, **250–251**
Role modeling eating habits, 300
Romano's Macaroni Grill
    and *Eat This, Not That!*, 16
    food, 206–207, **206–207**
    food swap, 27, **27**, 33, **33**
    frozen food, 275, **275**
Ruby Tuesday
    and *Eat This, Not That!*, 16
    food, 206–207, **206–207**
    food swap, 27, **27**, 33, **33**

S

7-Eleven, 38
Salads
  calories in, 64
  dressings for, 210–11, **210–11**
  food swap, 30, **30**
  homemade recipe
    Chinese Chicken Salad, 322, **323**
  house salad, 101
  paleo food, 71
  restaurant
    Applebee's, 116–117
    Arby's, 118–119
    Au Bon Pain, 120
    Baja Fresh, 122–123, **122–123**
    Bob Evans, 130
    Burger King, 135
    California Pizza Kitchen, 137, **137**
    The Cheesecake Factory, 140
    Chevy's Fresh Mex, 30, **30**
    Chick-fil-A, 143, **143**
    Chili's, 144–145
    Chipotle, 146–147
    Così, 151
    Domino's, 157
    Friendly's, 162–163
    IHOP, 77, 166–167
    Long John Silver's, 178
    McDonald's, 180
    Olive Garden, 182
    On the Border, 184
    Outback Steakhouse, 186–187
    Panera Bread, 190–191, **190–191**
    P.F. Chang's, 196
    Pizza Hut, 198
    Quizno's, 202–203
    Red Lobster, 204–205
    Romano's Macaroni Grill, 206
    Steak 'n Shake, 216–217
    Subway, 218–219, **218–219**
    Taco Bell, 223, **223**
    T.G.I. Friday's, 220–221, **220–221**
    Uno Pizzeria & Grill, 227
    Wendy's, 228
  tabouleh, 108
  taco salad, 99

  worst, 77, **77**
  worst, kids, 310
Salsa
  supermarket, 262–263, **262–263**
Salt
  average amount eaten, 73
  food swap, 32
  healthy version, 53
  in Applebee's food, 117
  in Blimpie food, 129
  in The Cheesecake Factory food, 141
  in Chili's food, 82, 144–145
  in Long John Silver's food, 179
  in On the Border food, 184
  in Papa John's food, 49
  in P.F. Chang's food, 196–197
  in Red Lobster food, 204
  in Ruby Tuesday food, 208
Sandwiches. See also Breakfast; Burgers
  at coffee chop, 96
  food swap, 32, **32**
  health, 23
  restaurant
    A&W, 114
    Applebee's, 116
    Arby's, 118–119, **118–119**
    Au Bon Pain, 120–121, **120–121**
    Blimpie, 128–129, **128–129**
    The Cheesecake Factory, 140, **141**,
      80, **80**
    Bob Evans, 131
    Burger King, 134–135
    Carl's Jr., 138–139, **138–139**
    The Cheesecake Factory, 140–141,
      140–141
    Chick-fil-A, 142–143, **142**
    Così, 150–151, **150**
    Denny's, 155, **155**
    Five Guys, 160
    Friendly's, 162–163, **162–163**
    Hardee's, 164–165
    In-N-Out Burger, 168–169
    Jack in the Box, 170–171, **170–171**
    Long John Silver's, 179
    McDonald's, 180–181, **180–181**
    Panera Bread, 190–191, **190**
    Perkins, 194–195

    Popeyes, 200–201, **200–201**
    Quiznos, 32, **32**, 202–203, **202–203**
    Sonic, 212–213, **212–213**
    Starbucks, 214
    Steak 'N Shake, 216, **217**
    Subway, 32, **32**, 218–219, **218–219**
    Tim Hortons, 224–225, **224–225**
    Wendy's, 229, **229**
  worst, 79, **79**
  worst, health-food fraud, 80, **80**
  worst, kids, 272, 275
  worst, peanut butter and jelly, 272, **272**
  wraps, 60
Saturated fats, 6, 19, 27, 35, 75, 79, 81,
      83, 84, 85, 88, 91, 115, 117, 127,
      129, 141, 149, 163, 168, 174, 183,
      193, 195, 199, 202, 207, 217, 253,
      255, 269, 272, 275, 285, 287,
      309, 326
Sauces
  chili, 198–99, **198–99**
  soy, 100
  spaghetti, 252–253, **252–253**
  supermarket, 252–253, **252–253**
  syrups and, for frozen yogurt, 105
  tahini, 108
  tomato, 252–253, **252–253**
Sausage
  Shiitake, Spinach & Goat Cheese
      Scramble, 290, **291**
  supermarket, 244–245, **244–245**
Serving sizes, 38
Shopping for food, 230–231
Shrimp
  food swap, 27, **27**
  restaurant
    Baja Fresh, 122–123
    California Pizza Kitchen, 136
    The Cheesecake Factory, 140–141
    Chili's, 144
    Long John Silver's, 188, **188**
    Olive Garden, 182
    Outback Steakhouse, 186–187
    Panda Express, 188–189
    P.F. Chang's, 196, **196**
    Popeyes, 201, **201**

Red Lobster, 204–205, **204**
Romano's Macaroni Grill, 207
Ruby Tuesday, 208–209
T.G.I. Friday's, 220–221
supermarket 276–277, **276–277**
Side dishes. *See also specific type*
frozen, 282–283, **282–283**
worst, kids, 304
Silk, 43, **43**
Smart Balance, 43, **43**
Smoothie King
smoothies, 34, **34**, 210–211, **210–211**
Smoothies
award winner, 44
cleanse, 66–67
food swap, 34, **34**
restaurant
Baskin-Robbins, 124–125
Ben & Jerry's, 126–127
Coldstone Creamery, 148
Jamba Juice, 172–173, **172–173**
McDonald's, 181
Smoothie King, 210–211, **210–211**
T.G.I. Friday's, 221
Tim Hortons, 225, **225**
Snacks. *See also* Appetizers
candy bars, 268–269, **268–269**
chips, 260–261, **260–261**
cookies, 266–267, **266–267**
dips, 262–263, **262–263**
Doritos, 63
energy bars, 256–257, **256–257**
Frito-Lay, 41
frozen, 282–283, **282–283**
frozen treats, 286–287, **286–287**
Natural Cheetos, 56
worst, 84, **84**
Sodium. *See* Salt
Sonic
abomination, 49
food, 212–213, **212–213**
Soups
homemade recipe
Grilled Cheese & Tomato Soup, 324, **325**
restaurants
Au Bon Pain, 120–121
California Pizza Kitchen, 136

Chick-fil-A, 142
Friendly's, 162–163
Olive Garden, 183
On the Border, 185
Panera Bread, 190
P.F. Chang's, 197
Quiznos, 202
Red Lobster, 205
Romano's Macaroni Grill, 206
Tim Hortons, 224
supermarket, 254–255, **254–255**
Spaghetti sauces, 252–253, **252–253**
Spinach, 13, 39, 52, 60, 70
homemade recipes
Shiitake, Spinach & Goat Cheese
Scramble, 318, **319**
Spinach-Artichoke Manicotti, 328, **329**
Spreads, 262–263, **262–263**. *See also* Dips
Starbucks
food and drink, 214–215, **214–215**
Menu Decoder, 96–97
social responsibility, 39
Steak 'n Shake
food, 216–217, **216–211**
food swap, 25, **25**
worst, fries, 76, **76**
Subs. *See* Sandwiches
Subway
food, 218–219, **218–219**
food swap, 32, **32**
wrap, 60
Sugar, 6, 8
homemade recipes
Vanilla-Bourbon French Toast, 314,
315
Chinese Chicken Salad, 322, **323**
Sundaes. *See* Ice cream
Supermarket food
beer, 294–295, **294–295**
biscuits, 249, **249**
breads, 248–249, **248–249**
breakfast breads, 236–237, **236–237**
candy bars, 268–269, **268–269**
cereals, 232–233, **232–233**, 234–235,
234–235
cheese, 240–241, **240–241**
chips, 260–261, **260–261**

condiments, 246–247, **246–247**
cookies, 266–267, **266–267**
crackers, 258–259, **258–259**
deli meats, 242–243, **242–243**
dips, 262–263, **262–263**
dressings, 264–265, **264–265**
energy bars, 256–257, **256–257**
frozen
beef entrées, 280–281, **280–281**
breakfast entrées, 270–271, **270–271**
chicken entrées, 278–279, **278–279**
fish entrées, 276–277, **276–277**
ice cream, 284–285, **284–285**
pasta entrées, 274–275, **274–275**
pizza, 272–273, **272–273**
sides, snacks & appetizers, 282–283,
282–283
treats, 286–287, **286–287**
grains, 250–251, **250–251**
hot dogs, 244–245, **244–245**
ice cream, 284–285, **284–285**
juices, 288–289, **288–289**
mixers, drink, 292–293, **292–293**
noodles, 250–251, **250–251**
pasta, 250–251, **250–251**
sauces, 252–253, **252–253**
sausage, 244–245, **244–245**
shopping for, 230–231
snacks, 282–283, **282–283**
soups, 254–255, **254–255**
spreads, 262–263, **262–263**
teas, 290–291, **290–291**
yogurt, 238–239, **238–239**

T

The 21-Day Belly Fix, 40
Taco Bell
abomination, 48
food, 222–223, **222–223**
Menu Decoder, 98
Tacos
kids, 311
Menu Decoder, 98
restaurants
Baja Fresh, 122–123
Chipotle Mexican Grill, 148–149,
148–149

Long John Silver's, 179, **179**
On the Border, 184–185, **184–185**
T.G.I. Friday's, 220
Taco Bell, 222–223, **222–223**
Tartar sauce, 248–249, **248–249**
Teas, 290–291, **290–291**
T.G.I. Friday's
    and *Eat This, Not That!*, 15
    food, 220–221, **220–221**
    worst, kids, 310
Tim Hortons food, 224–225, **224–225**
Tomatoes, 58
    Grilled Cheese & Tomato Soup, 324, **325**
    Jambalaya, 332, **333**
    Spinach-Artichoke Manicotti, 328, **329**
    Ultimate Club Sandwich, 320, **321**
Tortillas, 248–249, **248–249**
Trans fats, 48, 55, 57, 64, 88, 115, 122,
        158, 178, 180, 201, 228, 261, 279,
        280, 304, 306
Treats, frozen, 286–287, **286–287**
Tufts University research, 18
Turkey
    food swap, 32
    homemade recipes
        Ultimate Club Sandwich, 320, **321**
        Jambalaya, 332, **333**
    restaurant
        Applebee's, 116
        Arby's, 118, 119, **119**
        Au Bon Pain, 121, **121**
        Boston Market, 132, **132**
        Carl's Jr., 138
        Cosi, 150
        Dairy Queen, 153
        Hardee's, 164
        Panera Bread, 190-191
        Perkins, 195, **195**
        Quiznos, 202
        Ruby Tuesday, 209
        Subway, 218
    supermarket, 242–243, **242–243**
True Food Kitchen, 45
TV watching, limiting, 310

U

Udi's, 69, **69**
University of Western Australia, 11
Uno Pizzeria & Grill
    calories in, 5
    changes in, 17
    food, 226–227, **226–227**
    food swap 33, **33**
    worst, pizza, 93, **93**
USDA, 6, 60

V

Vegan, 41, 45, 64, 110–111
    worst, 65, **65**
Vegetables. *See also specific type*
    carotenoids, 13
    nutrition, 52
    homemade recipes
        Chinese Chicken Salad, 322, **323**
        Chicken & Dumplings, 330, **331**
        Jambalaya, 332, **333**
        Mile-High Omelets, 316, **317**
        Shiitake, Spinach & Goat Cheese
            Scramble, 318, **319**
        Spinach-Artichoke Manicotti, 328, **329**
        Ultimate Club Sandwich, 320, **321**
Vinaigrettes, 264–265, **264–265**
Vinegar. *See* Balsamic vinegar; Dressings
Vitalicious, 43, **43**, 44
Vitamin A, 254, 278, 283
Vitamin B, 11, 53, 64
Vitamin C, 58
Vitamin D, 70
Vitamin E, 98, 234
Vitamins. *See specific name*
Vitaminwater, 16

W

Waffles, frozen, 270–271, **270–271**
Walmart, 41, 231
Wake Forest Baptist Medical Center, 11
Weight loss
    blast belly fat, 18–19
    how to with this book, 20-23
    food swaps and, 24

Wendy's
    food, 228–229, **228–229**
William Paterson University, 13
Worst food
    in America, 51, **51**
    appetizers, 40, **40**, 47, **47**
    breakfast, 42, **42**
    burgers, 36, **36**, 45, **45**
    burrito, 43, **43**
    chicken, 44, **44**
    chips and dip, 40, **40**
    dessert, 37, **37**
    fish, 46, **46**
    French fries, 34, **34**
    grilled entrée, 50, **50**
    Health-Care Fraud, 41, **41**
    milk shake, 39, **39**
    pasta, 32, **32**, 49, **49**
    pastry, 33, **33**
    pizza, 48, **48**
    salad, 38, **38**
    sandwich, 35, **35**
    snack, 40, **40**
Wraps. *See* Sandwiches

X

Xanthan gum, 133

Y

Year in food, 36–41
Yogurt. *See also* Frozen yogurt
    abomination, 49
    gut health, 40, 54
    homemade recipes
        Grilled Cheese & Tomato Soup,
            234–235, **224–225**
    Menu Decoder, 104–105
    nutrition versus calories, 177
    sugar and, 64
    supermarket, 238–239, **238–239**

Z

Zoë's Kitchen, 45

EAT THIS.COM
The All-New EAT THIS, NOT THAT! Website

Authoritative advice, eye-opening food swaps, groundbreaking nutrition news and the world's most delicious collection of weight-loss recipes. It's the power of food—now at your fingertips.

WEIGHT LOSS
Blast belly fat fast with easy and effective no-diet secrets.

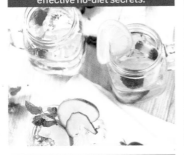

RESTAURANTS
Lose 10, 20, 30 pounds or more at all of your favorite spots!

SUPERMARKETS
Save hundreds of dollars on the very best fat-burning superfoods.

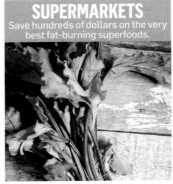

HEALTH
Protect yourself and your family with top doctors' best advice.

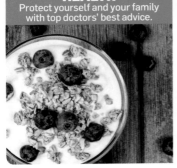

RECIPES
Indulge in delicious home-cooked, slimmed-down comforts.

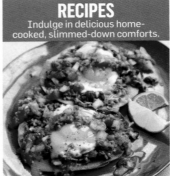

FAMILY
Make mealtime simple with 1,000s of tips and shortcuts.

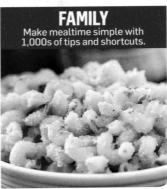